Respiratory Medicine

Series Editor:
Sharon I.S. Rounds

For further volumes:
http://www.springer.com/series/7665

Linda Nici · Richard ZuWallack

Editors

Chronic Obstructive Pulmonary Disease

Co-Morbidities and Systemic Consequences

Humana Press

Editors
Linda Nici, MD
Clinical Professor of Medicine
The Warren Alpert Medical
School of Brown University
Chief, Pulmonary
and Critical Care, Providence Veterans
Affairs Medical Center
Providence, RI, USA
linda_nici@brown.edu

Richard ZuWallack, MD
Clinical Professor of Medicine
University of Connecticut
School of Medicine
Associate Chief Pulmonary
and Critical Care
St. Francis Hospital and Medical Center
Hartford, CT, USA
rzuwalla@stfranciscare.org

ISBN 978-1-60761-672-6   e-ISBN 978-1-60761-673-3
DOI 10.1007/978-1-60761-673-3
Springer New York Dordrecht Heidelberg London

Library of Congress Control Number: 2011935361

Printed on acid-free paper

Humana Press is part of Springer Science+Business Media (www.springer.com)

Preface

Chronic Obstructive Pulmonary Disease (COPD) is a preventable and treatable disease with commonly associated co-morbidities and significant systemic consequences. It is the fourth leading cause of death worldwide and the only one of the top ten leading causes of death that has shown a steady increase in morbidity and mortality. A major challenge in controlling and treating COPD is understanding its complexity. While COPD can be simplistically defined as a disease characterized by airflow limitation, we now understand it as a multicomponent disease with many clinical phenotypes. Evidence is rapidly emerging that COPD has a potent inflammatory basis which likely plays a role in the systemic consequences of the disease, including peripheral muscle, cardiac, nutritional, and psycho-social dysfunction. These systemic consequences are responsible for a large portion of the morbidity from this disease. Furthermore, patients with COPD are more likely to have significant co-morbid conditions, such as cardiovascular disease, that contribute to morbidity and mortality and present challenges when designing treatment guidelines.

Chronic Obstructive Pulmonary Disease: Co-Morbidities and Systemic Consequences uses a wide angle lens to view COPD, bringing into focus the ever-important extrapulmonary aspects of this disease. The chapters included here were all prepared by internationally recognized thought leaders in the field. Our common purpose was to examine and understand the complex nature of COPD, recognize its common co-morbidities and systemic consequences, and offer suggestions for comprehensive treatment strategies.

The first section of the book provides an overview of the role of co-morbidities, the basis for systemic inflammation, and how these impact on the disablement process in COPD. The following two sections provide in-depth analysis of the most common co-morbidities and systemic consequences associated with COPD. The last section of this book addresses treatment of these medically complex patients by discussing the need for transcending disease-specific guidelines, providing novel pharmacologic treatment strategies, and giving comprehensive pulmonary rehabilitation. The book concludes with a look to the future, emphasizing the importance of integrating care for patients with COPD. The latter will necessitate a crucial paradigm shift as we encounter much more complex and chronically ill patients in an increasingly fragmented health care system.

We thank each of the authors for their participation and applaud their efforts toward pushing the envelope in our understanding of COPD, its co-morbidities, and systemic consequences. The book is intended for both the experienced clinician and the student whose goals are to understand the complex expressions of COPD and to offer rational, individualized therapy for these highly complex patients. It is our hope that it might also be useful to the research community working on COPD, as they struggle to understand and develop better treatment strategies. We look forward to future research in this area. It has been our pleasure and it has been a distinct honor to serve as editors and oversee such wonderful scholarly work.

Providence, RI   Linda Nici
Hartford, CT   Richard ZuWallack

Contents

Contributors

Ingrid M.L. Augustin CIRO, Center of Expertise for Chronic Organ Failure, Horn, The Netherlands

Kristina L. Bailey Department of Internal Medicine, Pulmonary, Critical Care, Sleep and Allergy Division, University of Nebraska Medical Center, Omaha, NE, USA

Bramvan den Borst Department of Respiratory Medicine, NUTRIM School for Nutrition, Toxicology and Metabolism, Maastricht University Medical Center+, Maastricht, The Netherlands

Cynthia M. Boyd Department of Geriatric Medicine and Gerontology, Johns Hopkins Bayview Medical Center, Baltimore, MD, USA

Marc-André Caron Department of Respirology, Institut Universitaire de Cardiologie et de Pneumologie de Québec, Québec, QC, Canada

Vincent Cunanan Internal Medicine/Ambulatory Services, University of Connecticut, Saint Francis Hospital and Medicine Center, Hartford, CT, USA

Richard Debigaré Department of Respirology, Institut Universitaire de Cardiologie et de Pneumologie de Québec, Quebec, QC, Canada

Luis F. Diez-Morales Internal Medicine/Ambulatory Services, University of Connecticut, Saint Francis Hospital and Medicine Center, Hartford, CT, USA

Rachael A. Evans Department of Respiratory Medicine, West Park Healthcare Centre, Toronto, ON, Canada

Vincent S. Fan Department of Medicine, VA Puget Sound Health Care System, University of Washington School of Medicine, Seattle, WA, USA

Kristina Frogale Johns Hopkins Bayview Medical Center, Baltimore, MD, USA

Judith Garcia-Aymerich Centre for Research in Environmental Epidemiology (CREAL), Barcelona, Spain

Nicholas D. Giardino Department of Psychiatry, VA Ann Arbor Healthcare System, University of Michigan, Ann Arbor, MI, USA

Roger S. Goldstein Department of Respiratory Medicine, West Park Healthcare Centre, Toronto, ON, Canada

Jadvinder Goraya Department of Internal Medicine, Pulmonary, Critical Care, Sleep and Allergy Division, University of Nebraska Medical Center, Omaha, NE, USA

Matthew D. Jankowich Division of Pulmonary Medicine, Department of Medicine, Providence VA Medical Center, Providence, RI, USA

François Maltais Department of Respirology, Institut Universitaire de Cardiologie et de Pneumologie de Québec, Québec, QC, Canada

Paula Meek Denver College of Nursing, University of Colorado, Aurora, CO, USA

Kambiz Mirzaei Department of Pharmacy, West Park Healthcare Centre, Toronto, ON, Canada

Michael D.L. Morgan Department of Respiratory Medicine, University Hospital of Leicester, Glenfield Hospital, Leicester, UK

Linda Nici The Warren Alpert Medical School of Brown University, Providence, RI, USA
Providence Veterans Affairs Medical Center, Providence, RI, USA

Stephen L. Rennard Department of Internal Medicine, Pulmonary, Critical Care, Sleep and Allergy Division, University of Nebraska Medical Center, Omaha, NE, USA

Kerry M. Schnell School of Medicine, Johns Hopkins University, Baltimore, MD, USA

Annemie M.W.J. Schols Department of Respiratory Medicine, NUTRIM School for Nutrition, Toxicology and Metabolism, Maastricht University Medical Center+, Maastricht, The Netherlands

Don D. Sin Department of Medicine, University of British Columbia, St. Paul's Hospital, Vancouver, BC, Canada

Marie-Eve Thériault Department of Respirology, Institut Universitaire de Cardiologie et de Pneumologie de Québec, Quebec, QC, Canada

Thierry Troosters Department of Pulmonary Rehabilitation, Respiratory Division, University Hospital Gasthuisberg, Leuven, Belgium

Robert G. Varadi Department of Respiratory Medicine, West Park Healthcare Centre, Toronto, ON, Canada

Emiel F.M. Wouters Department of Respiratory Medicine, Maastricht University Medical Center, Maastricht, The Netherlands

Richard ZuWallack University of Connecticut School of Medicine, Hartford, CT, USA

St. Francis Hospital and Medical Center, Hartford, CT, USA

Chapter 1
Mortality in COPD: The Role of Comorbidities

Don D. Sin

Abstract Although total mortality has decreased dramatically over the past 30 years, driven largely by successful reductions in deaths from cardiovascular diseases (CVDs), mortality from chronic obstructive pulmonary disease (COPD) has more than doubled. COPD is currently the 4th leading cause of mortality worldwide, accounting for more than three million deaths per year. Owing to increased prevalence of smoking in developing countries and the aging of the population across Western nations, COPD mortality is expected to more than double over the next 20 years, so that by 2030, it will be responsible for 10% of the world's total mortality (currently 7%), accounting for seven million deaths annually. Although these figures are truly alarming, they probably underestimate the global impact of COPD on overall mortality, because COPD contributes significantly to other major causes of mortality, such as ischemic heart disease (IHD), stroke, and lung cancer.

Keywords COPD • Mortality • Cardiovascular disease • Comorbidity • Heart disease • Smoking • Developing countries • Western nations • Global impact • Lung cancer

Introduction

Although total mortality has decreased dramatically over the past 30 years, driven largely by successful reductions in deaths from cardiovascular diseases (CVDs), mortality from chronic obstructive pulmonary disease (COPD) has more than doubled [1]. COPD is currently the 4th leading cause of mortality worldwide, accounting for more than three million deaths per year [2]. Owing to increased prevalence of

D.D. Sin (✉)
Department of Medicine, University of British Columbia, St. Paul's Hospital,
Vancouver, BC, Canada
e-mail: don.sin@hli.ubc.ca

L. Nici and R. ZuWallack (eds.), *Chronic Obstructive Pulmonary Disease: Co-Morbidities and Systemic Consequences*, Respiratory Medicine, DOI 10.1007/978-1-60761-673-3_1, © Springer Science+Business Media, LLC 2012

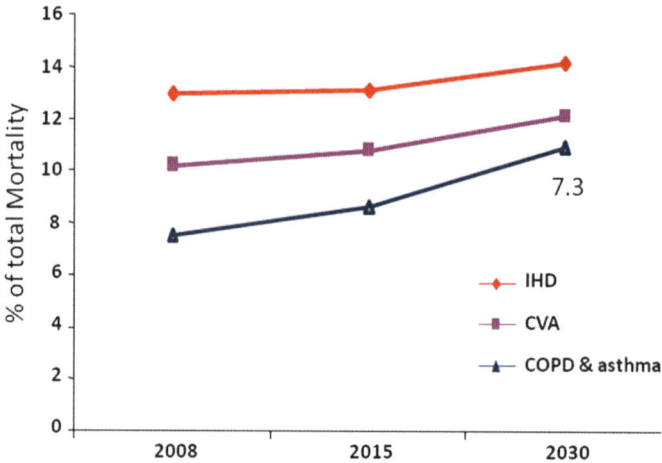

Fig. 1.1 Future worldwide mortality from chronic obstructive pulmonary disease. Projections based on estimates provided by the World Health organization. [3]. It is estimated that by 2030, 7.3 million people will die from COPD and asthma worldwide. *IHD* ischemic heart disease, *CVD* cerebrovascular disease, *COPD* chronic obstructive pulmonary disease

smoking in developing countries and the aging of the population across Western nations, COPD mortality is expected to more than double over the next 20 years, so that by 2030, it will be responsible for 10% of the world's total mortality (currently 7%), accounting for seven million deaths annually (Fig. 1.1) [3]. In China alone, if the current trends in cigarette smoking and solid fuel use persist, more than two million Chinese will die yearly from COPD by 2033 [4]. Although these figures are truly alarming, they probably underestimate the global impact of COPD on overall mortality, because COPD contributes significantly to other major causes of mortality, such as ischemic heart disease (IHD), stroke, and lung cancer. In this chapter, we will critically examine the relationship of COPD to total as well as disease-specific causes of mortality and explore possible mechanisms by which COPD may enhance the risk of mortality from CVD and offer potential strategies to abrogate the excess risk.

What Is the Overall Prognosis of COPD Patients?

The overall prognosis of patients with COPD is variable and modified by several key factors such as age, gender, body mass index (BMI), comorbidities, functional status, and severity of lung function impairment. There is general consensus that with progression of airflow limitation as defined by a reduction in forced expiratory volume in one second (FEV_1), mortality rates increase. However, there is tremendous heterogeneity in the mortality rates within a given severity of airflow limitation, suggesting the need to consider other factors. In a recent paper by Puhan et al., the investigators showed in a Spanish cohort of 342 patients that the 3-year mortality was 12%; whereas in a Swiss cohort of 232 patients, the 3-year mortality was nearly 22% [5]. The large discordance in the mortality rate between the two cohorts related to major differences in age (68 vs. 72 years of age), baseline FEV_1 (52 vs. 45%) and the presence of CVD (38 vs. 25%). Interestingly, the Swiss cohort had fewer current smokers (18 vs. 33%) and lower BMI (26 kg/m^2 vs. 28 kg/m^2) than the Spanish cohort. In the meta-analysis by Briggs and colleagues of 12 clinical trials of COPD involving 8,802 patients and over 6,000 person-years of follow-up performed by GlaxoSmithKline (GSK) in COPD, the single most significant predictor of total mortality in these patients with moderate to severe COPD, who enrolled in these trials, was the presence of CVD [6] with a hazard ratio (HR) of 2.5 ($p<0.001$), followed by age (HR of 1.05; $p=0.001$), BMI less than 20 kg/m^2 (HR, 2.08; $p=0.002$) and FEV_1 (HR, 0.98; $p=0.006$). Interestingly, in that study, neither gender ($p=0.35$) nor quality of life scores ($p=0.26$) were significantly associated with total mortality. Together, these data suggest that FEV_1 alone is only a weak (though statistically significant) predictor of total mortality in COPD patients. Other important predictors are advanced age, low BMI (less than 20 kg/m^2), and presence of CVD. While the data on gender are mixed [with some studies showing that women are at increased risk of mortality [4, 7] and others showing that they have reduced risk [8], the totality of data suggests that gender is not a significant predictor of mortality when other factors such as age, lung function, BMI and presence of CVD are included in the analysis [9], though women have more respiratory symptoms and have an enhanced risk of exacerbations [9].

One important life-changing event for COPD patients is hospitalization. The contemporary in-hospital mortality rate of COPD exacerbation is approximately 16% [10], though with mild exacerbations, the case fatality can be as low as 2% [11]. However, exacerbations associated with acute hypoxemia and hypercapnia have high case fatality rates, ranging from 20 to 30% [12]. Patients who require intubation and mechanical ventilation have the worst prognosis with most succumbing to their disease during their hospitalization [13]. Our group has shown previously, using a large administrative health database, that patients with COPD who are hospitalized and discharged successfully have a very guarded prognosis with a 3-year mortality rate approaching 50% [14], a finding that was replicated by other groups [7]. A more contemporaneous cohort study suggests, however, that the overall prognosis has improved over the past decade. The 3-year mortality rate now following discharge from hospital may be in the order of 38%, likely reflecting better in-hospital treatment [15].

What Do Patients with COPD Die from?

The answer to this question is dependent on the disease severity of patients. In the Lung Health Study (LHS), which enrolled more than 5,000 smokers with mild COPD (defined spirometrically using FEV_1 in the range between 60 and 90% of predicted) demonstrated that in this group of patients, the leading cause of mortality

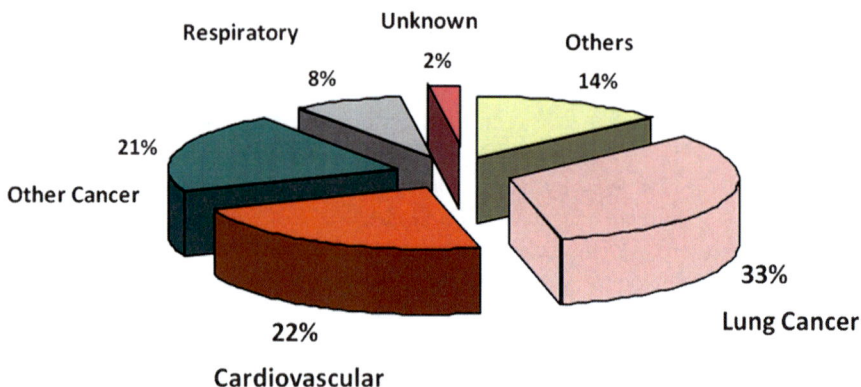

Fig. 1.2 Causes of mortality in the lung health study. The figure is drawn based on data reported by Anthonisen et al. [63]

was lung cancer, accounting for approximately 33% of the total mortality [16], followed by CVDs (at 22%), extrapulmonary cancers (at 21%), and respiratory failure (at 8%) (Fig. 1.2). In the more severe COPD patients (with FEV_1 less than 60% of predicted), however, the order changes. In the recently completed TORCH trial (Towards a Revolution in COPD Health), the leading cause of mortality was respiratory failure, accounting for 35% of the total mortality, which was then followed by CVDs at 26%, and then by cancer at 21% [17]. In terms of individual disease entities, COPD was the leading cause of death, accounting for 27% of the deaths, followed by sudden (cardiac) deaths at 16%, and lung cancer at 14% [17]. Interestingly, in this study, the risk of total mortality at 3 years of follow-up was just over 15% in the placebo arm, which had an average age of 65 years and FEV_1 of 44% of predicted post-bronchodilator [18]. In contrast, in the recently completed UPLIFT trial (Understanding Potential Long-Term Impacts on Function with Tiotropium), just over 10% of the patients died at 3 years of follow-up in the placebo arm which had similar demographic and clinical characteristics as those involved in the TORCH trial [19]. Although the reasons behind the discordance in the mortality rates between the two studies have not been fully elucidated, these data suggest that there are factors other than lung function and age that are important in the overall prognosis of patients with COPD. These factors may include smoking status, comorbidities such as CVD, and health status of the patients, which were different between the TORCH and UPLIFT studies.

The main criticism of the mortality data in LHS, TORCH, and UPLIFT was that the cause of death was not verified with autopsies. Although there are certain limitations with autopsies, they are nevertheless considered the gold standard for assigning causality to deaths. One study that used autopsy in addition to clinical information in assigning causality was the report by Zvezdin and colleagues (Fig. 1.3) [20]. In this study, the investigators examined the cause of death in 43 consecutive patients with COPD who died within 24 h of hospitalization. In all cases, the initial hospital diagnosis was COPD exacerbation. However, autopsy on these patients demonstrated

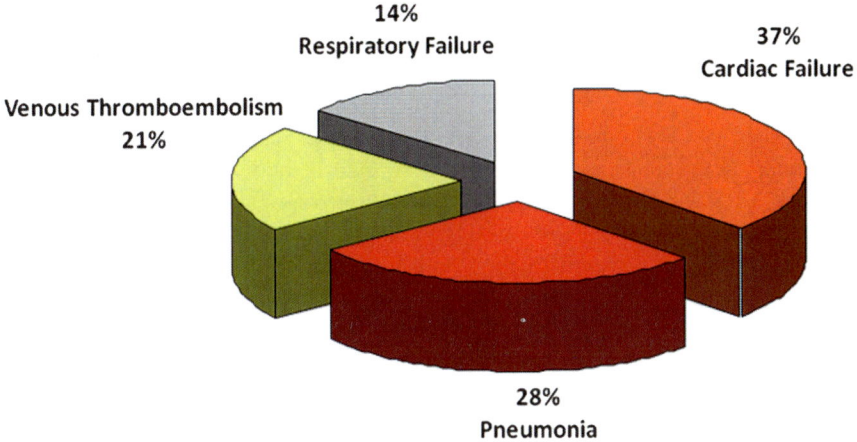

Fig. 1.3 Causes of mortality based on clinical features and autopsy of patients who expired within 24 h of hospitalization for COPD. The figure is drawn based on data reported by Zvezdin et al. [20]

that in 37% of these deaths, the likely cause of mortality was cardiac failure, followed by pneumonia (28%), and venous thromboembolic disease (21%). Only 14% of the patients in this study died from progressive respiratory failure secondary to COPD [20]. Together, these data suggest that in patients with GOLD (Global initiative for Obstructive Lung Disease) 1 or 2 disease (mild to moderate COPD with FEV_1 50% or greater), the predominant cause of mortality is lung cancer (and other forms of cancer), followed by CVD in about a quarter of the cases. Very few die from respiratory failure. On the other hand, in patients with GOLD 3 or 4 disease (FEV_1 less than 50% of predicted), respiratory failure related to COPD progression, pneumonia or cardiac failure is the predominant cause of mortality, followed by lung cancer in about 15% of the cases. In all stages of COPD, CVD is an important direct or comorbid contributor to the patients' mortality. Thus, it is essential that CVD comorbidities be identified early in the course of the patient's disease and be aggressively treated.

Possible Mechanistic Links Between COPD and CVD

How COPD increases the risk of poor cardiovascular outcomes is not well known. Patients with COPD patients have elevated resting heart rate and are at increased risk of arrhythmias [21]. Thus, some have suggested that altered neurohumoral signals may be the reason for the enhanced risk of CVD in COPD patients [22]. Indeed, studies that have evaluated autonomic tone in COPD patients have found evidence for excess sympathetic nervous activity and reduced vagal tone related largely to hypoxemia [23]. Bronchodilators in certain susceptible patients may further worsen the autonomic dysregulation, though in reality, the risk imposed by inhaled bronchodilators appears to be very modest.

The mechanism that has received most of the attention over the past 5 years has been the role of systemic inflammation. It is widely accepted that lung inflammation plays a prominent role in COPD pathogenesis [24] and that systemic inflammation exists in COPD [25–27]. Some have postulated that the systemic inflammatory process related to COPD may be responsible for the increased risk of CVD and, in particular, IHD related to COPD. However, exactly how systemic inflammation causes CVD is largely unknown. One major reason for the uncertainty is the lack of a standardized definition of systemic inflammation. In many studies, owing to widespread availability in measurements, circulating biomarkers of inflammation such as C-reactive protein (CRP) or fibrinogen have been used to indicate systemic inflammation. However, this case definition is neither specific nor sensitive as salient inflammatory pathways independent of these molecules will be easily missed and non-inflammatory stimuli such as oral contraceptives can elevate these biomarkers without inducing inflammation [28].

Notwithstanding these limitations, increases in plasma fibrinogen, CRP, interleukin-6 and, more recently, surfactant protein-D have all been associated with elevated risk of total mortality in COPD [29–31].

The source of systemic inflammation in COPD is not entirely clear. It is well accepted that with prolonged exposure to cigarettes or air pollution, lung injury, and inflammation ensues [32]. Lung inflammation persists following smoking cessation [33]. The intensity of the inflammatory reaction in the small airways relates to the severity of the underlying COPD [33]. In a mouse model, Mutlu et al. have shown that airway inflammation induced by environmental triggers such as air pollution particles spills into the systemic circulation and causes an acceleration of arterial thrombosis that is dependent on interleukin-6 [34]. Removal of alveolar macrophages from this model abrogated the increased risk of arterial thrombosis, suggesting that lung inflammation is critical to this process.

The systemic inflammatory reaction has adverse downstream effects on the systemic and coronary vasculature. Suwa and colleagues, using Watanabe Heritable Hyperlipidemic rabbits, which develop atherosclerosis naturally, showed that intratracheal exposure to air pollution particles induces a brisk systemic inflammatory response, which in turn accelerates the progression of atherosclerosis [35]. In this model, the atherosclerotic burden was directly proportional to the concentration of alveolar macrophages that contained the particulate matter. As well, with the induction of airway inflammation, the endothelium overlying the atherosclerotic plaques in these rabbits became activated with increased expression of adhesion molecules such as intercellular adhesion molecule-1 and vascular cell adhesion molecule-1 [36]. Because these molecules play critical roles in the recruitment of monocytes and lymphocytes into the atherosclerotic plaques, they further propagate the plaque and make them unstable, which contribute to plaque rupture, hemorrhage, and subsequent fibrosis [37].

Treatments that Modify Mortality in COPD

Treatment of Acute Exacerbations

Most respiratory deaths occur during periods of acute exacerbations defined as an event requiring the use of antibiotics or systemic corticosteroids or both. On an average, patients with COPD have one exacerbation per year [38]. The rate of exacerbation increases with increasing severity of disease, as measured by FEV_1. In GOLD 2 disease, the average number of exacerbations per year is 0.85; for GOLD 3, it is 1.34 per year; and for GOLD 4, it is 2 per year [38]. During these events, patients are vulnerable to mortality from both respiratory and CVD causes [39].

Most likely the use of bronchodilators in this setting enhances survival; however, there are insufficient data from high-quality clinical trials to support this notion. Similarly, although supplemental oxygen therapy is frequently provided to COPD patients during acute exacerbations, there is a paucity of data on survival. A recent meta-analysis suggests that the use of antimicrobial therapy in hospital can reduce mortality by nearly 80% [40]. However, it is notable that none of the randomized controlled trials included in this analysis was powered specifically on mortality as an endpoint. The most recently published clinical trial on this topic failed to demonstrate a significant survival advantage of patients on antibiotics over placebo [41]. Thus, it remains uncertain whether antibiotics used during acute exacerbations modify total mortality in patients with COPD. On the other hand, the survival data for the use of non-invasive mechanical ventilation (NIMV) during acute exacerbations are much more robust. Compared to standard therapy alone, the addition of NIMV to standard therapy resulted in > 50% relative risk reduction in total mortality [40]. The survival benefits are particularly notable in patients who demonstrate resting hypercapnia on arterial blood gases [40].

Chronic Management of COPD and Survival

Smoking Cessation

In the Western World, cigarette smoking accounts for ~70% of the cases of COPD. Accordingly, smoking cessation is of primary importance in improving long-term outcomes of patients with COPD. In a dose-dependent manner, smoking induces cough and dyspnea, and smoking cessation attenuates these symptoms [42]. Smoking cessation is a proven effective way to reduce mortality in COPD patients. In the LHS, smokers with mild COPD, who quit smoking, had mortality rates that were on average 45% lower than those who continued to smoke throughout the 14.5 years of follow-up. Intermittent quitters had 30% lower mortality than continued smokers but 28% higher mortality than those who quit smoke entirely (i.e., sustained quitters) [16]. Interestingly, in the LHS study, smoking cessation was associated with a rapid reduction in the risk of CVD. However, mortality from lung cancer was only significantly reduced in sustained quitters. Thus, smoking cessation is the single most important intervention for patients with COPD who also smoke.

Although the prevalence of smoking has declined over the past two decades in the U.S. and other industrialized nations, 20% of adults in the Western world are smokers. In the developing world, smoking rates are increasing with nearly 40% of adults smoking on a daily basis in certain countries [43]. General advice on smoking cessation is effective in inducing smoking cessation in only 5% of smokers [44]. A better way to foster smoking cessation is to tell patients about their "lung age." Lung age is defined as the age of the average person who has the same FEV_1 as that of the patient and can be estimated using the formula: lung age (for men) = 2.87×height (in inches) − 31.25×observed FEV_1 (l) − 39.375 and lung age (for women) = age = 3.56 × height (in inches) − 40×observed FEV_1 (l) − 77.28. [45]. In a randomized trial, smokers who received information regarding their "lung age" were twice as more likely to quit than smokers who received their raw FEV_1 data [46]. At 12 months of follow-up, the cessation rate was 14% in the lung age group versus 6% in the control group.

Recalcitrant smokers should be referred to a comprehensive multi-disciplinary smoking cessation clinic, which generally consists of medical advice coupled with cognitive and behavioral modification programs, and nicotine replacement therapy (NRT) [47]. Cognitive programs employ techniques such as distraction, positivism, relaxation, and mental imagery to modify patient's attitude towards smoking [47]. Behavioral interventions, on the other hand, focus on breaking the smoking habit by avoiding smoking triggers such as drinking coffee or alcohol or associating with friends who smoke. Collectively, these methods are effective in fostering quitting in about 10–15% of motivated smokers [48].

NRT is very effective especially if it is provided in a milieu that supports smoking cessation. The major goals of NRT are to (1) attenuate withdrawal symptoms, (2) eliminate craving, and (3) make smoking less rewarding. NRT generally doubles the cessation rate compared to physician advice alone [49]. High doses of NRT are more effective than lower doses but are fraught with more side effects [47]. However, for those patients refractory to the lower doses, higher doses should be considered. Side effects include insomnia, skin irritation (for patches), and early morning cravings for nicotine. There are 6 ways in which NRT can be administered: as a patch, gum, sublingual tablet, lozenge, nasal spray, or inhaler. The patches are the most common mode of delivery and are found in 16-h (5, 10, 15 mg) or 24-h (7, 14, 21 mg) formulations. The gums are also frequently used and they are packaged in 2 or 4 mg pieces.

Non-nicotine-based pharmacologic therapies are also available and are as effective as NRT in fostering smoking cessation. Anti-depressants and in particular bupropion significantly enhance cessation rates. Similar to NRTs, bupropion and nortryptyline double the quitting rates compared with advice alone [50]. Bupropion should be prescribed at least one week before the cessation date, so that adequate blood levels can be achieved and continued for 2–3 months following cessation. There is insufficient evidence to determine whether or not anti-depressants provide incremental benefits on cessation beyond that achieved by NRT alone. Serious side effects from anti-depressants are relatively uncommon. The risk of seizures is about 0.1% with the use of bupropion [50]. Thus, bupropion should be avoided in patients with a seizure disorder [47]. Although there are ongoing concerns regarding the possible increased risk of suicides among those who take bupropion, there is an insufficient body of evidence to support this notion.

α4β2 nicotinic acetylcholine receptor agonists (e.g., varenicline) are the most effective pharmacologic method of inducing smoking cessation [51]. Varenicline is a partial α4β2 nicotinic receptor agonist and is approximately three times more effective in effecting smoking cessation than is placebo [52]. It should be started at 0.5 mg daily while the patient is still smoking and then escalated to 1 mg per day by the second week. The patient should quit smoking completely by week 2 and the drug should be continued for another 12 weeks. The most common side effect of this drug is nausea, which can be mitigated by taking the drug following meals. Varenicline appears to be more effective than bupropion (odds ratio for smoking cessation, 1.66) [52]. However, it should be used with extreme caution (if at all) in patients with a past history of severe depression or a psychosis as it has been rarely associated with major psychiatric adverse effects [53].

Domiciliary Oxygen Therapy

According to the British MRC trial, supplemental oxygen therapy prolongs survival of COPD patients with resting hypoxemia by nearly 2.4-fold compared with no oxygen therapy [54] and according to the Nocturnal Oxygen Therapy Trial (NOTT), continuous supplemental oxygen therapy is better than nocturnal oxygen therapy in that continuous therapy extends survival by two-fold compared with nocturnal use only [55]. Oxygen therapy should thus be offered to COPD patients who demonstrate resting hypoxemia. Whether supplemental oxygen therapy benefits those COPD patients who have exertional or nocturnal hypoxemia is uncertain. However, in a small randomized clinical trial of 76 patients with nocturnal (but not resting) hypoxemia, supplemental oxygen therapy did not affect survival of COPD patients [56]. There is now a large multi-center clinical trial sponsored by the National Institutes of Health and the Centers for Medicare & Medicaid Services in the US currently underway that will provide clarity on the role of supplemental oxygen therapy for patients with exertional or nocturnal hypoxemia (http://www.nih.gov/news/pr/nov2006/nhlbi-20.htm).

Bronchodilators and Inhaled Corticosteroids

Inhaled medications are commonly used as symptomatic therapy in COPD. Long-acting bronchodilators and inhaled corticosteroids also reduce rates of exacerbation. However, none of these medications have been shown to reduce total mortality [18, 19]. Thus, these medications should be used largely to treat symptoms and to improve the quality of life of patients with COPD.

Statins and Beta-Blockers

With the increased recognition of the importance of cardiovascular comorbidities, there is a growing interest in using 3-hydroxy-3-methyl-glutaryl-CoA reductase (or "statins") as a disease-modifying agent in COPD. Observational studies suggest that they are of benefit in COPD [57] and may even reduce total mortality [57–59]. However, to date, there have been no large-scale clinical trials that have validated the findings of these observational studies. Currently, there is a large clinical trial sponsored by the US National Institutes of Health that may provide additional insights on the role of statins in COPD (http://clinicaltrials.gov/ct2/show/NCT01061671). Similarly, there is a growing body of literature on the use of beta-blockers in COPD. Contrary to classical teaching, beta-blockers are generally well tolerated by patients with COPD and importantly, may be associated with reduced mortality, especially in those with a cardiovascular comorbidity [60–62]. Thus, beta-blockers should not be withheld in patients with COPD who have a CVD indication for their use. In the future, they may be used as disease-modifying agents in COPD.

Summary and Future Directions

COPD is a growing health burden around the world. It is responsible for three million deaths per year worldwide and an important contributor to other causes of mortality such as CVD and lung cancer. By 2020, the worldwide mortality from COPD is expected to surpass seven million. The only effective interventions in reducing mortality are smoking cessation and domiciliary oxygen for patients who are hypoxemic. The pathophysiology linking COPD with CVD and lung cancer is not well known. However, systemic inflammation may play an important role in the pathogenesis of CVD. There is growing enthusiasm for using statins and beta-blockers to treat COPD patients, especially if they have underlying CVD indications for these drugs. In the future, with improved understanding of the pathogenesis, more targeted therapies will be introduced to treat patients for their underlying respiratory and cardiovascular problems and enhance survival of patients with COPD.

References

1. Jemal A, Ward E, Hao Y, Thun M. Trends in the leading causes of death in the United States, 1970–2002. JAMA. 2005;294(10):1255–9.
2. Murray CJ, Lopez AD. Alternative projections of mortality and disability by cause 1990–2020: Global Burden of Disease Study. Lancet. 1997;349(9064):1498–504.
3. Mathers CD, Loncar D. Projections of global mortality and burden of disease from 2002 to 2030. PLoS Med. 2006;3(11):e442.
4. Lin HH, Murray M, Cohen T, Colijn C, Ezzati M. Effects of smoking and solid-fuel use on COPD, lung cancer, and tuberculosis in China: a time-based, multiple risk factor, modelling study. Lancet. 2008;372(9648):1473–83.

5. Puhan MA, Garcia-Aymerich J, Frey M, ter Riet G, Anto JM, Agusti AG, et al. Expansion of the prognostic assessment of patients with chronic obstructive pulmonary disease: the updated BODE index and the ADO index. Lancet. 2009;374(9691):704–11.
6. Briggs A, Spencer M, Wang H, Mannino D, Sin DD. Development and validation of a prognostic index for health outcomes in chronic obstructive pulmonary disease. Arch Intern Med. 2008;168(1):71–9.
7. Almagro P, Calbo E, Ochoa de Echaguen A, Barreiro B, Quintana S, Heredia JL, et al. Mortality after hospitalization for COPD. Chest. 2002;121(5):1441–8.
8. Vestbo J, Prescott E, Lange P, Schnohr P, Jensen G. Vital prognosis after hospitalization for COPD: a study of a random population sample. Respir Med. 1998;92(5):772–6.
9. Celli B, Vestbo J, Jenkins CR, Jones PW, Ferguson GT, Calverley PM, et al. Gender differences in mortality and clinical expressions of patients with COPD: the TORCH experience. Am J Respir Crit Care Med. 2011;183:317–22.
10. Hoogendoorn M, Hoogenveen RT, Rutten-van Molken MP, Vestbo J, Feenstra TL. Case-fatality of COPD exacerbations: a meta-analysis and statistical modeling approach. Eur Respir J. 2011;37:508–15.
11. Tabak YP, Sun X, Johannes RS, Gupta V, Shorr AF. Mortality and need for mechanical ventilation in acute exacerbations of chronic obstructive pulmonary disease: development and validation of a simple risk score. Arch Intern Med. 2009;169(17):1595–602.
12. Brochard L, Mancebo J, Wysocki M, Lofaso F, Conti G, Rauss A, et al. Noninvasive ventilation for acute exacerbations of chronic obstructive pulmonary disease. N Engl J Med. 1995; 333(13):817–22.
13. Seneff MG, Wagner DP, Wagner RP, Zimmerman JE, Knaus WA. Hospital and 1-year survival of patients admitted to intensive care units with acute exacerbation of chronic obstructive pulmonary disease. JAMA. 1995;274(23):1852–7.
14. Sin DD, Man SF. Inhaled corticosteroids and survival in chronic obstructive pulmonary disease: does the dose matter? Eur Respir J. 2003;21(2):260–6.
15. Almagro P, Salvado M, Garcia-Vidal C, Rodriguez-Carballeira M, Delgado M, Barreiro B, et al. Recent improvement in long-term survival after a COPD hospitalisation. Thorax. 2010;65(4):298–302.
16. Anthonisen NR, Skeans MA, Wise RA, Manfreda J, Kanner RE, Connett JE. The effects of a smoking cessation intervention on 14.5-year mortality: a randomized clinical trial. Ann Intern Med. 2005;142(4):233–9.
17. McGarvey LP, John M, Anderson JA, Zvarich M, Wise RA. Ascertainment of cause-specific mortality in COPD: operations of the TORCH Clinical Endpoint Committee. Thorax. 2007;62(5):411–5.
18. Calverley PM, Anderson JA, Celli B, Ferguson GT, Jenkins C, Jones PW, et al. Salmeterol and fluticasone propionate and survival in chronic obstructive pulmonary disease. N Engl J Med. 2007;356(8):775–89.
19. Tashkin DP, Celli B, Senn S, Burkhart D, Kesten S, Menjoge S, et al. A 4-year trial of tiotropium in chronic obstructive pulmonary disease. N Engl J Med. 2008;359(15):1543–54.
20. Zvezdin B, Milutinov S, Kojicic M, Hadnadjev M, Hromis S, Markovic M, et al. A postmortem analysis of major causes of early death in patients hospitalized with COPD exacerbation. Chest. 2009;136(2):376–80.
21. Engstrom G, Wollmer P, Hedblad B, Juul-Moller S, Valind S, Janzon L. Occurrence and prognostic significance of ventricular arrhythmia is related to pulmonary function: a study from "men born in 1914," Malmo, Sweden. Circulation. 2001;103(25):3086–91.
22. Andreas S, Anker SD, Scanlon PD, Somers VK. Neurohumoral activation as a link to systemic manifestations of chronic lung disease. Chest. 2005;128(5):3618–24.
23. Heindl S, Lehnert M, Criee CP, Hasenfuss G, Andreas S. Marked sympathetic activation in patients with chronic respiratory failure. Am J Respir Crit Care Med. 2001;164(4):597–601.
24. Rabe KF, Hurd S, Anzueto A, Barnes PJ, Buist SA, Calverley P, et al. Global strategy for the diagnosis, management, and prevention of chronic obstructive pulmonary disease: GOLD executive summary. Am J Respir Crit Care Med. 2007;176(6):532–55.

25. Dahl M, Vestbo J, Lange P, Bojesen SE, Tybjaerg-Hansen A, Nordestgaard BG. C-reactive protein as a predictor of prognosis in chronic obstructive pulmonary disease. Am J Respir Crit Care Med. 2007;175(3):250–5.
26. Gan WQ, Man SF, Senthilselvan A, Sin DD. Association between chronic obstructive pulmonary disease and systemic inflammation: a systematic review and a meta-analysis. Thorax. 2004;59(7):574–80.
27. Sin DD, Man SF. Why are patients with chronic obstructive pulmonary disease at increased risk of cardiovascular diseases? The potential role of systemic inflammation in chronic obstructive pulmonary disease. Circulation. 2003;107(11):1514–9.
28. van Rooijen M, Hansson LO, Frostegard J, Silveira A, Hamsten A, Bremme K. Treatment with combined oral contraceptives induces a rise in serum C-reactive protein in the absence of a general inflammatory response. J Thromb Haemost. 2006;4(1):77–82.
29. Danesh J, Lewington S, Thompson SG, Lowe GD, Collins R, Kostis JB, et al. Plasma fibrinogen level and the risk of major cardiovascular diseases and nonvascular mortality: an individual participant meta-analysis. JAMA. 2005;294(14):1799–809.
30. Lomas DA, Silverman EK, Edwards LD, Locantore NW, Miller BE, Horstman DH, et al. Serum surfactant protein D is steroid sensitive and associated with exacerbations of COPD. Eur Respir J. 2009;34(1):95–102.
31. Man SF, Connett JE, Anthonisen NR, Wise RA, Tashkin DP, Sin DD. C-reactive protein and mortality in mild to moderate chronic obstructive pulmonary disease. Thorax. 2006;61(10): 849–53.
32. Hogg JC. Pathophysiology of airflow limitation in chronic obstructive pulmonary disease. Lancet. 2004;364(9435):709–21.
33. Hogg JC, Chu F, Utokaparch S, Woods R, Elliott WM, Buzatu L, et al. The nature of small-airway obstruction in chronic obstructive pulmonary disease. N Engl J Med. 2004;350(26): 2645–53.
34. Mutlu GM, Green D, Bellmeyer A, Baker CM, Burgess Z, Rajamannan N, et al. Ambient particulate matter accelerates coagulation via an IL-6-dependent pathway. J Clin Invest. 2007; 117(10):2952–61.
35. Suwa T, Hogg JC, Quinlan KB, Ohgami A, Vincent R, van Eeden SF. Particulate air pollution induces progression of atherosclerosis. J Am Coll Cardiol. 2002;39(6):935–42.
36. Cybulsky MI, Iiyama K, Li H, Zhu S, Chen M, Iiyama M, et al. A major role for VCAM-1, but not ICAM-1, in early atherosclerosis. J Clin Invest. 2001;107(10):1255–62.
37. Ross R. Atherosclerosis – an inflammatory disease. N Engl J Med. 1999;340(2):115–26.
38. Hurst JR, Vestbo J, Anzueto A, Locantore N, Mullerova H, Tal-Singer R, et al. Susceptibility to exacerbation in chronic obstructive pulmonary disease. N Engl J Med. 2010;363(12): 1128–38.
39. Donaldson GC, Hurst JR, Smith CJ, Hubbard RB, Wedzicha JA. Increased risk of myocardial infarction and stroke following exacerbation of COPD. Chest. 2010;137(5):1091–7.
40. Quon BS, Gan WQ, Sin DD. Contemporary management of acute exacerbations of COPD: a systematic review and metaanalysis. Chest. 2008;133(3):756–66.
41. Daniels JM, Snijders D, de Graaff CS, Vlaspolder F, Jansen HM, Boersma WG. Antibiotics in addition to systemic corticosteroids for acute exacerbations of chronic obstructive pulmonary disease. Am J Respir Crit Care Med. 2010;181(2):150–7.
42. Stein MD, Weinstock MC, Herman DS, Anderson BJ. Respiratory symptom relief related to reduction in cigarette use. J Gen Intern Med. 2005;20(10):889–94.
43. Ezzati M, Lopez AD. Estimates of global mortality attributable to smoking in 2000. Lancet. 2003;362(9387):847–52.
44. Bailey WC. Smoking cessation. Chest. 1985;88(3):322–4.
45. Morris JF, Temple W. Spirometric "lung age" estimation for motivating smoking cessation. Prev Med. 1985;14(5):655–62.
46. Parkes G, Greenhalgh T, Griffin M, Dent R. Effect on smoking quit rate of telling patients their lung age: the Step2quit randomised controlled trial. BMJ. 2008;336(7644):598–600.
47. Schroeder SA. What to do with a patient who smokes. JAMA. 2005;294(4):482–7.

48. Kanner RE, Connett JE, Williams DE, Buist AS. Effects of randomized assignment to a smoking cessation intervention and changes in smoking habits on respiratory symptoms in smokers with early chronic obstructive pulmonary disease: the Lung Health Study. Am J Med. 1999; 106(4):410–6.
49. Molyneux A. Nicotine replacement therapy. BMJ. 2004;328(7437):454–6.
50. Hughes JR, Stead LF, Lancaster T. Antidepressants for smoking cessation. Cochrane Database Syst Rev. 2007;2007(1):CD000031.
51. Gonzales D, Rennard SI, Nides M, Oncken C, Azoulay S, Billing CB, et al. Varenicline, an alpha4beta2 nicotinic acetylcholine receptor partial agonist, vs sustained-release bupropion and placebo for smoking cessation: a randomized controlled trial. JAMA. 2006;296(1): 47–55.
52. Cahill K, Stead LF, Lancaster T. Nicotine receptor partial agonists for smoking cessation. Cochrane Database Syst Rev. 2007;2007(1):006103.
53. Pumariega AJ, Nelson R, Rotenberg L. Varenicline-induced mixed mood and psychotic episode in a patient with a past history of depression. CNS Spectr. 2008;13(6):511–4.
54. Long term domiciliary oxygen therapy in chronic hypoxic cor pulmonale complicating chronic bronchitis and emphysema. Report of the Medical Research Council Working Party. Lancet. 1981;1(8222):681–6.
55. Continuous or nocturnal oxygen therapy in hypoxemic chronic obstructive lung disease: a clinical trial. Nocturnal Oxygen Therapy Trial Group. Ann Intern Med. 1980;93(3):391–8.
56. Chaouat A, Weitzenblum E, Kessler R, Charpentier C, Enrhart M, Schott R, et al. A randomized trial of nocturnal oxygen therapy in chronic obstructive pulmonary disease patients. Eur Respir J. 1999;14(5):1002–8.
57. Janda S, Park K, FitzGerald JM, Etminan M, Swiston J. Statins in COPD: a systematic review. Chest. 2009;136(3):734–43.
58. van Gestel YR, Hoeks SE, Sin DD, Simsek C, Welten GM, Schouten O, et al. Effect of statin therapy on mortality in patients with peripheral arterial disease and comparison of those with versus without associated chronic obstructive pulmonary disease. Am J Cardiol. 2008;102(2): 192–6.
59. Soyseth V, Brekke PH, Smith P, Omland T. Statin use is associated with reduced mortality in COPD. Eur Respir J. 2007;29(2):279–83.
60. Dransfield MT, Rowe SM, Johnson JE, Bailey WC, Gerald LB. Use of beta blockers and the risk of death in hospitalised patients with acute exacerbations of COPD. Thorax. 2008;63(4): 301–5.
61. Rutten FH, Zuithoff NP, Hak E, Grobbee DE, Hoes AW. Beta-blockers may reduce mortality and risk of exacerbations in patients with chronic obstructive pulmonary disease. Arch Intern Med. 2010;170(10):880–7.
62. van Gestel YR, Hoeks SE, Sin DD, Welten GM, Schouten O, Witteveen HJ, et al. Impact of cardioselective beta-blockers on mortality in patients with chronic obstructive pulmonary disease and atherosclerosis. Am J Respir Crit Care Med. 2008;178(7):695–700.
63. Anthonisen NR, Connett JE, Kiley JP, Altose MD, Bailey WC, Buist AS, et al. Effects of smoking intervention and the use of an inhaled anticholinergic bronchodilator on the rate of decline of FEV1. The Lung Health Study. JAMA. 1994;272(19):1497–505.

Chapter 2
The Role of Systemic Inflammation in COPD

Kristina L. Bailey, Jadvinder Goraya, and Stephen L. Rennard

Abstract Chronic obstructive pulmonary disease (COPD) is defined as a preventable and treatable disease with significant extrapulmonary effects. Many of the extra-pulmonary effects of COPD are thought to be mediated by systemic inflammation. Local inflammation has always been appreciated as part of the COPD disease process; however, it is becoming clear that the inflammatory response is also systemic. There are multiple theories about the mechanisms driving the systemic inflammation associated with COPD. However, there is no consensus on which theory is correct. The systemic inflammation likely contributes to systemic mani-festations of COPD, including cardiovascular disease, lung cancer, weight loss, osteoporosis and diabetes.

Keywords COPD • Extrapulmonary effects • Disease severity • Local inflammation • Lung parenchyma • Cytokines • Systemic • Tumor necrosis alpha • Interleukin • C-reactive proteins

Introduction

Chronic obstructive pulmonary disease (COPD) is defined as a preventable and treatable disease with significant extrapulmonary effects that may contribute to dis-ease severity in individual patients [1]. Many of the extrapulmonary effects of COPD are believed to be mediated by systemic inflammation. Local inflammation

K.L. Bailey (✉) • J. Goraya • S.L. Rennard
Department of Internal Medicine, Pulmonary, Critical Care, Sleep and Allergy Division,
University of Nebraska Medical Center, Omaha, NE, USA
e-mail: kbailey@unmc.edu; srennard@unmc.edu

L. Nici and R. ZuWallack (eds.), *Chronic Obstructive Pulmonary Disease: Co-Morbidities and Systemic Consequences*, Respiratory Medicine, DOI 10.1007/978-1-60761-673-3_2, © Springer Science+Business Media, LLC 2012

of the airways and lung parenchyma has always been acknowledged as part of the COPD disease process; however, it is becoming clear that the inflammatory response is systemic [2].

Many studies demonstrate that there is an increase in inflammatory cytokines not only in the lung, but systemically. There is an increase in tumor necrosis factor alpha (TNF-α) [3] interleukin (IL)-6, and IL-8 [4]. Inflammatory markers such as C-reactive protein (CRP) are also elevated [5]. This chapter will review the origins, clinical consequences, pathogenesis, and the treatment of systemic inflammation in COPD.

Origins of Systemic Inflammation

There are multiple theories about the mechanisms driving the systemic inflammation associated with COPD. There is no consensus on which theory is correct, although it is likely that several mechanisms may contribute.

One proposed mechanism suggests that the inflammatory process originates in the airways and lung parenchyma, then "spills over" into the systemic circulation [6]. One may then assume that the systemic inflammation should directly correlate with pulmonary inflammation. This, however, has not been demonstrated. Specifically, there is no consistent relationship between sputum neutrophil numbers and systemic neutrophil numbers or systemic biomarkers of inflammation such as CRP [7, 8]. Likewise, pulmonary inflammatory cytokine concentrations such as TNF-α and IL-8 do not show a correlation with systemic concentrations [9, 10].

Another proposed mechanism is that systemic inflammation is caused by tobacco smoke. This is an attractive theory because tobacco smoke has been implicated as a cause of other systemic inflammatory diseases such as atherosclerosis and coronary artery disease [11]. Indeed, in passive smoke exposure, there is increased systemic oxidative stress and peripheral vascular endothelial dysfunction [12]. However, multiple studies demonstrate that ex-smokers have evidence of persistent inflammation [9]. This implies that tobacco smoking may initiate inflammation, but does not explain the sustained inflammation seen in COPD.

It is also possible that the pathophysiologic changes that occur in the lung with COPD may lead to systemic inflammation. Processes that have been implicated include hypoxia and hyperinflation. Hypoxia is a common problem in COPD. In patients with mild COPD who undergo hypoxic challenge, there is an increase in serum IL-6 levels [13]. There is also a correlation between serum TNF-α levels and degree of hypoxemia in COPD patients [14]. Likewise, in animal experiments, hypoxia leads to increased TNF-α, macrophage inflammatory protein (MIP)-1β, and monocyte chemoattractant protein (MCP)-1 MrnA [15]. Hyperinflation is also a common finding in COPD that results from chronic airway obstruction. Dynamic hyperinflation can lead to increases in systemic TNF-α and IL-8 [16], IL-6, and IL-1β [17]. The presence of dynamic hyperinflation predicts a higher mortality for COPD patients [18].

It has been suggested that the increases in systemic inflammation observed in conjunction with COPD are at least in part due to the normal aging process. COPD is a chronic disease, which progresses very slowly, and the majority of patients are older. Normal aging is associated with increases in low-grade systemic inflammation, including production of cytokines such as IL-6 and TNF-α [19]. There is also an increase in nitric oxide and reactive oxygen species [20]. Aging cannot account for all COPD-related systemic inflammation, as most studies examining COPD include age-matched controls and the systemic inflammation in COPD patients is still greater.

It has been suggested that COPD may trigger the production of systemic inflammatory mediators in other parts of the body such as skeletal muscle and the bone marrow. For instance, compared to healthy controls, patients with COPD have increases in systemic inflammation, including TNF-α production, after exercise [21]. It was initially thought that the source of this inflammation might be the skeletal muscle itself [22]. However, in a well-controlled study, it was shown that the muscular TNF-α in COPD subjects was actually less than that of control subjects [23]. Another possibility is that the bone marrow may be involved in the initiation of systemic inflammation. This is an attractive theory because the bone marrow is the site of production of inflammatory cells. Smoking or air pollution may indirectly stimulate the bone marrow, which results in an accelerated release of mature and immature cells [24].

In summary, there are many theories regarding the origin of systemic inflammation in COPD. The true origin of systemic inflammation is likely to be multifactorial and more research is necessary to identify the different contributory factors and their relative importance.

Consequences of Systemic Inflammation

The systemic inflammation associated with COPD can contribute to the development of other disease states. The systemic manifestations of COPD are widespread and can affect nearly every system in the body. Disease states that are commonly related to the systemic inflammation seen in COPD include: cardiovascular disease, lung cancer, weight loss, osteoporosis, and diabetes.

Cardiovascular Disease

Cardiovascular disease has long been associated with COPD. Smoking is a major risk factor for both diseases, so it is not surprising that many patients with COPD also have cardiovascular disease. In fact, the majority of patients with COPD die from cardiovascular disorders [25, 26]. Although COPD and cardiovascular disease share smoking as a risk factor, there is an increased risk of fatal myocardial infarction, independent of smoking status, in COPD patients [27]. There is also an increased risk of cardiovascular disease in smokers who develop COPD than in smokers that do not develop COPD [27]. Likewise, those with more severe COPD are also more likely to have cardiovascular disease [28] even when corrected for smoking. These studies suggest that it is not smoking alone that leads to the increased risk of cardiovascular disease. Importantly, having both COPD and cardiovascular disease increases mortality and hospitalizations over either condition separately [29].

The mechanisms for the synergistic interaction between COPD and cardiovascular disease are not well defined. It has been suggested that the chronic low-grade systemic inflammation seen with both diseases may drive both processes.

Lung Cancer

Lung cancer is a common cause of death in patients with COPD. Patients with COPD are four times more likely to develop lung cancer than smokers who have not developed COPD [30]. Smoking cessation does not diminish the risk of developing lung cancer [31]. Even in individuals who have never smoked, there is an increased risk of lung cancer with decreasing lung function and COPD [32].

The mechanism(s) of how COPD increases the risk for lung cancer is not well defined. However, there is emerging evidence that chronic inflammation may play a significant role in the pathogenesis of lung cancer as a tumor promoter. Inflammatory mechanisms have been shown to induce a tumor-promoting effect in lung cancer in mice. In this model, tobacco smoke promotes lung tumorigenesis by triggering IKKβ- and JNK1-dependent inflammation [33]. There are also links between NF-κB and lung cancer, including resistance to chemotherapy and induction of pro-metastatic, pro-angiogenic, and anti-apoptotic genes [34]. Likewise, epidermal growth factor, which promotes epithelial proliferation, is present in higher levels in COPD patients [35].

Weight Loss/Muscle Wasting

Many studies have shown nutritional abnormalities in patients with COPD. These include changes in caloric intake, basal metabolic rate, and body composition [36, 37]. Unexplained weight loss occurs in about 50% of patients with severe COPD, but it also occurs in 10–15% of those with mild to moderate disease [38]. Unexplained weight loss is a poor prognostic indicator in COPD, and is independent of FEV1 or hypoxia [39]. Likewise, malnutrition predicts longer hospitalization and more readmissions after acute exacerbation of COPD [40].

The weight loss seen in COPD is not due to decreased caloric intake. In fact, caloric intake in patients with COPD is often normal or increased [41]. This increase in caloric intake is often not enough to offset the increased basal metabolic rate in COPD [42]. The weight loss seen in COPD, which is likely due to cachexia, does not respond as well to nutritional supplementation as simple malnutrition [43].

However, if body weight is regained, the overall prognosis is improved, despite lack of change in lung function [39].

Skeletal muscle atrophy is the major cause of weight loss in COPD, with fat mass contributing only a small part of the total weight loss [38]. The remaining muscle is often weak [44], contributing to the limited exercise capacity in COPD.

The mechanisms of weight loss and skeletal muscle atrophy are also likely linked to systemic inflammation. There is a correlation between metabolic derangement and increased levels of inflammatory mediators in COPD [45]. TNF-α production is increased in COPD patients with weight loss [46], TNF-α, as well as other inflammatory cytokines, activates NFκB, which can upregulate inducible nitric oxide synthase (iNOS) and lead to degradation of myosin [47], ultimately resulting in decreased skeletal muscle mass.

Osteoporosis

The prevalence of osteoporosis is very high in patients with COPD. Over half of the patients recruited for the large TORCH (Towards a Revolution in COPD Health) trial had osteopenia or osteoporosis [48]. In patients with severe COPD, the prevalence of osteoporosis goes up to 75%. In this study the use of steroids alone could not explain the high prevalence of osteoporosis in patients with COPD [49].

Osteoporosis adds significant morbidity to COPD. With progressive loss of bone mass, the patient is at high risk for vertebral or hip fractures. Vertebral compression fractures can cause kyphosis, which can result in worsened pulmonary function. Hip fractures cause significant morbidity such as pain, decreased mobility, and even mortality [50].

Osteoporosis associated with COPD is multifactorial in its etiology. It is most commonly seen in individuals who are elderly, are on steroids, have a history of smoking, or have chronic illness [51]. Patients who have moderate-to-severe COPD have nearly all of these clinical features that predispose them to osteoporosis. However, COPD itself may be a risk factor for osteoporosis and this may be related to systemic inflammation. The mechanism through which systemic inflammation leads to increased osteoporosis is very poorly understood. It is known that increased production of pro-inflammatory cytokines such as IL-1, TNF-α, and IL-6 is associated with osteoclastic bone resorption in a number of inflammatory disease states including rheumatoid arthritis [52]. In addition, the inflammatory mediator, circulating MMP-9, has also been related to the presence of osteoporosis in patients with COPD and not to lung function [53].

Diabetes

Type II diabetes is also frequently seen in conjunction with COPD. There is nearly a twofold increase in prevalence of type II diabetes in patients with COPD, even in those with mild disease [54]. In the Women's Health Study, asthma and COPD were independently associated with an increased risk of type II diabetes [55]. This indicates that chronic airway inflammation may contribute to diabetes pathogenesis. The reason for this association is not yet fully understood, but it likely involves systemic inflammation. It does appear that there is an increase in insulin resistance in patients with COPD compared with healthy subjects. In this study, insulin resistance was related to higher serum IL-6, and TNF-α soluble receptor, suggesting that insulin resistance is related to systemic inflammation [56]. In patients with Type II diabetes, more severe systemic inflammation (elevated levels of TNF-α, fibrinogen, ferritin, and CRP) may be associated with both inadequate glucose control and worsening lung function [57]. Another possible cause of Type II diabetes in patients with COPD could be the use of inhaled steroids. Inhaled corticosteroid use was associated with a 34% increase in the rate of diabetes. The risk was greatest with the highest inhaled corticosteroid doses, equivalent to fluticasone 1,000 μg per day or more [58].

Pathophysiology of Systemic Inflammation

The systemic inflammation associated with COPD has many different mediators. They include circulating inflammatory cells, inflammatory mediators such as cytokines, oxidative stress, and growth factors.

Circulating Inflammatory Cells

An integral part of systemic inflammatory response is the activation of bone marrow, which results in the release of leukocytes into the circulation [6], including neutrophils, monocytes/macrophages, and lymphocytes. Patients with COPD have various abnormalities in these circulating leukocytes. The abnormalities seen may have effects on organs other than the lung and therefore contribute to the systemic inflammation observed in COPD patients.

Neutrophils

Circulating neutrophils are an important component of host defense in the lung. In patients with COPD, circulating neutrophils do not function normally, which contributes to the systemic inflammatory response. In COPD, neutrophils have an increased chemotactic response, increased ability to digest connective tissue, and increased expression of cell surface adhesion molecules [59].

Although increased numbers of neutrophils are seen in the airway of patients with COPD, this does not necessarily translate to increased numbers of circulating neutrophils compared to healthy nonsmokers. There is, however, an inverse correlation between FEV_1 and neutrophil numbers in circulation [60]. An inflammatory stimulus can trigger increased production of neutrophils from the bone marrow but also result in increased numbers of neutrophils in the lung parenchyma [61].

One important pathogenic mechanism responsible for abnormal neutrophil function in patients with COPD is that their neutrophils produce more reactive oxygen species (ROS) than smokers with normal lung function, and healthy nonsmokers [59, 62]. Systemic oxidative stress can upregulate the expression of adhesion molecules, facilitating recruitment into the lung [63].

We have a clear understanding that neutrophils play an integral part in the inflammatory response generated in COPD. The lack of differences in neutrophil activation and function among smokers with COPD and nonsmoker healthy subjects suggests that smoke itself is not responsible for this effect. Rather, these abnormalities are characteristic of COPD itself.

Lymphocytes

Lymphocytes play a prominent role in the systemic inflammation seen in patients with COPD. Nonsmoking COPD patients had higher number of CD^{8+} lymphocytes than nonsmoking healthy controls [64]. Studies also demonstrate that a higher CD^{8+} lymphocyte count is associated with both low CD^4/CD^8 ratio and a higher degree of airflow obstruction and lower FEV_1 [64–67]. Whether this abnormality is mirrored in the systemic circulation is unclear. Changes in the circulating lymphocytes are difficult to interpret because they may reflect a recruitment of circulating lymphocytes into the lung.

Current thinking suggests that abnormal lymphocyte regulation has a role in the pathogenesis of COPD. Proposed mechanisms include abnormalities in the apoptosis of T-cells. There is an increase in apoptosis along with an increase in T-cell migration/recruitment and a decrease in airways clearance by defective macrophages [68]. Apoptosis is under the control of Fas proteins, tissue growth factor (TGFβ), and tumor necrosis factor (TNFα) [66, 67, 69]. Fas protein belongs to the TNF family and is upregulated upon T-cell activation. The Fas/FasL (ligand) system induces apoptosis and regulates elimination of activated lymphocytes [70]. Higher numbers of CD^{8+} T-cells exhibiting Fas expression have been reported in COPD smokers as compared to healthy smokers and nonsmokers [67]. Similarly, TNFα and TGFβ have been shown to induce apoptosis in CD^{8+} T-cells in COPD patients [71]. Combined, these studies shed light on possible dysregulation in mechanisms that control apoptosis and may bear some responsibility in the pathogenesis of COPD.

Monocytes/Macrophages

Macrophages play an important role in the inflammatory response responsible for the pathophysiology of COPD. Monocytes circulating in the peripheral blood are recruited into the lungs, where they mature into macrophages. This recruitment is upregulated in COPD. Monocyte-selective chemokines produced in the lungs are the signal for the migration of monocytes. In particular, macrophage chemotactic protein (MCP-1), a monocyte selective chemokine belonging to the CC chemokine family, is increased in the sputum and BAL of patients with COPD [72]. MCP-1 binds to the chemokine receptor (CCR-2) on the monocytes and mediates recruitment into the airway epithelium and the lung parenchyma. Chemokines from the CXC subfamily have also been shown to act as monocyte chemoattractants via the CXC receptor (CXCR-2). Similar to MCP-1, the CXC chemokine, GRO-α, exists in higher concentration in the sputum and BAL of smokers with COPD compared to healthy smokers and nonsmokers [73]. Interestingly, CXCR-2 expression is not present on all monocytes. Traves et al. postulates that there is upregulation of the recycling of the CXCR-2 receptor only in the COPD population compared to non-smokers and healthy smokers, which could be the reason for increased migration of monocytes in COPD [73].

Under normal circumstances, macrophages have a tissue lifespan of many months. In former smokers, cigarette particulates persist in the alveolar macrophages over 2 years after smoking cessation, indicating that macrophages in smokers persist for abnormally long durations [74]. Expression of anti-apoptotic protein Bcl-X_L and p21$^{CIP/WAF1}$ in smokers could be one mechanism for this prolonged survival [56, 75]. Impaired mucocilliary clearance or inadequate lymphatic drainage may also impair the ability to clear macrophages from the airways in COPD patients.

Inflammatory Mediators

Patients with COPD have elevated levels of circulating cytokines, chemokines, and growth factors in their peripheral circulation. The components of this systemic inflammation may account for the systemic manifestations of COPD and may worsen comorbid conditions.

Cytokines

IL-6

IL-6 is increased in the systemic circulation of COPD patients. This is particularly true during acute exacerbations. The downstream effects of elevated levels of IL-6 are not yet clearly defined because of its pleiotrophic effects. It is clear that IL-6 levels track with markers of systemic inflammation. For instance, increased circulating IL-6 has been shown to induce the acute phase reactant CRP production from the liver [76]. Increased IL-6 levels have also been shown to be associated with many of the systemic comorbidities of COPD. Elevated IL-6 may play a role in the development of pulmonary hypertension [77] insulin resistance [56], and osteoporosis [78].

TNF-α

Elevated levels of TNF-α are seen in the sputum of patients with COPD, especially during exacerbations. Many cells make TNF-α, including epithelial cells, T-cells, and mast cells, but the major source is macrophages. Macrophages from patients with COPD produce more TNF-α in vitro than macrophages from normal controls [79]. Elevated TNF-α levels are associated with systemic effects of COPD such as weight loss. Because of this association, TNF-α blocking antibodies, such as infliximab, have been studied as a treatment for COPD. Unfortunately, they have not been able to show any differences in inflammatory markers [80], Chronic Respiratory Questionnaire score, FEV1, or 6-min walk [81]. There is evidence, however, that etanercept, another TNF-α antagonist, decreases COPD hospitalizations [82].

IL-1β

IL-1β is also elevated in the sputum of patients with COPD [83]. IL-1β activates macrophages to secrete inflammatory cytokines. IL-1β correlates with disease severity and FEV_1 [83] It has also been linked to cachexia.

Chemokines

The first chemokine to be discovered in COPD is CXCL-8. Elevated levels of CXCL-8 are found in the sputum, BAL fluid, and the circulation of patients with COPD versus normal smokers and nonsmoking controls. CXCL8 activates CSCL1 (GRO-α) and CXCR2. CXCL-8 and CXCR2 play an important role in neutrophil and monocyte recruitment in COPD.

Growth Factors

Granulocyte-Macrophage Colony Stimulating Factor (GM-CSF)

GM-CSF is secreted predominantly by macrophages in response to inflammatory stimuli and plays a role in the differentiation and survival of neutrophils. There are increased levels of GM-CSF in the BAL fluid of patients with COPD particularly during exacerbations [84].

Transforming Growth Factor-β (TGF-β)

TGF-β expression is increased in the airway epithelial cells and macrophages of the small airways of patients with COPD [85]. It can induce proliferation of fibroblasts and airway smooth muscle cells. It also can lead to suppression of the regulatory T cells such as Th1, Th2, and Th17 cells [86].

Treatment

Because systemic inflammation can lead to many of the comorbidities associated with COPD, it is important to consider how to best treat systemic inflammation. Although research into how best to treat the systemic inflammation associated with COPD is in its infancy, we do have some information. Some of the therapies we have traditionally used to treat COPD may also have an effect on systemic inflammation. In addition, drugs used to treat the comorbidities of COPD may also may have unexpected positive effects on systemic inflammation.

Inhaled Steroids

A small study of inhaled steroids shows a reduction in CRP levels in COPD patients [87]. However, a much larger controlled trial of high-dose inhaled steroids in COPD patients (TORCH trial) shows no reduction in IL-6 and CRP levels and no reduction in mortality, although these results may have been affected by withdrawal bias [88]. One of the advantages of inhaled corticosteroids is that they are delivered locally to the lung to avoid the systemic side effects of oral steroids. Perhaps it is not surprising then that inhaled steroids have little or no effect on systemic inflammation. Despite this fact, they still have positive effects on the overall care of COPD patients, such as reduced exacerbation frequency, improved health status, and spirometric values [89].

Anticholinergics

It has been suggested that anticholinergics such as tiotroprium may have a role in decreasing systemic inflammation. This is because airway epithelial cells and macrophages can release acetycholine, and this may activate neutrophils and macrophages. Theoretically, by antagonizing this pathway, there is a potential to decrease inflammation. However, in practice, tiotroprium has no effect on serum IL-6 and CRP in COPD patients, although it does decrease the number of exacerbations [90].

Exercise/Pulmonary Rehabilitation

Pulmonary rehabilitation improves functional capacity, perception of dyspnea, BODE index, and health care utilization [91]. Because pulmonary rehabilitation has a positive effect on the overall health of COPD patients, one would think it may do so through decreasing systemic inflammation. However, to date, this has not been shown. There is no difference in systemic inflammatory markers such as CRP and IL-6 [92] after pulmonary rehabilitation. In fact, in one study, there was an increase in production of IL-6 and TNF-α in muscle cells after exercise training [93]. Although there have not been differences in systemic inflammatory markers with pulmonary rehabilitation alone, there may be benefits when combined with nutritional therapy [94]. In this study there was a decrease in CRP, IL-6, IL-8, and TNFα after 12 weeks of low intensity exercise and nutritional supplementation of 400 kcal/day.

Smoking Cessation

Smoking cessation is always recommended for patients with COPD. It not only helps slow the progression of COPD, but also has beneficial effects on comorbidities such as cardiovascular disease and lung cancer. Smoking cessation also leads to decreases in systemic inflammation as measured by CRP [95].

Statins

3-Hydroxy-3-methylglutaryl-coenzyme A (*HMG-CoA*) *reductase* inhibitors, also known as statins, were developed to reduce cholesterol. However, statins are now known to have pleiotropic effects, including anti-inflammatory and immunomodulatory effects that may be important in the treatment of systemic inflammation from COPD.

Statins have been shown to decrease mortality after COPD exacerbation, even in the absence of ischemic heart disease in retrospective studies [96]. This is especially relevant, given the number of COPD patients who also have ischemic heart disease. Statins also decrease the number of COPD exacerbations in retrospective studies [97]. The mechanism(s) through which statins impart their beneficial effects are not completely understood. However, it is likely that at least part of their action is through decreasing systemic inflammation. Statins decrease markers of systemic inflammation such as CRP [98] and chemokines, such as CCL2 and CXCL8 [99].

Statins also may have beneficial effects on the comorbidities of COPD that are mediated by systemic inflammation. Statins are associated with a decreased risk of developing lung cancer in COPD patients [100]. They may also have a beneficial effect on diabetes and osteoporosis [101].

Prospective, randomized, controlled studies are needed to evaluate whether statins have a beneficial effect on the systemic inflammation related to COPD.

Summary

In summary, COPD can no longer be considered a disease only of the lungs. It is associated with systemic effects that are related to systemic inflammation. A better understanding of the origins of systemic inflammation in COPD will allow for better therapy for COPD and improved outcomes.

References

1. Rabe KF, Hurd S, Anzueto A, Barnes PJ, Buist SA, Calverley P, et al. Global strategy for the diagnosis, management, and prevention of chronic obstructive pulmonary disease: GOLD executive summary. Am J Respir Crit Care Med. 2007;176(6):532–55.
2. Gan WQ, Man SF, Senthilselvan A, Sin DD. Association between chronic obstructive pulmonary disease and systemic inflammation: a systematic review and a meta-analysis. Thorax. 2004;59(7):574–80.
3. Tanni SE, Pelegrino NR, Angeleli AY, Correa C, Godoy I. Smoking status and tumor necrosis factor-alpha mediated systemic inflammation in COPD patients. J Inflamm (Lond). 2010; 9(7):29.
4. Pinto-Plata VM, Livnat G, Girish M, Cabral H, Masdin P, Linacre P, et al. Systemic cytokines, clinical and physiological changes in patients hospitalized for exacerbation of COPD. Chest. 2007;131(1):37–43.
5. Karadag F, Kirdar S, Karul AB, Ceylan E. The value of C-reactive protein as a marker of systemic inflammation in stable chronic obstructive pulmonary disease. Eur J Int Med. 2008;19(2):104–8.
6. Agusti AG, Noguera A, Sauleda J, Sala E, Pons J, Busquets X. Systemic effects of chronic obstructive pulmonary disease. Eur Respir J. 2003;21(2):347–60.
7. Singh D, Edwards L, Tal-Singer R, Rennard S. Sputum neutrophils as a biomarker in COPD: findings from the ECLIPSE study. Respir Res. 2010;11:77.
8. Roy K, Smith J, Kolsum U, Borrill Z, Vestbo J, Singh D. COPD phenotype description using principal components analysis. Respir Res. 2009;10:41.
9. Vernooy JH, Kucukaycan M, Jacobs JA, Chavannes NH, Buurman WA, Dentener MA, et al. Local and systemic inflammation in patients with chronic obstructive pulmonary disease: soluble tumor necrosis factor receptors are increased in sputum. Am J Respir Crit Care Med. 2002;166(9):1218–24.
10. Michel O, Dentener M, Corazza F, Buurman W, Rylander R. Healthy subjects express differences in clinical responses to inhaled lipopolysaccharide that are related with inflammation and with atopy. J Allergy Clin Immunol. 2001;107(5):797–804.
11. Hansson GK. Inflammation, atherosclerosis, and coronary artery disease. N Engl J Med. 2005;352(16):1685–95.
12. Dietrich M, Block G, Benowitz NL, Morrow JD, Hudes M, 3rd Jacob P, et al. Vitamin C supplementation decreases oxidative stress biomarker f2-isoprostanes in plasma of nonsmokers exposed to environmental tobacco smoke. Nutr Cancer. 2003;45(2):176–84.
13. Sabit R, Thomas P, Shale DJ, Collins P, Linnane SJ. The effects of hypoxia on markers of coagulation and systemic inflammation in patients with COPD. Chest. 2010;138(1):47–51.
14. Takabatake N, Nakamura H, Abe S, Inoue S, Hino T, Saito H, et al. The relationship between chronic hypoxemia and activation of the tumor necrosis factor-alpha system in patients with chronic obstructive pulmonary disease. Am J Respir Crit Care Med. 2000;161(4 Pt 1):1179–84.
15. Madjdpour C, Jewell UR, Kneller S, Ziegler U, Schwendener R, Booy C, et al. Decreased alveolar oxygen induces lung inflammation. Am J Physiol Lung Cell Mol Physiol. 2003;284(2): L360–7.
16. Pini L, Valsecchi A, Boni E, Guerini M, Tantucci C. Acute dynamic hyperinflation and systemic inflammation in stable COPD patients. Am J Respir Crit Care Med. 2010;181:A2907.
17. Vassilakopoulos T, Katsaounou P, Karatza MH, Kollintza A, Zakynthinos S, Roussos C. Strenuous resistive breathing induces plasma cytokines: role of antioxidants and monocytes. Am J Respir Crit Care Med. 2002;166(12 Pt 1):1572–8.
18. Casanova C, Cote C, de Torres JP, Aguirre-Jaime A, Marin JM, Pinto-Plata V, et al. Inspiratory-to-total lung capacity ratio predicts mortality in patients with chronic obstructive pulmonary disease. Am J Respir Crit Care Med. 2005;171(6):591–7.
19. Sharma G, Hanania NA, Shim YM. The aging immune system and its relationship to the development of chronic obstructive pulmonary disease. Proc Am Thorac Soc. 2009;6(7): 573–80.

20. Ito K, Barnes PJ. COPD as a disease of accelerated lung aging. Chest. 2009;135(1):173–80.
21. Rabinovich RA, Figueras M, Ardite E, Carbo N, Troosters T, Filella X, et al. Increased tumour necrosis factor-alpha plasma levels during moderate-intensity exercise in COPD patients. Eur Respir J. 2003;21(5):789–94.
22. Montes de Oca M, Torres SH, De Sanctis J, Mata A, Hernandez N, Talamo C. Skeletal muscle inflammation and nitric oxide in patients with COPD. Eur Respir J. 2005;26(3):390–7.
23. Barreiro E, Schols AM, Polkey MI, Galdiz JB, Gosker HR, Swallow EB, et al. Cytokine profile in quadriceps muscles of patients with severe COPD. Thorax. 2008;63(2):100–7.
24. Terashima T, Wiggs B, English D, Hogg JC, van Eeden SF. The effect of cigarette smoking on the bone marrow. Am J Respir Crit Care Med. 1997;155(3):1021–6.
25. Hansell AL, Walk JA, Soriano JB. What do chronic obstructive pulmonary disease patients die from? A multiple cause coding analysis. Eur Respir J. 2003;22(5):809–14.
26. Mannino DM, Watt G, Hole D, Gillis C, Hart C, McConnachie A, et al. The natural history of chronic obstructive pulmonary disease. Eur Respir J. 2006;27(3):627–43.
27. Sin DD, Man SF. Chronic obstructive pulmonary disease as a risk factor for cardiovascular morbidity and mortality. Proc Am Thorac Soc. 2005;2(1):8–11.
28. Black-Shinn JL, Kinney GL, Wise A, Regan E, Make BJ, Krants M, et al. Cardiovascular disease is associated with COPD severity and reduced functional capacity. Am J Respir Crit Care Med. 2010;181:A5918.
29. Mannino DM, Thorn D, Swensen A, Holguin F. Prevalence and outcomes of diabetes, hypertension and cardiovascular disease in COPD. Eur Respir J. 2008;32(4):962–9.
30. Tockman MS, Anthonisen NR, Wright EC, Donithan MG. Airways obstruction and the risk for lung cancer. Ann Intern Med. 1987;106(4):512–8.
31. Anthonisen NR, Skeans MA, Wise RA, Manfreda J, Kanner RE, Connett JE, et al. The effects of a smoking cessation intervention on 14.5-year mortality: a randomized clinical trial. Ann Intern Med. 2005;142(4):233–9.
32. Turner MC, Chen Y, Krewski D, Calle EE, Thun MJ. Chronic obstructive pulmonary disease is associated with lung cancer mortality in a prospective study of never smokers. Am J Respir Crit Care Med. 2007;176(3):285–90.
33. Takahashi H, Ogata H, Nishigaki R, Broide DH, Karin M. Tobacco smoke promotes lung tumorigenesis by triggering IKKbeta- and JNK1-dependent inflammation. Cancer Cell. 2010;17(1):89–97.
34. Dennis PA, Van Waes C, Gutkind JS, Kellar KJ, Vinson C, Mukhin AG, et al. The biology of tobacco and nicotine: bench to bedside. Cancer Epidemiol Biomarkers Prev. 2005;14(4):764–7.
35. de Boer WI, Hau CM, van Schadewijk A, Stolk J, van Krieken JH, Hiemstra PS. Expression of epidermal growth factors and their receptors in the bronchial epithelium of subjects with chronic obstructive pulmonary disease. Am J Clin Pathol. 2006;125(2):184–92.
36. Creutzberg EC, Schols AM, Weling-Scheepers CA, Buurman WA, Wouters EF. Characterization of nonresponse to high caloric oral nutritional therapy in depleted patients with chronic obstructive pulmonary disease. Am J Respir Crit Care Med. 2000;161(3 Pt 1):745–52.
37. Schols AM, Wouters EF. Nutritional abnormalities and supplementation in chronic obstructive pulmonary disease. Clin Chest Med. 2000;21(4):753–62.
38. Schols AM, Soeters PB, Dingemans AM, Mostert R, Frantzen PJ, Wouters EF. Prevalence and characteristics of nutritional depletion in patients with stable COPD eligible for pulmonary rehabilitation. Am Rev Respir Dis. 1993;147(5):1151–6.
39. Schols AM, Slangen J, Volovics L, Wouters EF. Weight loss is a reversible factor in the prognosis of chronic obstructive pulmonary disease. Am J Respir Crit Care Med. 1998;157(6 Pt 1):1791–7.
40. Giron R, Matesanz C, Garcia-Rio F, de Santiago E, Mancha A, Rodriguez-Salvanes F, et al. Nutritional state during COPD exacerbation: clinical and prognostic implications. Ann Nutr Metab. 2009;54(1):52–8.

41. Baarends EM, Schols AM, Pannemans DL, Westerterp KR, Wouters EF. Total free living energy expenditure in patients with severe chronic obstructive pulmonary disease. Am J Respir Crit Care Med. 1997;155(2):549–54.
42. Schols AM, Fredrix EW, Soeters PB, Westerterp KR, Wouters EF. Resting energy expenditure in patients with chronic obstructive pulmonary disease. Am J Clin Nutr. 1991;54(6): 983–7.
43. Ferreira IM, Brooks D, Lacasse Y, Goldstein RS. Nutritional support for individuals with COPD: a meta-analysis. Chest. 2000;117(3):672–8.
44. Gosker HR, Kubat B, Schaart G, van der Vusse GJ, Wouters EF, Schols AM. Myopathological features in skeletal muscle of patients with chronic obstructive pulmonary disease. Eur Respir J. 2003;22(2):280–5.
45. Schols AM, Buurman WA, Staal van den Brekel AJ, Dentener MA, Wouters EF. Evidence for a relation between metabolic derangements and increased levels of inflammatory mediators in a subgroup of patients with chronic obstructive pulmonary disease. Thorax. 1996;51(8): 819–24.
46. Di Francia M, Barbier D, Mege JL, Orehek J. Tumor necrosis factor-alpha levels and weight loss in chronic obstructive pulmonary disease. Am J Respir Crit Care Med. 1994;150(5 Pt 1): 1453–5.
47. Agusti A, Morla M, Sauleda J, Saus C, Busquets X. NF-kappaB activation and iNOS upregulation in skeletal muscle of patients with COPD and low body weight. Thorax. 2004;59(6): 483–7.
48. Ferguson GT, Calverley PM, Anderson JA, Jenkins CR, Jones PW, Willits LR, et al. Prevalence and progression of osteoporosis in patients with COPD: results from the towards a revolution in COPD health study. Chest. 2009;136(6):1456–65.
49. Jorgensen NR, Schwarz P, Holme I, Henriksen BM, Petersen LJ, Backer V. The prevalence of osteoporosis in patients with chronic obstructive pulmonary disease: a cross sectional study. Respir Med. 2007;101(1):177–85.
50. Block JE, Stubbs H. Hip fracture-associated mortality reconsidered. Calcif Tissue Int. 1997;61(1):84.
51. Robbins J, Aragaki AK, Kooperberg C, Watts N, Wactawski-Wende J, Jackson RD, et al. Factors associated with 5-year risk of hip fracture in postmenopausal women. JAMA. 2007;298(20):2389–98.
52. Mundy GR. Osteoporosis and inflammation. Nutr Rev. 2007;65(12 Pt 2):S147–51.
53. Bolton CE, Stone MD, Edwards PH, Duckers JM, Evans WD, Shale DJ. Circulating matrix metalloproteinase-9 and osteoporosis in patients with chronic obstructive pulmonary disease. Chron Respir Dis. 2009;6(2):81–7.
54. Rana JS, Mittleman MA, Sheikh J, Hu FB, Manson JE, Colditz GA, et al. Chronic obstructive pulmonary disease, asthma, and risk of type 2 diabetes in women. Diabet Care. 2004;27(10): 2478–84.
55. Song Y, Klevak A, Manson JE, Buring JE, Liu S. Asthma, chronic obstructive pulmonary disease, and type 2 diabetes in the women's health study. Diabet Res Clin Pract. 2010;90(3): 365–71.
56. Bolton CE, Evans M, Ionescu AA, Edwards SM, Morris RH, Dunseath G, et al. Insulin resistance and inflammation - a further systemic complication of COPD. COPD. 2007;4(2): 121–6.
57. Dennis RJ, Maldonado D, Rojas MX, Aschner P, Rondon M, Charry L, et al. Inadequate glucose control in type 2 diabetes is associated with impaired lung function and systemic inflammation: a cross-sectional study. BMC Pulm Med. 2010;10:38.
58. Suissa S, Kezouh A, Ernst P. Inhaled corticosteroids and the risks of diabetes onset and progression. Am J Med. 2010;123(11):1001–6.
59. Noguera A, Batle S, Miralles C, Iglesias J, Busquets X, MacNee W, et al. Enhanced neutrophil response in chronic obstructive pulmonary disease. Thorax. 2001;56(6):432–7.
60. Sparrow D, Glynn RJ, Cohen M, Weiss ST. The relationship of the peripheral leukocyte count and cigarette smoking to pulmonary function among adult men. Chest. 1984;86(3):383–6.

61. van Eeden SF, Lawrence E, Sato Y, Kitagawa Y, Hogg JC. Neutrophils released from the bone marrow by granulocyte colony-stimulating factor sequester in lung microvessels but are slow to migrate. Eur Respir J. 2000;15(6):1079–86.
62. Noguera A, Busquets X, Sauleda J, Villaverde JM, MacNee W, Agusti AG. Expression of adhesion molecules and G proteins in circulating neutrophils in chronic obstructive pulmonary disease. Am J Respir Crit Care Med. 1998;158(5 Pt 1):1664–8.
63. Agusti A. Systemic effects of chronic obstructive pulmonary disease: what we know and what we don't know (but should). Proc Am Thorac Soc. 2007;4(7):522–5.
64. de Jong JW, van der Belt-Gritter B, Koeter GH, Postma DS. Peripheral blood lymphocyte cell subsets in subjects with chronic obstructive pulmonary disease: association with smoking, IgE and lung function. Respir Med. 1997;91(2):67–76.
65. Kim WD, Kim WS, Koh Y, Lee SD, Lim CM, Kim DS, et al. Abnormal peripheral blood T-lymphocyte subsets in a subgroup of patients with COPD. Chest. 2002;122(2):437–44.
66. Hodge SJ, Hodge GL, Reynolds PN, Scicchitano R, Holmes M. Increased production of TGF-beta and apoptosis of T lymphocytes isolated from peripheral blood in COPD. Am J Physiol Lung Cell Mol Physiol. 2003;285(2):L492–9.
67. Domagala-Kulawik J, Hoser G, Dabrowska M, Chazan R. Increased proportion of Fas positive CD8+ cells in peripheral blood of patients with COPD. Respir Med. 2007;101(6):1338–43.
68. Barnes PJ, Shapiro SD, Pauwels RA. Chronic obstructive pulmonary disease: molecular and cellular mechanisms. Eur Respir J. 2003;22(4):672–88.
69. Sauleda J, Garcia-Palmer FJ, Gonzalez G, Palou A, Agusti AG. The activity of cytochrome oxidase is increased in circulating lymphocytes of patients with chronic obstructive pulmonary disease, asthma, and chronic arthritis. Am J Respir Crit Care Med. 2000;161(1):32–5.
70. Varadhachary AS, Salgame P. CD95 mediated T cell apoptosis and its relevance to immune deviation. Oncogene. 1998;17(25):3271–6.
71. Blobe GC, Schiemann WP, Lodish HF. Role of transforming growth factor beta in human disease. N Engl J Med. 2000;342(18):1350–8.
72. de Boer WI, Sont JK, van Schadewijk A, Stolk J, van Krieken JH, Hiemstra PS. Monocyte chemoattractant protein 1, interleukin 8, and chronic airways inflammation in COPD. J Pathol. 2000;190(5):619–26.
73. Traves SL, Smith SJ, Barnes PJ, Donnelly LE. Specific CXC but not CC chemokines cause elevated monocyte migration in COPD: a role for CXCR2. J Leukoc Biol. 2004;76(2):441–50.
74. Marques LJ, Teschler H, Guzman J, Costabel U. Smoker's lung transplanted to a nonsmoker. Long-term detection of smoker's macrophages. Am J Respir Crit Care Med. 1997;156(5):1700–2.
75. Tomita K, Caramori G, Lim S, Ito K, Hanazawa T, Oates T, et al. Increased p21(CIP1/WAF1) and B cell lymphoma leukemia-x(L) expression and reduced apoptosis in alveolar macrophages from smokers. Am J Respir Crit Care Med. 2002;166(5):724–31.
76. Bhowmik A, Seemungal TA, Sapsford RJ, Wedzicha JA. Relation of sputum inflammatory markers to symptoms and lung function changes in COPD exacerbations. Thorax. 2000;55(2):114–20.
77. Chaouat A, Savale L, Chouaid C, Tu L, Sztrymf B, Canuet M, et al. Role for interleukin-6 in COPD-related pulmonary hypertension. Chest. 2009;136(3):678–87.
78. Bon JM, Zhang Y, Duncan SR, Pilewski JM, Zaldonis D, Zeevi A, et al. Plasma inflammatory mediators associated with bone metabolism in COPD. COPD. 2010;7(3):186–91.
79. de Godoy I, Donahoe M, Calhoun WJ, Mancino J, Rogers RM. Elevated TNF-alpha production by peripheral blood monocytes of weight-losing COPD patients. Am J Respir Crit Care Med. 1996;153(2):633–7.
80. Dentener MA, Creutzberg EC, Pennings HJ, Rijkers GT, Mercken E, Wouters EF. Effect of infliximab on local and systemic inflammation in chronic obstructive pulmonary disease: a pilot study. Respiration. 2008;76(3):275–82.
81. Rennard SI, Fogarty C, Kelsen S, Long W, Ramsdell J, Allison J, et al. The safety and efficacy of infliximab in moderate to severe chronic obstructive pulmonary disease. Am J Respir Crit Care Med. 2007;175(9):926–34.

82. Suissa S, Ernst P, Hudson M. TNF-alpha antagonists and the prevention of hospitalisation for chronic obstructive pulmonary disease. Pulm Pharmacol Ther. 2008;21(1):234–8.

83. Sapey E, Ahmad A, Bayley D, Newbold P, Snell N, Rugman P, et al. Imbalances between interleukin-1 and tumor necrosis factor agonists and antagonists in stable COPD. J Clin Immunol. 2009;29(4):508–16.

84. Balbi B, Bason C, Balleari E, Fiasella F, Pesci A, Ghio R, et al. Increased bronchoalveolar granulocytes and granulocyte/macrophage colony-stimulating factor during exacerbations of chronic bronchitis. Eur Respir J. 1997;10(4):846–50.

85. de Boer WI, van Schadewijk A, Sont JK, Sharma HS, Stolk J, Hiemstra PS, et al. Transforming growth factor beta1 and recruitment of macrophages and mast cells in airways in chronic obstructive pulmonary disease. Am J Respir Crit Care Med. 1998;158(6):1951–7.

86. Wan YY, Flavell RA. Regulatory T cells, transforming growth factor-beta, and immune suppression. Proc Am Thorac Soc. 2007;4(3):271–6.

87. Sin DD, Lacy P, York E, Man SF. Effects of fluticasone on systemic markers of inflammation in chronic obstructive pulmonary disease. Am J Respir Crit Care Med. 2004;170(7):760–5.

88. Vestbo J, Anderson JA, Calverley PM, Celli B, Ferguson GT, Jenkins C, et al. Bias due to withdrawal in long-term randomised trials in COPD: evidence from the TORCH study. Clin Respir J. 2011;5(1):44–9.

89. Calverley PM, Anderson JA, Celli B, Ferguson GT, Jenkins C, Jones PW, et al. Salmeterol and fluticasone propionate and survival in chronic obstructive pulmonary disease. N Engl J Med. 2007;356(8):775–89.

90. Powrie DJ, Wilkinson TM, Donaldson GC, Jones P, Scrine K, Viel K, et al. Effect of tiotropium on sputum and serum inflammatory markers and exacerbations in COPD. Eur Respir J. 2007;30(3):472–8.

91. Lacasse Y, Goldstein R, Lasserson TJ, Martin S. Pulmonary rehabilitation for chronic obstructive pulmonary disease. Cochrane Database Syst Rev. 2006;18(4):CD003793.

92. Bolton CE, Broekhuizen R, Ionescu AA, Nixon LS, Wouters EF, Shale DJ, et al. Cellular protein breakdown and systemic inflammation are unaffected by pulmonary rehabilitation in COPD. Thorax. 2007;62(2):109–14.

93. Vogiatzis I, Stratakos G, Simoes DC, Terzis G, Georgiadou O, Roussos C, et al. Effects of rehabilitative exercise on peripheral muscle TNFalpha, IL-6, IGF-I and MyoD expression in patients with COPD. Thorax. 2007;62(11):950–6.

94. Sugawara K, Takahashi H, Kasai C, Kiyokawa N, Watanabe T, Fujii S, et al. Effects of nutritional supplementation combined with low-intensity exercise in malnourished patients with COPD. Respir Med. 2010;104(12):1883–9.

95. Wannamethee SG, Lowe GD, Shaper AG, Rumley A, Lennon L, Whincup PH. Associations between cigarette smoking, pipe/cigar smoking, and smoking cessation, and haemostatic and inflammatory markers for cardiovascular disease. Eur Heart J. 2005;26(17):1765–73.

96. Soyseth V, Brekke PH, Smith P, Omland T. Statin use is associated with reduced mortality in COPD. Eur Respir J. 2007;29(2):279–83.

97. Blamoun AI, Batty GN, DeBari VA, Rashid AO, Sheikh M, Khan MA. Statins may reduce episodes of exacerbation and the requirement for intubation in patients with COPD: evidence from a retrospective cohort study. Int J Clin Pract. 2008;62(9):1373–8.

98. Melbye H, Halvorsen DS, Hartz I, Medbo A, Brox J, Eggen AE, et al. Bronchial airflow limitation, smoking, body mass index, and statin use are strongly associated with the C-reactive protein level in the elderly. The Tromso Study 2001. Respir Med. 2007;101(12):2541–9.

99. Hothersall E, McSharry C, Thomson NC. Potential therapeutic role for statins in respiratory disease. Thorax. 2006;61(8):729–34.

100. Khurana V, Bejjanki HR, Caldito G, Owens MW. Statins reduce the risk of lung cancer in humans: a large case-control study of US veterans. Chest. 2007;131(5):1282–8.

101. Paraskevas KI, Tzovaras AA, Briana DD, Mikhailidis DP. Emerging indications for statins: a pluripotent family of agents with several potential applications. Curr Pharm Des. 2007;13(35):3622–36.

Chapter 3
The Disablement Process in COPD

Michael D.L. Morgan

Abstract It is, to some extent, still understandable that chronic obstructive pulmonary disease (COPD) is seen as a one-dimensional problem where airway inflammation caused by cigarette smoking leads to airway obstruction, dyspnoea and activity limitation. In this model, the problem can be simply solved by the avoidance of cigarette smoking or a cure for airway inflammation. Whilst this theory may have continuing appeal for politicians, public health doctors and those scientists interested in airway inflammation, we now realise that it is a misleading over-simplification. The pathway that leads to incapacity in COPD begins with airway damage but becomes increasingly complex as it incorporates factors of influence in a multi system disease.

Keywords COPD • Airway inflammation • Smoking • Airway obstruction • Dyspnoea • Airway inflammation • Incapacity • Airway damage • Multi-system disease

Introduction

It is, to some extent, still understandable that chronic obstructive pulmonary disease (COPD) is seen as a one-dimensional problem, where airway inflammation caused by cigarette smoking leads to airway obstruction, dyspnoea and activity limitation. In this model, the problem can be simply solved by the avoidance of cigarette smoking or a cure for airway inflammation. Whilst this theory may have continuing appeal for politicians, public health doctors and those scientists interested in airway inflammation, we now realise that it is a misleading over-simplification. The pathway that

M.D.L. Morgan (✉)
Department of Respiratory Medicine, University Hospital of Leicester, Glenfield Hospital, Leicester, UK
e-mail: mike.morgan@uhl-tr.nhs.uk

L. Nici and R. ZuWallack (eds.), *Chronic Obstructive Pulmonary Disease: Co-Morbidities and Systemic Consequences*, Respiratory Medicine, DOI 10.1007/978-1-60761-673-3_3, © Springer Science+Business Media, LLC 2012

leads to incapacity in COPD begins with airway damage but becomes increasingly complex as it incorporates factors of influence in a multisystem disease. Ultimately, the degree of disability resulting from COPD cannot be predicted from the degree of airflow limitation alone. Other important contributors to disability include the direct impact of dyspnoea on the skeletal muscles, the natural ageing process and the development of other co-morbid conditions. Even if there is a common origin, the impact of COPD-engendered disability will also vary in relation to the social and cultural context of the individual. Disability, as we shall see, is not solely defined by functional limitation but also by expectations and personal needs. The societal impact of COPD is a function of the cost of care and patients who lose their independence find it expensive, particularly if they are admitted to hospital during exacerbations. The governments of most nations now realise that the battleground for health has moved towards the management of chronic diseases. This means that we have to understand the nature and development of disability in COPD. While it may not be possible to reverse abnormal lung function, there may be an opportunity to correct or prevent some of the reversible factors that lead to disability. Recognition of this new approach opens the way to improving the quality of care at the same time as reducing the cost.

The Nomenclature of Disability

The taxonomy of disability can be confusing but it is important to be precise in order to understand the subject. The word "disability" is widely used but is an imprecise term implying some form of barrier to normal healthy physical functioning. The original World Health Organization (WHO) classification of impairments, disabilities and handicaps in 1980 used the term as description of activity limitation that results from a physical impairment. The specific descriptor was removed from the 2001 ICF revision and replaced by the term "activity limitation" to recognise that overall disability results from an interaction between the consequences of the disease and social and environmental factors beyond the illness itself (Fig. 3.1) [1]. The term handicap was replaced with "participation restriction." It is also possible in this framework to explain how nonphysical illnesses like depression can lead to activity limitation. There are several theoretical descriptive models that can be used to understand the process. For COPD, the medical model of disability that assumes that organ damage (impairment) leads directly to activity limitation is a reasonable framework to adopt. However, there are social aspects to the development of overall disability in COPD that may have an impact, as we shall see later. For the purposes of this chapter, it will be best to restrict the term disability (or disablement) to the constraints placed on people with COPD that limit their physical activity and may subsequently disadvantage them in the society that they live. Obviously, this requires a further discussion about the nature of physical activity and its measurement.

Fig. 3.1 The schematic World Health Organisation (WHO) description of activity limitation (disability). The revised version from 2001 now acknowledges that factors other than physiological impairments may have a role in the development of activity limitation

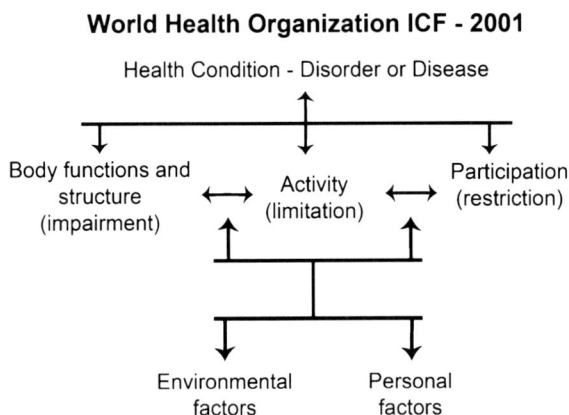

Assessing Disability in COPD

The ability to perform daily activities, particularly those concerned with self-care, is a fundamental necessity for people especially if they have chronic disease. To perform physical activities, a person requires a physiological capacity for exercise and a willingness to use the physical capacity. This distinction between the capacity for exercise (what people can do) and what they actually do spontaneously (what people do) is important because it is an exploitable gap between the limits of abnormal physiology of irreversible chronic disease and the potential for improvement through rehabilitation. The overall estimation of disability in COPD will involve both a measurement of capacity and an assessment of what people do in terms of spontaneous physical activity.

The Measurement of Exercise Capacity

The measurement of this bodily function usually involves the performance of a task under supervision, so it is important to be specific about the nature of the exercise. Not all exercise tests measure the same thing. In the laboratory, whole body exercise performance is usually measured during a symptom-limited incremental cycle ergometer or treadmill. Maximal exercise capacity is usually expressed as oxygen uptake at peak performance (VO_{2Max}). In health, this is defined by the limit of skeletal muscle uptake of oxygen from circulation. In early COPD, the same limits to maximal capacity may apply but, as the disease progresses, exercise may be terminated by the ventilatory limit imposed by dynamic hyperinflation (VO_{2peak}). The performance here sets the upper limit for maximal performance that is unlikely to be influenced subsequently by treatment or volition. In the distinction between performance and capacity, it is important to understand that a person's performance is both a function of their capacity and their ability to use a significant proportion of that capacity. A measure of capacity usage is the endurance (or constant workload) cycle ergometer test, where the subject is asked to sustain a proportion of their peak performance (say 75% VO_{2max}) for as long as possible. This measure is much more sensitive to change following intervention, though perhaps not as sensitive as endurance walking in COPD [2].

Access to exercise laboratories is not always available, so field tests of maximal and endurance capacity have been developed as a practical substitute. Walking is an important human activity and therefore both an appropriate exercise challenge and outcome measure. There are two categories of field walking tests, depending upon whether the walking speed is externally controlled (paced) or whether the subject is free to set their own pace. Examples of paced walking tests include the incremental and endurance shuttle walk tests, whilst the most popular un-paced test is the 6-min walk test.

The shuttle walk tests were developed to provide field equivalents for the laboratory incremental symptom limited test and the laboratory endurance (constant) workload equivalent [3, 4]. They are both relatively simple to conduct around a 10 m course where the pace is set by an external audio signal. In the incremental version (ISWT), the pace increases every minute until the patient cannot keep up. In the endurance version (ESWT), the pace is set from the outset at a proportion (80%) of peak performance and the patient continues at that pace until they have to stop. The shuttle walk tests reflect similar properties to their laboratory counterparts. The ISWT is a test of maximal walking capacity whilst the ESWT is a reflection of the ability to effectively use that maximal capacity and is more sensitive to intervention.

The 6-min walk test is a very popular exercise assessment and seen as an apparently simple concept where the patient walks as far as they can in their own time in 6 min. This is thought to reflect a safer real life exercise challenge and has been shown to be responsive to rehabilitation and other interventions. In spite of its apparent simplicity, it does, however, have some complex characteristics depending upon the patient's approach and the tester's behaviour [5]. Some patients who set off quickly can rapidly reach their VO_{2peak} unintentionally [6]. Nevertheless, the 6-min walk test is proving durable and has been incorporated into multi-dimensional assessment tools such as the BODE (body mass index, airflow obstruction, dyspnoea, exercise capacity) index [7].

There are a large number of subjective measures of functional capacity that have been used in COPD. Possibly, the most popular is the self reported view of the limitation of exercise by dyspnoea captured by the MRC Dyspnoea Scale. This simple five-point scale relates well to objective measures of exercise performance such as the shuttle walk test and provides a complementary guide to disability as well as a meaningful but relatively insensitive outcome measure [8, 9].

Assessment of Spontaneous Physical Activity

The World Health Organization's definition of physical activity is "any bodily movement produced by skeletal muscles that requires energy expenditure." Obviously, physical activity so described, is a fundamental human activity common to all. In the context of COPD, physical activity can be sub-divided into general physical activity that can be linked to the usual wider health benefits and the more specific activities of daily living that may become impaired by illness. The opportunities for assessment here include patient reported outcomes (questionnaires), objective observed task performance and the direct measurement of spontaneous activity with motion sensors.

Patient reported outcomes come in two categories. The first are the generic physical activity questionnaires that have generally been developed to assess cardiovascular risk. Some of these have been used in elderly or COPD populations but none are disease-specific. Most attention has been paid to the use of questionnaires that specifically reflect either basic activities of daily living or slightly broader functional status (Table 3.1) [10]. Examples of specific activities of daily living questionnaires include the Manchester Respiratory ADL (activities of daily living) Questionnaire and the London Chest ADLQ (activities of daily living questionnaire) [11, 12].

Objective assessment of the ability to perform daily activities is also possible in the form of task batteries or timed obstacle courses. Some objective task performance tests have been used in COPD. These include the Short Physical Performance Battery and the Timed Up and Go test [13, 14]. Neither, however, has yet been repeated following an intervention. Some instruments take a broader approach to the assessment of functional incapacity, that include some social restrictions as well

Table 3.1 Assessing physical capacity and activity

Physiological capacity	Functional (task) performance –field tests and self report	Spontaneous physical (domestic) activity – physical activity monitors and self report
Cardiopulmonary exercise test (VO_{2Max})	Incremental shuttle walk test	Physical activity monitors (accelerometers)
Constant workload cycle ergometer laboratory test (endurance)	Endurance shuttle walk test	Pedometers
	6 min walk test	Minnesota leisure Time Physical Activity Questionnaire
	MRC Dyspnoea Score	Physical Activity Scale for the Elderly (PASE)
	PFSDQ, etc.	
	ADL Questionnaires	

ADL activities of daily living, *MRC* medical research council, *PFSDQ* pulmonary functional status and dyspnoea questionnaire as the more restricted limitation of daily activities. These include functional status questionnaires and some domains of the more popular disease-specific quality-of-life questionnaires. A good example of the former would be the Pulmonary Functional Status and Dyspnoea Questionnaire (PFSDQ) [15].

Collecting information about patterns of spontaneous daily activity is quite difficult. There are some questionnaires that have been used in the COPD age group. Examples include the Minnesota Leisure Time Physical Activity Questionnaire and the physical activity scale for the elderly (PASE) [16, 17]. Recently, the direct observation of spontaneous physical activity has become possible with motion sensors [18, 19]. These are usually accelerometers worn on the arm or leg that capture movement in more than one plane. Some are also capable of measuring energy expenditure in addition. The data from these sensors is usually expressed as arbitrary counts and therefore cannot be compared between systems.

The Background Effect of Ageing

In common with all animals, the ageing process in humans begins when growth has ceased. In humans, this means that from the age of about 30, function and activity tend to decline. The mechanism for the decline includes increased fatigability, muscle weakness, decreased muscle bulk and oxygen uptake. This leads in turn to a reduced spontaneous physical activity, insulin resistance and obesity. However, the reduction in faculties is not inevitable and an individual can maintain physical activity and fitness by remaining active and training. Unfortunately, the majority of modern populations do not remain sufficiently active to prevent the decline in function. Apart from the impact of the disease, people with COPD will be vulnerable to the effect of these "normal" age-related changes. Importantly, the health messages surrounding the maintenance of physical activity are just as relevant in people with chronic disease.

Factors that Curtail Activity in COPD

In the struggle to maintain or improve physical activity, a patient with COPD may be impeded by dyspnoea, fatigue or the unpredictable effects of exacerbations. The key factors are the impact of dyspnoea and the progression of skeletal muscle weakness. In most cases of COPD, physical activity is terminated by dyspnoea. With time, the intensity of task-limiting dyspnoea does not change, but the frequency of occurrence increases and the threshold for limitation reduces. [20]. As dyspnoea begins to interfere with activities of daily living, it also begins to impede the quality of life. Naturally, people with COPD will try to avoid the unpleasant stimulus, and spontaneous physical activity levels will subsequently diminish. This runs the risk of inducing skeletal muscle weakness through de-conditioning. This potentially reversible process can then accelerate the downward spiral into disability.

Fatigue is another limiting symptom that is reported frequently by patients but rather more difficult to measure or pin down to a cause. However, recent studies suggest that fatigue is certainly a frequent occurrence and is associated with exercise limitation. [21, 22]. A new disease-specific fatigue questionnaire may be helpful in this respect [23].

Skeletal muscle weakness may be the key additional factor in the decline of function and the development of fatigue. Muscle bulk and function naturally declines with age unless the individual takes steps to recover or prevent the deterioration [24]. The loss of muscle function is particularly noticeable in patients with COPD and is more marked in the lower limb musculature associated with the muscles of ambulation. Loss of quadriceps muscle strength in COPD is a stronger predictor of mortality than age or lung function [25]. The nature of limb muscle damage in COPD remains relatively unexplained and, to date, descriptions of a generalised inflammatory process are unconvincing and simple inactivity-induced de-conditioning is a more likely explanation. The latter would also explain the relative preservation of upper limb function which is more likely to be retained in daily activities.

The Trajectory of Disability

While we know something about the decline in FEV1 in people with COPD, the epidemiology of disability is a subject in infancy. The temporal relationship between various impairments and the onset of activity limitation or reduction in spontaneous physical activity is only beginning to be explored. Information is available from cross-sectional studies of impairment and physical activity and, to a limited degree, there are longitudinal examinations of some outcomes. The long term relationship between impairments and the development of physical inactivity is still largely unclear. Lack of physical activity may either be the consequence of impairment or even the cause of disability [26].

Several studies have now examined the degree of physical inactivity in people with COPD and also compared their position to those with other chronic diseases [19]. Using the activity monitors over week-long periods, it is possible to build up a picture of people's lives compared to healthy subjects. It is clear that patients with COPD demonstrate consistently about half of the spontaneous physical activity across the whole week compared to control subjects [27]. Those who use long term oxygen treatment are even less active at about one-sixth of the normal pattern of activity. More sophisticated examination using physical activity monitors can also determine that people with COPD come to spend more time lying and sitting than standing and walking [28]. There are also seasonal reductions in spontaneous physical activity as vulnerable people with chronic illness are reluctant to leave their homes in the winter months [29]. While this reduction in physical activity is to be expected in people with chronic disease, it is clear from recent comparative studies that people with COPD are much more inactive than those with other common illnesses. In a recent pedometer comparison, people with COPD had sedentary levels of daily step counts that were worse than any other chronic disease group, including those with heart failure or neuromuscular disease [30].

It is reasonable to assume that reduction in physical activity follows on from the damage to airway function. While increasing dyspnoea may well lead to activity avoidance and loss of fitness, it may not necessarily be the whole story. In the same way that healthy people who keep active reduce their cardiovascular risk, those people with COPD who have higher levels of self-reported physical activity are less likely to be readmitted to hospital , have better lung function and are less likely to die than those who report lower levels [31, 32].

Several longitudinal studies show that age and lung function are good prognostic indicators. This is ingrained in the management of COPD, as evidenced by the main staging systems such as GOLD that use FEV1 as the yardstick. While this has broad utility, the prognostic process can be refined by adding other factors, including exercise to a multi-dimensional model. A good example of this is the BODE index that combines airflow obstruction (FEV1), body composition [body mass index (BMI)], dyspnoea (MRC) and exercise (6MWT) to provide a better prediction of prognosis than the individual components can provide. While survival can be reflected in The BODE index, the exercise factor is probably the most influential component in the composite and also most amenable to change. Background studies using individual components have shown that various exercise parameters can singularly demonstrate better prognostic ability than other measurements. For example, over a 5-year period, the relative reduction in VO_{2peak} and VE_{max} shows much greater relative decline than FEV1 and a strong correlation with declining MRC Dyspnoea score [33]. The same is also true with field exercise tests where function declines with time and there appears to a threshold effect that predicts survival. In the case of the 6MWT, this threshold is around 350 m and the field test is a stronger predictor of mortality than the laboratory cardiopulmonary exercise testing [34]. A similar study has been performed for the incremental shuttle walk test and this identifies a distance of 170 m as a critical threshold of performance associated with increased mortality [35].

While lung function in COPD declines in a relatively predictable and linear fashion, it does not seem likely that either exercise performance or activity limitation behaves in the same manner. The implication of many of the cross-sectional or observational studies is that once a certain threshold is passed, the impact of the disease on people's lives or daily activities is suddenly worsened. This is conceptually attractive because the idea that people gradually use up their reserve of lung function without much penalty is easy to comprehend. Once they have reached the point where their ventilatory limitation or skeletal muscle weakness begins to impinge on activities of daily living, then further decline is likely to be associated with significant impact. To date, no longitudinal studies have confirmed this pattern of events, but information is becoming available from examination of the broad range of severity. In a large, cross-sectional study, Watz and colleagues examined the relationship between FEV1, 6MWD and spontaneous physical activity using a multi sensor armband. The authors had the opportunity to study patients across the range of GOLD staging and also carried out comparisons with a separate group of people without significant airflow obstruction (GOLD 0) [36, 37]. They also linked their observations to measures of inflammation but found no relationship. In spite of the lack of a genuine control group, it seemed as if reductions in spontaneous activity occur before there is an impact on functional capacity, though eventually GOLD three to four stages are associated with sedentary behaviour and activity limitation. Clearly, if spontaneous activity starts to diminish before it is curtailed by physiological limitation, then there must be an element of behaviour modification in the generation of disability.

A recent study examined the evolution of disability in a well characterised group of younger COPD patients over a 2 year period. This confirmed that lung function alone does not fully describe the risk of disability [38]. Other nonrespiratory factors such as body composition and lower limb strength, together with functional limitation, carry an increased risk of disability development above and beyond respiratory impairment.

The Impact of Exacerbations

The downward course of COPD is not smooth but punctuated by temporary periods of worsening symptoms called exacerbations that become more frequent as the disease progresses. The impact of exacerbations can be severe and will lead to reduced lung function, accelerated impairment of health status, enhanced systemic inflammation and a limitation on physical activity. Population studies suggest that, in the community, the effect of an exacerbation will be to limit activities outside the home for up to a month after the event [39]. Furthermore, if patients are unlucky enough to be admitted to hospital, then the associated immobility may have a significant effect on skeletal muscle strength and function [40]. Reductions in quadriceps strength have been demonstrated in patients who have been admitted to hospital for exacerbations. Studies in healthy people suggest that lean muscle mass can be lost very quickly following immobilisation but then takes at least four times as long to recover once full activity is restored [41]. The implication of this is that hospital admission for exacerbation is likely to have a significant deleterious effect on muscle function that will not be repaired in time for discharge. Consequently, exacerbations can identified as a cause of step-wise deterioration in function which will speed up the onset of disability. Fortunately, this has now been recognised and methods of preserving muscle function by electrical stimulation or employing early rehabilitation have been described [42–44].

The Additional Effect of Co-morbidity on Physical Activity

Over half the patients with COPD who are eligible to attend a pulmonary rehabilitation programme will have another chronic disease that will contribute to overall disability. Broadly, these are cardiovascular diseases (hypertension, heart failure or ischaemic heart disease), metabolic diseases (diabetes, obesity and hypercholesterolemia), musculoskeletal disease (arthritis) and psychiatric illness (depression and anxiety). These co-morbid conditions will clearly make a contribution to the development of disability and they are described in detail in other chapters. There are no studies that quantify this contribution but some insight can be gained from the observations of the effect of rehabilitation on patients with COPD and co-morbid conditions. In a recent paper from Italy, Crisafulli and colleagues examined the impact of one or more co-morbidities on the ability to benefit from a rehabilitation programme [45]. A large number of people with significant COPD (GOLD II & III) had a co-morbid condition (62%), but the presence of one or more other conditions did not seem to affect the baseline 6 min walk distance or the St. Georges Respiratory Questionnaire score. The presence of either one or more co-morbid conditions did not seem to offset the benefit of the rehabilitation programme with the possible exception of a negative correlation with osteoporosis. This is an encouraging position because it does appear as if multiple conditions may compound disability from COPD to some degree but, overall, may not prevent improvement following rehabilitation.

Social and Cultural Aspects of Disability

We have focussed on activity limitation as the core of disability in COPD but this does not really reflect a picture of broader disability which could be considered as "difficulty in performing activities or roles that are normal for one's age and sex." There are cultural and environmental aspects of disability that will clearly influence how people with COPD will be able to function effectively in their world. For the individual, the impact of COPD worldwide will be broadly similar in terms of symptoms but may be modified by the local culture or geography. There are very few cross-cultural studies of COPD that explore the comparative onset of disability. One such study has examined the activity patterns of COPD patients in Europe and South America [46]. In this case, well matched patients from Austria were compared from a similar sample from a climatically similar part of Brazil. The group from Austria had significantly lower walking time and movement intensity and a 50% lower chance of achieving at least 30 min activity in a day. This evidence suggests that all other things being equal, socioeconomic factors can influence the pattern of daily activity and hence the risk of disability (Table 3.2).

So far, in this chapter, we have considered disability primarily from the perspective of the physiological impairment of dyspnoea leading to activity limitation. This physical model is not the only perspective on the broader perception of disability. The social model of disability holds that society's perception of the person and defines their disability. In the case of COPD, this might involve negative attitudes towards cigarette smokers or even failure to appreciate the severity of limiting dyspnoea in a person who has no obvious disability and no symptoms at rest. We know that is far from the truth and people with COPD who have limiting dyspnoea

Table 3.2 Factors that may influence the development of disability

Lung function
Age
Co-morbidity
Physiological exercise capacity
Habitual physical activity
Geography and affluence
Skeletal muscle dysfunction
Psychology/health status
Exacerbations
Body composition/nutrition

after a few steps undergo similar sensations and metabolic challenges that athletes experience when they face much greater challenges [47]. This apparent lack of visible disability to others has been pointed out by patient support groups in their campaigns for better recognition. It has also been observed in other situations, where those with COPD and equivalent levels of disability to other more obviously disabled groups such as those with neurological disability receive a much lower level of assessed social support [48]. This suggests that there is an institutional factor in the way that social services are less amenable to patients with disability due to lung disease.

Summary

As COPD develops, airway function is steadily lost as FEV1 declines. The initial impact of loss of FEV1 may go unnoticed for some time while the reserve of lung function is eroded. Once it appears, the progression of activity limitation might subsequently progress rapidly. Once people become symptomatic, they compound the problem by avoiding activities that make them breathless. This will eventually lead to lower limb muscle weakness primarily through inactivity. Habitual inactivity is itself a risk factor for mortality and hospital admission during exacerbations. Hospital-induced inactivity during exacerbations may further impact on the ability to recover from the episode and increase the risk of future hospital re-admission. Age and co-morbidity will complicate the progressive decline. Social and cultural factors may not only influence the speed of the onset of disability but may also modify the response of society towards the disabled person (Fig. 3.2). On an optimistic note, many patients do not use the capacity available to them. Therefore, improving the level of habitual activity or providing pulmonary rehabilitation programmes may slow the onset of disability or reverse some of its effects.

AIRWAY DAMAGE

Dyspnoea

General deconditoning
Lower limb muscle weakness
Ageing process

Habitual activity
Co-morbid conditions
Exacerbations

Activity Limitation

Activities of Daily Living

Culture and environment

Societal response

Disability

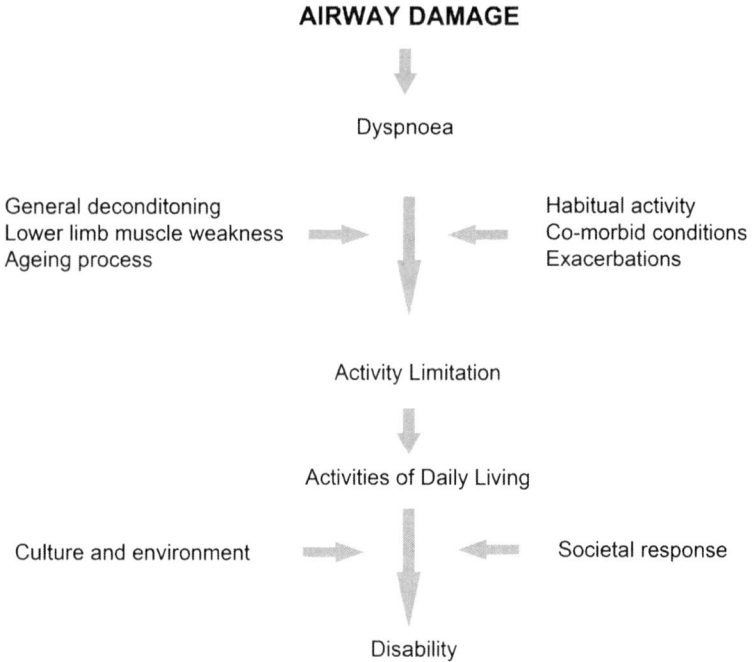

Fig. 3.2 Factors in the development of wider disability in COPD

Summary Points

- Significant disability may not be apparent until lung damage is well advanced.
- Once apparent, the reductions in exercise capacity and health status may be rapid.
- Disability may be compounded by natural age-related changes and co-morbidity.
- Some people do not use all the capacity available to them.
- There are some potentially modifiable factors that contribute to disability (unlike airway function).

References

1. International Classification of Functioning, Disability and Health (ICF). World Health Organisation, Geneva 2001.
2. Pepin V, Saey D, Whittom F, LeBlanc P, Maltais F. Walking versus cycling: sensitivity to bronchodilation in chronic obstructive pulmonary disease. Am J Respir Crit Care Med. 2005;172(12):1517–22.
3. Revill SM, Morgan MD, Singh SJ, Williams J, Hardman AE. The endurance shuttle walk: a new field test for the assessment of endurance capacity in chronic obstructive pulmonary disease. Thorax. 1999;54(3):213–22.

4. Singh SJ, Morgan MD, Scott S, Walters D, Hardman AE. Development of a shuttle walking test of disability in patients with chronic airways obstruction. Thorax. 1992;47(12):1019–24.

5. ATS Committee on Proficiency Standards for Clinical Pulmonary Function Laboratories. ATS statement: guidelines for the six-minute walk test. Am J Respir Crit Care Med. 2002;166(1): 111–7.

6. Onorati P, Antonucci R, Valli G, Berton E, De Marco F, Serra P, et al. Non-invasive evaluation of gas exchange during a shuttle walking test vs. a 6-min walking test to assess exercise tolerance in COPD patients. Eur J Appl Physiol. 2003;89(3–4):331–6.

7. Celli BR, Cote CG, Marin JM, Casanova C, Montes dO, Mendez RA, et al. The body-mass index, airflow obstruction, dyspnea, and exercise capacity index in chronic obstructive pulmonary disease. N Engl J Med. 2004;350(10):1005–12.

8. Bestall JC, Paul EA, Garrod R, Garnham R, Jones PW, Wedzicha JA. Usefulness of the Medical Research Council (MRC) dyspnoea scale as a measure of disability in patients with chronic obstructive pulmonary disease. Thorax. 1999;54(7):581–6.

9. Evans RA, Singh SJ, Collier R, Williams JE, Morgan MD. Pulmonary rehabilitation is successful for COPD irrespective of MRC dyspnoea grade. Respir Med. 2009;103(7):1070–5.

10. Leidy NK. Subjective measurement of activity in chronic obstructive pulmonary disease. COPD. 2007;4(3):243–9.

11. Yohannes AM, Roomi J, Winn S, Connolly MJ. The manchester respiratory activities of daily living questionnaire: development, reliability, validity, and responsiveness to pulmonary rehabilitation. J Am Geriatr Soc. 2000;48(11):1496–500.

12. Garrod R, Bestall JC, Paul EA, Wedzicha JA, Jones PW. Development and validation of a standardized measure of activity of daily living in patients with severe COPD: the London Chest Activity of Daily Living scale (LCADL). Respir Med. 2000;94(6):589–96.

13. Guralnik JM, Simonsick EM, Ferrucci L, Glynn RJ, Berkman LF, Blazer DG, et al. A short physical performance battery assessing lower extremity function: association with self-reported disability and prediction of mortality and nursing home admission. J Gerontol. 1994;49(2): M85–94.

14. Butcher SJ, Meshke JM, Sheppard MS. Reductions in functional balance, coordination, and mobility measures among patients with stable chronic obstructive pulmonary disease. J Cardiopulm Rehabil. 2004;24(4):274–80.

15. Lareau SC, Meek PM, Roos PJ. Development and testing of the modified version of the pulmonary functional status and dyspnea questionnaire (PFSDQ-M). Heart Lung. 1998;27(3):159–68.

16. Richardson MT, Leon AS, Jacobs Jr DR, Ainsworth BE, Serfass R. Comprehensive evaluation of the Minnesota Leisure Time Physical Activity Questionnaire. J Clin Epidemiol. 1994;47(3):271–81.

17. Washburn RA, McAuley E, Katula J, Mihalko SL, Boileau RA. The physical activity scale for the elderly (PASE): evidence for validity. J Clin Epidemiol. 1999;52(7):643–51.

18. Benzo R. Activity monitoring in chronic obstructive pulmonary disease. J Cardiopulm Rehabil Prev. 2009;29(6):341–7.

19. Pitta F, Troosters T, Probst VS, Spruit MA, Decramer M, Gosselink R. Quantifying physical activity in daily life with questionnaires and motion sensors in COPD. Eur Respir J. 2006;27(5): 1040–55.

20. Meek PM. Measurement of dyspnea in chronic obstructive pulmonary disease: what is the tool telling you? Chron Respir Dis. 2004;1(1):29–37.

21. Baghai-Ravary R, Quint JK, Goldring JJ, Hurst JR, Donaldson GC, Wedzicha JA. Determinants and impact of fatigue in patients with chronic obstructive pulmonary disease. Respir Med. 2009;103(2):216–23.

22. Gagnon P, Saey D, Vivodtzev I, Laviolette L, Mainguy V, Milot J, et al. Impact of preinduced quadriceps fatigue on exercise response in chronic obstructive pulmonary disease and healthy subjects. J Appl Physiol. 2009;107(3):832–40.

23. Alshair K, Kolsum U, Berry P, Smith J, Caress A, Singh D, et al. Development, dimensions, reliability and validity of the novel Manchester COPD fatigue scale. Thorax. 2009;64(11):950–5.

24. Nair KS. Aging muscle. Am J Clin Nutr. 2005;81(5):953–63.
25. Swallow EB, Reyes D, Hopkinson NS, Man WD, Porcher R, Cetti EJ, et al. Quadriceps strength predicts mortality in patients with moderate to severe chronic obstructive pulmonary disease. Thorax. 2007;62(2):115–20.
26. Polkey MI, Rabe KF. Chicken or egg: physical activity in COPD revisited. Eur Respir J. 2009;33(2):227–9.
27. Sandland CJ, Singh SJ, Curcio A, Jones PM, Morgan MD. A profile of daily activity in chronic obstructive pulmonary disease. J Cardiopulm Rehabil. 2005;25(3):181–3.
28. Pitta F, Troosters T, Spruit MA, Probst VS, Decramer M, Gosselink R. Characteristics of physical activities in daily life in chronic obstructive pulmonary disease. Am J Respir Crit Care Med. 2005;171(9):972–7.
29. Sewell L, Singh SJ, Williams JE, Morgan MD. Seasonal variations affect physical activity and pulmonary rehabilitation outcomes. J Cardiopulm Rehabil Prev. 2010;30(5):329–33.
30. Tudor-Locke C, Washington TL, Hart TL. Expected values for steps/day in special populations. Prev Med. 2009;49(1):3–11.
31. Garcia-Aymerich J, Lange P, Benet M, Schnohr P, Anto JM. Regular physical activity reduces hospital admission and mortality in chronic obstructive pulmonary disease: a population based cohort study. Thorax. 2006;61(9):772–8.
32. Garcia-Aymerich J, Lange P, Benet M, Schnohr P, Anto JM. Regular physical activity modifies smoking-related lung function decline and reduces risk of chronic obstructive pulmonary disease: a population-based cohort study. Am J Respir Crit Care Med. 2007;175(5):458–63.
33. Oga T, Nishimura K, Tsukino M, Sato S, Hajiro T, Mishima M. Exercise capacity deterioration in patients with COPD: longitudinal evaluation over 5 years. Chest. 2005;128(1):62–9.
34. Casanova C, Cote CG, Marin JM, de Torres JP, Aguirre-Jaime A, Mendez R, et al. The 6-min walking distance: long-term follow up in patients with COPD. Eur Respir J. 2007;29(3):535–40.
35. Ringbaek T, Martinez G, Brondum E, Thogersen J, Morgan M, Lange P. Shuttle walking test as predictor of survival in chronic obstructive pulmonary disease patients enrolled in a rehabilitation program. J Cardiopulm Rehabil Prev. 2010;30(6):409–14.
36. Watz H, Waschki B, Meyer T, Magnussen H. Physical activity in patients with COPD. Eur Respir J. 2009;33(2):262–72.
37. Watz H, Waschki B, Boehme C, Claussen M, Meyer T, Magnussen H. Extrapulmonary effects of chronic obstructive pulmonary disease on physical activity: a cross-sectional study. Am J Respir Crit Care Med. 2008;177(7):743–51.
38. Eisner MD, Iribarren C, Blanc PD, Yelin EH, Ackerson L, Byl N, et al. Development of disability in chronic obstructive pulmonary disease: beyond lung function. Thorax. 2011;66(2):108–14.
39. Donaldson GC, Wilkinson TM, Hurst JR, Perera WR, Wedzicha JA. Exacerbations and time spent outdoors in chronic obstructive pulmonary disease. Am J Respir Crit Care Med. 2005;171(5):446–52.
40. Spruit MA, Gosselink R, Troosters T, Kasran A, Gayan-Ramirez G, Bogaerts P, et al. Muscle force during an acute exacerbation in hospitalised patients with COPD and its relationship with CXCL8 and IGF-I. Thorax. 2003;58(9):752–6.
41. Jones SW, Hill RJ, Krasney PA, O'Conner B, Peirce N, Greenhaff PL. Disuse atrophy and exercise rehabilitation in humans profoundly affects the expression of genes associated with the regulation of skeletal muscle mass. FASEB J. 2004;18(9):1025–7.
42. Vivodtzev I, Lacasse Y, Maltais F. Neuromuscular electrical stimulation of the lower limbs in patients with chronic obstructive pulmonary disease. J Cardiopulm Rehabil Prev. 2008;28(2):79–91.
43. Neder JA, Sword D, Ward SA, Mackay E, Cochrane LM, Clark CJ. Home based neuromuscular electrical stimulation as a new rehabilitative strategy for severely disabled patients with chronic obstructive pulmonary disease (COPD). Thorax. 2002;57(4):333–7.
44. Seymour JM, Moore L, Jolley CJ, Ward K, Creasey J, Steier JS, et al. Outpatient pulmonary rehabilitation following acute exacerbations of COPD. Thorax. 2010;65(5):423–8.

45. Crisafulli E, Gorgone P, Vagaggini B, Pagani M, Rossi G, Costa F, et al. Efficacy of standard rehabilitation in COPD outpatients with comorbidities. Eur Respir J. 2010;36(5):1042–8.
46. Pitta F, Breyer MK, Hernandes NA, Teixeira D, Sant'anna TJ, Fontana AD, et al. Comparison of daily physical activity between COPD patients from Central Europe and South America. Respir Med. 2009;103(3):421–6.
47. Steiner MC, Evans R, Deacon SJ, Singh SJ, Patel P, Fox J, et al. Adenine nucleotide loss in the skeletal muscles during exercise in chronic obstructive pulmonary disease. Thorax. 2005;60(11):932–6.
48. Yohannes AM, Roomi J, Connolly MJ. Elderly people at home disabled by chronic obstructive pulmonary disease. Age Ageing. 1998;27(4):523–5.

Chapter 4
Cardiovascular Disease

Thierry Troosters

Abstract Many patients who suffer from chronic obstructive pulmonary disease (COPD) also suffer or even die from cardiovascular morbidity. Some authors have estimated the percentage of patients with COPD who die of cardiovascular reasons to be in the range of 12–37%. The most prevalent cardiovascular comorbidities are acute myocardial infarction, arrhythmia, chronic heart failure, peripheral vascular disease, and stroke, all of which are more prevalent in patients with COPD compared to the non-COPD population. It is no surprise that patients who suffer from COPD have increased risk of developing cardiovascular disease.

Keywords COPD • Cardiovascular disease • Comorbidity • Acute myocardial infarction • Arrhythmia • Chronic heart failure • Peripheral vascular disease • Stroke

Introduction

Many patients who suffer from chronic obstructive pulmonary disease (COPD) also suffer or even die from cardiovascular morbidity. Sin et al. estimated the percentage of patients with COPD who die of cardiovascular reasons to be in the range of 12–37% [1]. The most prevalent cardiovascular comorbidities are acute myocardial infarction, arrhythmia, chronic heart failure, peripheral vascular disease, and stroke, all of which are more prevalent in patients with COPD compared to the non-COPD population. It is no surprise that patients who suffer from COPD have increased risk of developing cardiovascular disease. In the large NHANES (National Health and

T. Troosters (✉)
Department of Pulmonary Rehabilitation, Respiratory Division,
University Hospital Gasthuisberg, Leuven, Belgium
e-mail: thierry.troosters@med.kuleuven.be

L. Nici and R. ZuWallack (eds.), *Chronic Obstructive Pulmonary Disease: Co-Morbidities and Systemic Consequences*, Respiratory Medicine, DOI 10.1007/978-1-60761-673-3_4, © Springer Science+Business Media, LLC 2012

Nutrition Examination Survey) III, subject with the lowest quintile of FEV1 values had a fivefold increased risk of death from ischemic heart disease, compared to patients with the highest quintile of FEV1. Similarly, at least two studies have reported an association of FEV1-decline and an increased risk of cardiovascular disease [2, 3]. In addition, patients with coronary artery disease have a worse survival rate when hospitalized with acute exacerbations of COPD [4]. When patients with COPD are admitted with an exacerbation of COPD and have elevated levels of NT-proBNP and/or troponin T, they compromise their 30 day survival [5]. The data are in line with the observation that for patients with COPD who die within the first day of a hospital admission for an acute exacerbation, the cause of death is heart failure (as confirmed by autopsy) in 37% of cases [6]. This points again to an intimate relation between cardiovascular and respiratory factors during exacerbations.

COPD shares several risk factors with cardiovascular disease. Smoking or even second hand smoke exposure [7] is an obvious risk factor for COPD and is also well-recognized as a dose-dependent risk for cardiovascular diseases [8]. Another potential risk factor is low grade systemic inflammation. Persistent systemic inflammation has been associated with ischemic heart disease, heart failure, atherosclerosis, and stroke. Although it is tempting to speculate that systemic inflammation may be the consequence of spill-over from the pulmonary inflammation to the systemic circulation, it is unclear to what extent COPD-induced systemic inflammation contributes to the development of cardiovascular disease. Recently, it was shown that platelet activation was increased in patients with COPD, particularly during acute exacerbations [9]. Along the same lines, Marchetti et al. [10] noted the vascular endothelium to be less responsive during exacerbations, indicating that the vascular smooth muscle function is further impaired during exacerbations. During exacerbations, patients have increased circulating inflammatory cytokines, indicative of systemic inflammation [11]. This feeds the hypothesis that systemic inflammation could be causally related to the development of cardiovascular disease in COPD.

Despite the observation that systemic inflammation is present both in patients with COPD and patients with cardiovascular disease, it remains particularly difficult to disentangle the many risk factors for the development of cardiovascular disease patients with COPD are exposed to. Physical inactivity has also recently been recognized as a potential risk factor for COPD, by showing accelerated lung function decline in smokers who are physically inactive, compared to physically active smokers [12]. Physical activity has been recognized as an important risk factor for the development of cardiovascular diseases for more than half a century. There is a wealth of data supporting the causal link between physical activity and the development of cardiovascular disease [13]. After measuring physical activity for a complete year, Aoyagi and coworkers recently demonstrated that there was an increased arterial stiffness with decreasing physical activity levels. In patients with less than 6,518 steps per day (the median observed in the study) the pulse wave velocity was significantly reduced [14]. The recent insight that patients with COPD become inactive very early in the disease [15, 16] may help our understanding of the link between CV disease and COPD. Figure 4.1 depicts the potential direct and indirect association between COPD and the development of cardiovascular disease.

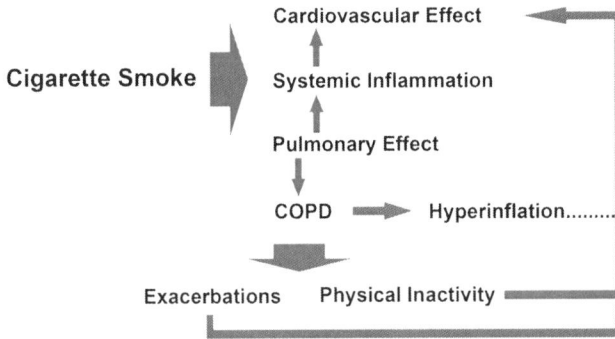

Fig. 4.1 The relation between cigarette smoke and its pulmonary and cardiovascular effects. The *dashed line* indicates a less studied, but likely relation

The present chapter does not intend to review the mechanisms by which COPD and cardiovascular disease can develop simultaneously. We refer to excellent and open access review papers on the subject [17]. Due to the shared risk factors, all patients with COPD should likely be regarded as at risk of developing cardiovascular disease and should be screened accordingly, across all lines of health care. Integrated care of patients with COPD should therefore ensure proper cardiac and vascular screening. This chapter will briefly discuss the prevalence of cardiac and vascular morbidity in patients with COPD, the prevalence of COPD, and its consequences in patients with significant cardiovascular disease to raise the awareness of clinicians for the co-existence of cardiac and vascular pathology in patients with COPD. Subsequently, the implications for the management of patients with COPD will be discussed. Pulmonary vascular morbidity will not be discussed although the prevalence of pulmonary hypertension should not be underestimated in COPD. Although at rest pulmonary hypertension is rarely severe, pulmonary artery pressures may rise during exercise and start limiting adequate oxygen delivery to the skeletal muscle. Excellent reviews on the topic however exist to which the interested reader is directed [18].

Prevalence of Cardiovascular Disease in Patients with COPD

When patients with COPD die during an exacerbation, autopsies confirm the presence of heart failure in 58% of the cases [6]. Several studies have investigated the prevalence of cardiovascular disease in patients suffering from COPD. In over a million patients included in a large database of primary care medical records collected at general practices throughout the UK, 2.5% of patients with physician-diagnosed COPD (61% confirmed by spirometry) had 5 times more chance of having cardiovascular morbidity [19]. These patients also had a threefold higher incidence rate of developing myocardial infarction in the 3 years of follow-up. Interestingly this was particularly true in the lowest age group.

In a more systematic study including just over 400 patients recruited in primary care without a prior diagnosis of heart failure, 83 (20%) new cases of heart failure were identified upon thorough diagnostic work-up [20]. Roughly half of these cases were systolic and the other half isolated diastolic heart failure. None of the patients had isolated right heart failure in this study. Compared to patients without heart failure, these patients had a larger smoking exposure, had higher NT-ProBNP levels, more systemic inflammation (as evidenced by increased C-reactive protein). In patients recruited from an outpatient chest clinic, 23% had elevated NT-ProBNP values (>125 pg ml⁻¹). This percentage was seen across all GOLD stages. It should be noted, however, that echographic evidence of severe heart failure was limited to less than 5% of patients. Vascular function was assessed in this study by the ankle-brachial index, a marker of peripheral arterial disease, and was impaired in 25% of subjects again independently of the GOLD stage. Similarly, several studies reported increased arterial stiffness an important predictor of cardiovascular morbidity (i.e., acute myocardial infarction and stroke) [21] in patients with COPD [22, 23]. Interestingly, also in patients with alpha 1 antitripsin deficiency, and a limited smoking exposure, an increased arterial stiffness was reported compared to smoking matched control subjects [24].

The Impact of COPD on Cardiac Function

Few, if any, large cohort studies looked at the prevalence of spirometry diagnosed COPD in patients with cardiovascular disease. When COPD diagnosis is obtained by patient report or the use of concomitant medication use, the prevalence is very much underestimated. Two large cohort studies, using this technique reported a prevalence of reported COPD in patients with acute myocardial infarction to be 8.6% [25], 11.1% [26]. In patients with heart failure, the prevalence of (self-) reported COPD was 11% in one study [27] and 23% in another [28]. All these studies found that COPD was an independent risk factor for adverse outcome of the cardiovascular condition. Nevertheless, it is reasonable to assume that all these studies have significantly underestimated the prevalence of COPD in these patients. Two studies systematically performed spirometry in patients with congestive heart failure and found the prevalence of COPD to be 35% in patients admitted to hospital with heart failure [29]. Interestingly in only 43% of these patients, the diagnosis of COPD was known before the spirometry was conducted. The information obtained from formal lung function testing showed to provide independent prognostic information to the "self-reported" COPD diagnosis. Per 10% predicted decrease in FEV1, the hazard rate was 14% (8–20%) increased [30]. These data were mirrored by a smaller cohort (n = 186) of patients followed in a heart failure clinic where 39.2% of patients had spirometry proven COPD [31]. A last study investigated over 3,000 patients that underwent vascular surgery, confirmed the 39% of spirometry proven COPD [32]. In the latter study, patients with COPD had worse survival. Altogether, there is strong evidence that COPD is much more prevalent in patients with cardiovascular conditions than in the general population and even in smokers without cardiovascular disease. COPD contributes independently to an adverse outcome of cardiovascular conditions. The reasons why COPD worsens cardiac disease remain largely unexplored. COPD, and particularly the associated dynamic hyperinflation, and increased thoracic pressure swings may further compromise cardiovascular function and as such may aggravate cardiac conditions. Hyperinflation imposes stress on the cardiovascular system and reduced cardiac chamber size has been reported with increased hyperinflation [33]. Similarly during exercise, dynamic hyperinflation may further compromise cardiac function. Lower oxygen pulse (i.e., the oxygen consumption per heart beat, an indirect measure of stroke volume), has been reported in patients with hyperinflation [34]. The causality of the impairment has been convincingly shown by the improved cardiac response to exercise upon administration of different types of bronchodilators [35] and of other interventions (HELIOX) [36, 37] with a direct impact on dynamic hyperinflation. The presence of COPD does further worsen the exercise tolerance of patients with heart failure. In patients with severe heart failure (Ejection Fraction 34%), the peak oxygen consumption was reduced 26% more in patients with concomitant COPD (FEV1 73% pred), compared to CHF matched patients without COPD. Similarly, the CHF patients with COPD had a 6 min walking distance that was 71 m less than those without COPD [38].

Although large studies are missing, it is not unlikely that even mild COPD, when associated with (dynamic) hyperinflation [39] would aggravate symptoms of heart disease, particularly during exercise, by imposing additional stress to heart.

Treating Cardiovascular Function to Improve Outcome in COPD

Guidelines for treating cardiovascular conditions are widely available and most guidance can be adapted to patients with COPD. Two pharmacological interventions, frequently used in the primary or secondary prevention, have recently received specific attention in patients with COPD and merit some specific discussion here. Lastly, rehabilitation is a comprehensive intervention which is evidence based therapy for patients with COPD, ischemic heart disease, chronic heart failure, peripheral vascular disease, and stroke. Pulmonary rehabilitation, including exercise therapy, may have the potential to prevent the onset or worsening of cardiovascular morbidity in patients at risk.

Statin Treatment

Statins (3-hydroxy-3-methylglutaryl coenzyme A reductase inhibitors) were originally directed to reducing cholesterol levels and improving peripheral vascular perfusion. Statin therapy reduces the incidence of coronary and cerebro-vascular events and is a first line cardiovascular therapy in patients at risk [40]. Recently, however, reports have proposed that statins would have a protective effect in patients with COPD. A systematic review suggested benefits of statin therapy in terms of mortality, exacerbation rate, exercise tolerance, and lung function [41]. Unfortunately, only one of the studies described was a randomized controlled study. Most other studies were case-control or cohort studies. The effects of statins in COPD are rather attributed to the anti-inflammatory and immune modulating effects of statin therapy. Van Gestel and coworkers have shown better survival in patients with COPD who underwent cardiovascular surgery and were on statins [32]. Statin therapy is of particular interest in patients with increased systemic and pulmonary inflammation. Cohort studies suggest benefits of statin therapy to prevent exacerbation associated mortality [42]. Again larger randomized controlled studies are not yet available to provide a solid proof of principle. In animal models of smoking induced emphysema, the mechanisms through which statins may exert a beneficial effect were recently investigated. Statins seem to have an effect on the pulmonary vascular pressures and the pulmonary vascular remodeling, observed in this model [43]. These effects are confirmed in very severe COPD (pre-lung transplantation) [44]. In the animal model, Simvastatin did slow down the development of emphysema (as judged by the morphometric analysis of the airspaces) but did not prevent the small airway remodeling. Excellent reviews are on the topic are available [45]. A word of caution is needed, as statins have been associated with the development of skeletal muscle weakness [46]. In patients with COPD, at risk to develop muscle weakness, which in terms has devastating effects on exercise tolerance, function, and survival, it should be advised to carefully monitor muscle function, when statin therapy is initiated. Clearly, large randomized controlled studies will need to provide the final answers to the question whether statin treatment should be rigorously used in patients with COPD outside the current label in patients with COPD. Potential future indications may be the use of these drugs as an adjuvant after acute exacerbations.

Beta Blockers

Beta blockers are first line pharmacotherapy in patients with hypertension, angina, myocardial infarction, cardiac arrhythmias, and heart failure, and as prophylaxis against cardiovascular events after high-risk surgery [47]. Historically, clinicians are reluctant to use beta blockers in patients with COPD. The combined use of beta-blockers and beta-agonists indeed seems counter-intuitive. Cardio-selective beta-blockers, however, can be safely used in patients with COPD, without impact on the lung function [48]. Rutten and coworkers [49] suggested from a cohort study that the use of β-blockers may reduce mortality as well as the risk of exacerbations of COPD, treated in primary care. Similarly, a study by Dransfield [50] suggested that patients receiving beta blockers were more likely to survive a hospital admission for an acute exacerbation. In univariate analysis, however, this interaction was not significant, so caution is warranted when interpreting the data. The mechanisms through which beta-blockers exert their possible benefits in COPD are not yet very clear. Whether there is an additional mechanism beyond the prevention of cardiovascular events by using beta-blockers needs to be studied from large randomized controlled trials. In the current state of knowledge, it is safe to conclude that cardioselective beta-blockers can be safely used in patients with COPD when there is a cardiovascular condition prompting the use.

Rehabilitation

Exercise training is an evidence-based therapy for patients with cardiovascular and respiratory disease. In addition, the adoption of a more active life style is an important goal to prevent cardiovascular morbidity. Unfortunately there is currently no direct evidence that patients with COPD who engaged in pulmonary rehabilitation programs develop less cardiovascular morbidity. Limited evidence showed that arterial stiffness – an important risk factor for the development of cardiovascular morbidity – is improved after exercise training [51]. The improvement in carotid-brachial pulse wave velocity was consistently reduced, observed after as little as 4 weeks of exercise training. The training program consisted of daily cycle endurance training (5 days/week) and exercise volume was increased from 18 min of cycling at 38% of the initial baseline peak work rate to 30 min at 65% of the initial peak work rate towards the end of the program. These data were recently replicated in a 7-week cohort study using multidisciplinary outpatient rehabilitation [52]. In patients with coronary artery disease, recent data support the acute beneficial effects of relatively short walking programs (30 min) on arterial stiffness, when assessed 24 h after a walking around [53]. Similar improvements in arterial stiffness are made in patients with diabetes undergoing an aerobic exercise training program by some authors [54], whereas another study, using a combination of unsupervised aerobic training (2 days/week) and twice weekly supervised resistance training tended to slow down the increase in PWV in patients with diabetes. This, however, did not reach significance. It is currently unknown whether the benefits observed after an exercise training program can be maintained afterwards, provided patients engage in a more active life style. Exercise training has been shown to nitric oxide production and circulating endothelial progenitor cells in patients with coronary artery disease [55–57] and in patients with peripheral vascular disease [58]. These factors are known to enhance angiogenesis and promote vascular repair in patients with (coronary) vascular problems. Other effects of endurance exercise training that may promote cardiovascular health include an improved endothelial function and blood coagulation [59].

Exercise training yields several benefits in patients with COPD, including an increase in exercise tolerance, a reduction in (exercise related) symptoms, an increase in health related quality [60] of life, and enhanced physical activity levels. [61].

Table 4.1 Nutritional advice provided in cardiac rehabilitation programs

Assessment of daily caloric intake and dietary content of fat, saturated fat, sodium, and other nutrients. Assessment of eating habits

Education of the patient and family members regarding salt intake, lipid use and water content of common foods. Healthy food choices including wide variety of foods, low salt foods, Mediterranean diet: fruits, vegetables, wholegrain cereals and bread, fish (especially oily), lean meat, low fat dairy products

Replace saturated fat with the above foods and with monounsaturated and polyunsaturated fats from vegetable (oleic acid as in olive oil and rapeseed oil) and marine sources to reduce total fat to less than 30% of energy, of which less than 1 of 3 is saturated

Avoidance of overweight, particularly by avoidance of beverages and foods with added sugars and salty food. In patients with COPD and cardiovascular risk these nutritional guidelines should be followed, and if needed combined with the nutritional counseling specific for COPD

Practice guidelines for exercise training in patients with COPD exist [62]. In order to yield significant physiological benefits programs need to be of high intensity, conducted with adequate supervision and carried out for several weeks with a training frequency of three times per week training [63]. It has currently not been studied as to which forms of exercise training would be best to treat or prevent cardiovascular events. Nevertheless, it seems that programs typically applied in COPD only marginally differ from those in patients with peripheral vascular disease (where the emphasis is slightly more on walking) [64], or programs applied to patients with ischemic cardiovascular disease [65]. In the latter program, there is an important place for nutritional counseling (Table 4.1).

Screening for Exercise Participation in COPD

Given the increased risk of cardiovascular morbidity, it is important to screen patients with COPD before they participate in training programs of high intensity. Recent guidelines of the European Association of Cardiovascular Prevention and Rehabilitation [59] suggest that sedentary subjects wanting to participate in moderate and high intense activity (such as that induced by training) need to be screened by a physician. A maximal incremental exercise test is recommended when patients have one of the following:

- A positive personal or family history of cardiovascular disease
- Suggestive clinical exam
- A risk SCORE (a composite score including region, gender, age, smoking history, systolic blood pressure and lipid profile) (66) above 5% or
- A positive resting ECG

In practice, this means that it is advised for most patients with COPD to undergo clinical exercise testing prior to enrolling in rehabilitation as these programs envisage high-intensity exercise training and an enhanced engagement in moderate to high exercise at home as part of the daily life.

Table 4.2 Proposed assessment for patients with cardiovascular disease when entering a cardiac rehabilitation program aiming at secondary prevention [65]

Clinical history	Screening for cardiovascular risk factors, co-morbidities and disabilities
Symptoms	Cardiovascular disease (NYHA class for dyspnoea and CCS class for angina)
Adherence	To the medical regime and self-monitoring (weight, blood pressure, symptoms)
Physical examination	General health status, heart failure signs, cardiac and carotid murmurs, blood pressure control, extremities for presence of arterial pulses and orthopedic pathology, cardiovascular accidents with/without neurological sequelae
Electrocardiogram	Heart rate, rhythm, repolarization
Cardiac imaging (two-dimensional and Doppler echocardiography)	In particular ventricular functions and valve heart diseases where appropriate
Blood testing	Routine biochemical assay, fasting blood glucose (HbA1C if fasting blood glucose is elevated), total cholesterol, LDL-C, HDL-C, triglycerides
Physical activity level	Domestic, occupational, and recreational needs, activities relevant to age, gender, and daily life, readiness to change behavior, self-confidence, barriers to increased physical activity, and social support in making positive changes
Peak exercise capacity	Symptom-limited exercise testing, either on bicycle ergometer, or on treadmill
Education	Clear, comprehensible information on the basic purpose of the CR program and the role of each component

NYHA New York Heart Association, *CCS* Canadian Cardiovascular Society

It should be mentioned that the exercise limitation of patients may change over the course of a rehabilitation program. It is not rare for patients to be limited by dyspnea at the outset of the rehabilitation program. When these symptoms improve as a consequence of the rehabilitation, they may become limited by peripheral vascular problems. Multidisciplinary screening involving cardiac screening, vascular screening, and thorough assessment of the cardiovascular risk factors (including lipid profile, resting ECG, and blood pressure, and exercise stress test) should be available to the rehabilitation team. For patients with cardiovascular problems, the proposed patient assessment by the Cardiac Rehabilitation Section of the European Association of Cardiovascular Prevention and Rehabilitation is given in Table 4.2.

Summary

Cardiovascular morbidity is frequent in patients with COPD and is linked to a significant part of the morbidity and mortality of COPD. Appropriate multidisciplinary screening of patients should include cardiovascular assessment. Smoking cessation, attention for nutrition, and exercise training or stimulating a physically active life style may prevent cardiovascular morbidity. Similarly, adequate pharmacological approaches can be set up according to guidelines for cardiac patients. For statins, there is limited evidence that support that these drugs may have additional effects, beyond their cardio-protective effects. More studies are, however, needed to support this hypothesis. Until more convincing evidence becomes available patients with COPD should be treated according to their cardiovascular risk profile with preventive therapy. Cardio-selective beta-blockers can be used in that respect safely in patients with COPD and this may prevent morbidity in patients with COPD and an enhanced cardiovascular risk profile.

References

1. Sin DD, Anthonisen NR, Soriano JB, Agusti AG. Mortality in COPD: role of comorbidities. Eur Respir J. 2006;28:1245–57.
2. Engstrom G, Hedblad B, Janzon L, Valind S. Respiratory decline in smokers and ex-smokers – an independent risk factor for cardiovascular disease and death. J Cardiovasc Risk. 2000;7:267–72.
3. Tockman MS, Pearson JD, Fleg JL, Metter EJ, Kao SY, Rampal KG, et al. Rapid decline in FEV1. A new risk factor for coronary heart disease mortality. Am J Respir Crit Care Med. 1995;151:390–8.
4. Roca B, Almagro P, Lopez F, Cabrera FJ, Montero L, Morchon D, et al. Factors associated with mortality in patients with exacerbation of chronic obstructive pulmonary disease hospitalized in General Medicine departments. Intern Emerg Med. 2011;6:47–54.
5. Chang CL, Robinson SC, Mills GD, Sullivan GD, Karalus NC, McLachlan JD, Hancox RJ. Biochemical markers of cardiac dysfunction predict mortality in acute exacerbations of COPD. Thorax. 2011;66(9):764–8. Epub 2011 Apr 7. PMID: 21474497.
6. Zvezdin B, Milutinov S, Kojicic M, Hadnadjev M, Hromis S, Markovic M, et al. A postmortem analysis of major causes of early death in patients hospitalized with COPD exacerbation. Chest. 2009;136(2):376.
7. Eisner MD, Wang Y, Haight TJ, Balmes J, Hammond SK, Tager IB. Secondhand smoke exposure, pulmonary function, and cardiovascular mortality. Ann Epidemiol. 2007;17:364–73.
8. Yusuf S, Hawken S, Ounpuu S, Dans T, Avezum A, Lanas F, et al. Effect of potentially modifiable risk factors associated with myocardial infarction in 52 countries (the INTERHEART study): case-control study. Lancet. 2004;364:937–52.
9. Maclay JD, McAllister DA, Johnston S, Raftis J, McGuinnes C, Deans A, Newby DE, Mills NL, Macnee W. Increased platelet activation in patients with stable and acute exacerbation of COPD. Thorax. 2011;66(9):769–74. Epub 2011 Apr 20.
10. Marchetti N, Ciccolella DE, Jacobs MR, Crookshank A, Gaughan JP, Kashem MA, et al. Hospitalized acute exacerbation of COPD impairs flow and nitroglycerin-mediated peripheral vascular dilation. COPD. 2011;8:60–5.
11. Spruit M, Gosselink R, Troosters T, Kasran A, Gayan-Ramirez G, Bogaerts P, et al. Muscle force during an acute exacerbation in hospitalised COPD patients and its relationship with CXCL8 and IGF-1. Thorax. 2003;58:752–6.
12. Garcia-Aymerich J, Lange P, Benet M, Schnohr P, Anto JM. Regular physical activity modifies smoking-related lung function decline and reduces risk of chronic obstructive pulmonary disease: a population-based cohort study. Am J Respir Crit Care Med. 2007;175:458–63.
13. Booth FW, Chakravarthy MV, Gordon SE, Spangenburg EE. Waging war on physical inactivity: using modern molecular ammunition against an ancient enemy. J Appl Physiol. 2002;93: 3–30.

14. Aoyagi Y, Park H, Kakiyama T, Park S, Yoshiuchi K, Shephard RJ. Yearlong physical activity and regional stiffness of arteries in older adults: the Nakanojo Study. Eur J Appl Physiol. 2010;109:455–64.
15. Watz H, Waschki B, Meyer T, Magnussen H. Physical activity in patients with COPD. Eur Respir J. 2009;33:262–72.
16. Troosters T, Sciurba F, Battaglia S, Langer D, Valluri SR, Martino L, et al. Physical inactivity in patients with COPD, a controlled multi-center pilot-study. Respir Med. 2010; 104(7):1005–111.
17. MacNee W, Maclay J, McAllister D. Cardiovascular injury and repair in chronic obstructive pulmonary disease. Proc Am Thorac Soc. 2008;5:824–33.
18. Remy-Jardin M, Remy J. Vascular disease in chronic obstructive pulmonary disease. Proc Am Thorac Soc. 2008;5:891–9.
19. Feary JR, Rodrigues LC, Smith CJ, Hubbard RB, Gibson JE. Prevalence of major comorbidities in subjects with COPD and incidence of myocardial infarction and stroke: a comprehensive analysis using data from primary care. Thorax. 2010;65:956–62.
20. Rutten FH, Moons KG, Cramer MJ, Grobbee DE, Zuithoff NP, Lammers JW, et al. Recognising heart failure in elderly patients with stable chronic obstructive pulmonary disease in primary care: cross sectional diagnostic study. BMJ. 2005;331:1379.
21. Mattace-Raso FU, van der Cammen TJ, Hofman A, van Popele NM, Bos ML, Schalekamp MA, et al. Arterial stiffness and risk of coronary heart disease and stroke: the Rotterdam Study. Circulation. 2006;113:657–63.
22. Maclay JD, McAllister DA, Mills NL, Paterson FP, Ludlam CA, Drost EM, et al. Vascular dysfunction in chronic obstructive pulmonary disease. Am J Respir Crit Care Med. 2009;180: 513–20.
23. Sabit R, Bolton CE, Edwards PH, Pettit RJ, Evans WD, McEniery CM, et al. Arterial stiffness and osteoporosis in chronic obstructive pulmonary disease. Am J Respir Crit Care Med. 2007; 175:1259–65.
24. Duckers JM, Shale DJ, Stockley RA, Gale NS, Evans BA, Cockcroft JR, et al. Cardiovascular and musculskeletal co-morbidities in patients with alpha 1 antitrypsin deficiency. Respir Res. 2010;11:173.
25. Hawkins NM, Huang Z, Pieper KS, Solomon SD, Kober L, Velazquez EJ, et al. Chronic obstructive pulmonary disease is an independent predictor of death but not atherosclerotic events in patients with myocardial infarction: analysis of the Valsartan in Acute Myocardial Infarction Trial (VALIANT). Eur J Heart Fail. 2009;11:292–8.
26. Wakabayashi K, Gonzalez MA, Delhaye C, Ben-Dor I, Maluenda G, Collins SD, et al. Impact of chronic obstructive pulmonary disease on acute-phase outcome of myocardial infarction. Am J Cardiol. 2010;106:305–9.
27. Kjoller E, Kober L, Iversen K, Torp-Pedersen C. Importance of chronic obstructive pulmonary disease for prognosis and diagnosis of congestive heart failure in patients with acute myocardial infarction. Eur J Heart Fail. 2004;6:71–7.
28. Macchia A, Monte S, Romero M, D'Ettorre A, Tognoni G. The prognostic influence of chronic obstructive pulmonary disease in patients hospitalised for chronic heart failure. Eur J Heart Fail. 2007;9:942–8.
29. Iversen KK, Kjaergaard J, Akkan D, Kober L, Torp-Pedersen C, Hassager C, et al. Chronic obstructive pulmonary disease in patients admitted with heart failure. J Intern Med. 2008;264:361–9.
30. Iversen KK, Kjaergaard J, Akkan D, Kober L, Torp-Pedersen C, Hassager C, et al. The prognostic importance of lung function in patients admitted with heart failure. Eur J Heart Fail. 2010;12:685–91.
31. Mascarenhas J, Lourenco P, Lopes R, Azevedo A, Bettencourt P. Chronic obstructive pulmonary disease in heart failure. Prevalence, therapeutic and prognostic implications. Am Heart J. 2008;155:521–5.
32. van Gestel YR, Hoeks SE, Sin DD, Simsek C, Welten GM, Schouten O, et al. Effect of statin therapy on mortality in patients with peripheral arterial disease and comparison of those with

versus without associated chronic obstructive pulmonary disease. Am J Cardiol. 2008;102: 192–6.

33. Watz H, Waschki B, Meyer T, Kretschmar G, Kirsten A, Claussen M, et al. Decreasing cardiac chamber sizes and associated heart dysfunction in COPD: role of hyperinflation. Chest. 2010;138:32–8.

34. Vassaux C, Torre-Bouscoulet L, Zeineldine S, Cortopassi F, Paz-Diaz H, Celli BR, et al. Effects of hyperinflation on the oxygen pulse as a marker of cardiac performance in COPD. Eur Respir J. 2008;32:1275–82.

35. Berton DC, Barbosa PB, Takara LS, Chiappa GR, Siqueira AC, Bravo DM, et al. Bronchodilators accelerate the dynamics of muscle O_2 delivery and utilisation during exercise in COPD. Thorax. 2010;65:588–93.

36. Laveneziana P, Palange P, Ora J, Martolini D, O'Donnell DE. Bronchodilator effect on ventilatory, pulmonary gas exchange, and heart rate kinetics during high-intensity exercise in COPD. Eur J Appl Physiol. 2009;107:633–43.

37. Laveneziana P, Valli G, Onorati P, Paoletti P, Ferrazza AM, Palange P. Effect of heliox on heart rate kinetics and dynamic hyperinflation during high-intensity exercise in COPD. Eur J Appl Physiol. 2011;111:225–34.

38. Guazzi M, Myers J, Vicenzi M, Bensimhon D, Chase P, Pinkstaff S, et al. Cardiopulmonary exercise testing characteristics in heart failure patients with and without concomitant chronic obstructive pulmonary disease. Am Heart J. 2010;160:900–5.

39. Ofir D, Laveneziana P, Webb KA, Lam YM, O'Donnell DE. Mechanisms of dyspnea during cycle exercise in symptomatic patients with GOLD stage I chronic obstructive pulmonary disease. Am J Respir Crit Care Med. 2008;177:622–9.

40. Mills EJ, Rachlis B, Wu P, Devereaux PJ, Arora P, Perri D. Primary prevention of cardiovascular mortality and events with statin treatments: a network meta-analysis involving more than 65,000 patients. J Am Coll Cardiol. 2008;52:1769–81.

41. Janda S, Park K, Fitzgerald JM, Etminan M, Swiston J. Statins in COPD: a systematic review. Chest. 2009;136:734–43.

42. Mortensen EM, Copeland LA, Pugh MJ, Restrepo MI, de Molina RM, Nakashima B, et al. Impact of statins and ACE inhibitors on mortality after COPD exacerbations. Respir Res. 2009;10:45.

43. Wright JL, Zhou S, Preobrazhenska O, Marshall C, Sin DD, Laher I, et al. Statin reverses smoke-induced pulmonary hypertension and prevents emphysema but not airway remodeling. Am J Respir Crit Care Med. 2011;183:50–8.

44. Reed RM, Iacono A, Defilippis A, Jones S, Eberlein M, Lechtzin N, et al. Statin therapy is associated with decreased pulmonary vascular pressures in severe COPD. COPD. 2011;8: 96–102.

45. Young RP, Hopkins R, Eaton TE. Pharmacological actions of statins: potential utility in COPD. Eur Respir Rev. 2009;18:222–32.

46. Thompson PD, Clarkson P, Karas RH. Statin-associated myopathy. JAMA. 2003;289: 1681–90.

47. Can beta-blockers be used for people with COPD? Drug Ther Bull 2011;49:2–5.

48. Salpeter S, Ormiston T, Salpeter E. Cardioselective beta-blockers for chronic obstructive pulmonary disease. Cochrane Database Syst Rev. 2005;4:CD003566.

49. Rutten FH, Zuithoff NP, Hak E, Grobbee DE, Hoes AW. Beta-blockers may reduce mortality and risk of exacerbations in patients with chronic obstructive pulmonary disease. Arch Intern Med. 2010;170:880–7.

50. Dransfield MT, Rowe SM, Johnson JE, Bailey WC, Gerald LB. Use of beta blockers and the risk of death in hospitalised patients with acute exacerbations of COPD. Thorax. 2008;63: 301–5.

51. Vivodtzev I, Minet C, Wuyam B, Borel JC, Vottero G, Monneret D, et al. Significant improvement in arterial stiffness after endurance training in patients with COPD. Chest. 2010;137: 585–92.

52. Gale NS, Duckers JM, Enright S, Cockcroft JR, Shale DJ, Bolton CE. Does pulmonary rehabilitation address cardiovascular risk factors in patients with COPD? BMC Pulm Med. 2011;11:20.
53. Michaelides AP, Soulis D, Antoniades C, Antonopoulos AS, Miliou A, Ioakeimidis N, et al. Exercise duration as a determinant of vascular function and antioxidant balance in patients with coronary artery disease. Heart. 2011;97:832–7.
54. Madden KM, Lockhart C, Cuff D, Potter TF, Meneilly GS. Short-term aerobic exercise reduces arterial stiffness in older adults with type 2 diabetes, hypertension, and hypercholesterolemia. Diabetes Care. 2009;32:1531–5.
55. Laufs U, Werner N, Link A, Endres M, Wassmann S, Jurgens K, et al. Physical training increases endothelial progenitor cells, inhibits neointima formation, and enhances angiogenesis. Circulation. 2004;109:220–6.
56. Richter B, Niessner A, Penka M, Grdic M, Steiner S, Strasser B, et al. Endurance training reduces circulating asymmetric dimethylarginine and myeloperoxidase levels in persons at risk of coronary events. Thromb Haemost. 2005;94:1306–11.
57. Steiner S, Niessner A, Ziegler S, Richter B, Seidinger D, Pleiner J, et al. Endurance training increases the number of endothelial progenitor cells in patients with cardiovascular risk and coronary artery disease. Atherosclerosis. 2005;181:305–10.
58. Schlager O, Giurgea A, Schuhfried O, Seidinger D, Hammer A, Groger M, et al. Exercise training increases endothelial progenitor cells and decreases asymmetric dimethylarginine in peripheral arterial disease: a randomized controlled trial. Atherosclerosis. 2011;217:240–8.
59. Borjesson M, Urhausen A, Kouidi E, Dugmore D, Sharma S, Halle M, Heidbüchel H, Björnstad HH, Gielen S, Mezzani A, Corrado D, Pelliccia A, Vanhees L. Cardiovascular evaluation of middle-aged/senior individuals engaged in leisure-time sport activities: position stand from the sections of exercise physiology and sports cardiology of the European Association of Cardiovascular Prevention and Rehabilitation. Eur J Cardiovasc Prev Rehabil. 2011 Jan 28. [Epub ahead of print] PMID: 21450560 [PubMed - as supplied by publisher].
60. Troosters T, Casaburi R, Gosselink R, Decramer M. Pulmonary rehabilitation in chronic obstructive pulmonary disease. Am J Respir Crit Care Med. 2005;172:19–38.
61. Troosters T, Gosselink R, Janssens W, Decramer M. Exercise training and pulmonary rehabilitation: new insights and remaining challenges. Eur Respir Rev. 2010;19:24–9.
62. Nici L, Donner C, Wouters E, ZuWallack R, Ambrosino N, Bourbeau J, et al. American thoracic society/European respiratory society statement on pulmonary rehabilitation. Am J Respir Crit Care Med. 2006;173:1390–413.
63. Casaburi R, ZuWallack R. Pulmonary rehabilitation for management of chronic obstructive pulmonary disease. N Engl J Med. 2009;360:1329–35.
64. McDermott MM, Ades P, Guralnik JM, Dyer A, Ferrucci L, Liu K, et al. Treadmill exercise and resistance training in patients with peripheral arterial disease with and without intermittent claudication: a randomized controlled trial. JAMA. 2009;301:165–74.
65. Piepoli MF, Corra U, Benzer W, Bjarnason-Wehrens B, Dendale P, Gaita D, et al. Secondary prevention through cardiac rehabilitation: from knowledge to implementation. A position paper from the Cardiac Rehabilitation Section of the European Association of Cardiovascular Prevention and Rehabilitation. Eur J Cardiovasc Prev Rehabil. 2010;17:1–17.
66. Graham I, Atar D, Borch-Johnsen K, Boysen G, et al. European guidelines on cardiovascular disease prevention in clinical practice: executive summary: fourth joint task force of the european society of cardiology and other societies on cardiovascular disease prevention in clinical practice (constituted by representatives of nine societies and by invited experts). Eur Heart J. 2007;28(19):2375–414.

Chapter 5
Osteoporosis

Luis F. Diez-Morales and Vincent Cunanan

Abstract Osteoporosis, a condition that is described by a decrease in bone mass, is further defined by the WHO as a bone mineral density (BMD) that is 2.5 standard deviations less than that of a young and healthy group of people. This is typically measured using a dual energy X-ray absorptiometry or (DXA) and is expressed as a T-score wherein a score of less than −2.5 is defined as osteoporosis and a score between −1 and −2.5 is defined as osteopenia. The T-score is a measure of standard deviation compared to young, healthy sex-matched controls. A Z-score, on the other hand, is a standard deviation measurement with age- and sex-matched controls as a point of comparison. Osteoporosis can further be diagnosed clinically in the presence of an osteoporotic fracture. Chronic obstructive pulmonary disease has been widely studied as a risk factor for the development of osteoporosis in both males and females and several mechanisms that address them have been suggested and investigated. Awareness of this relationship should prompt osteoporosis-screening initiatives for COPD patients and lead to early recognition and treatment.

Keywords Osteoporosis • COPD • Bone mineral density • Dual energy X-ray absorptiometry • Osteopenia • T-score • Z-score

Introduction

Osteoporosis, a condition that is described by a decrease in bone mass, is further defined by the World Health Organization (WHO) as a bone mineral density (BMD) that is 2.5 standard deviations less than that of a young and healthy group of people.

L.F. Diez-Morales(✉) • V. Cunanan
Internal Medicine/Ambulatory Services, University of Connecticut,
Saint Francis Hospital and Medicine Center, Hartford, CT, USA
e-mail: LDiez@stfranciscare.org; cunsper@yahoo.com

L. Nici and R. ZuWallack (eds.), *Chronic Obstructive Pulmonary Disease: Co-Morbidities and Systemic Consequences*, Respiratory Medicine, DOI 10.1007/978-1-60761-673-3_5, © Springer Science+Business Media, LLC 2012

This is typically measured using a dual energy X-ray absorptiometry (DXA) and is expressed as a T-score wherein a score of less than −2.5 is defined as osteoporosis and a score between −1 and −2.5 is defined as osteopenia [1]. The T-score is a measure of standard deviation compared to young, healthy sex-matched controls. A Z-score, on the other hand, is a standard deviation measurement with age and sex-matched controls as a point of comparison. Osteoporosis can further be diagnosed clinically in the presence of an osteoporotic fracture. Chronic obstructive pulmonary disease (COPD) has been widely studied as a risk factor for the development of osteoporosis in both males and females and several mechanisms that address them have been suggested and investigated. Awareness of this relationship should prompt osteoporosis-screening initiatives for COPD patients and lead to early recognition and treatment.

Epidemiology

An increased frequency of osteoporosis in adults with COPD has been described in several studies, although the relationship has not been ascribed to one single risk factor or pathophysiologic mechanism but rather a combination of multiple factors. A European study described an increased prevalence of osteoporosis in COPD compared to the general population (10.8% vs. 14.8%). Women had a higher prevalence of osteoporosis compared to men (18.4% vs. 1.7%) in the general population and the prevalence of osteoporosis increased in both genders with COPD (30.5% vs. 4.6%) [2]. It was noted, however, that the prevalence of osteoporosis regardless of the presence of COPD increased after the age of 75. In a study by Jorgensen et al., the prevalence of osteoporosis in patients with severe COPD was noted to be as high as 44.8% and 22.4% were osteopenic [3]. It has also been shown that bone mineral density also diminishes as the severity of COPD increases [4]. A low bone mineral density has been observed in 26% of GOLD stage II patients, 49.9% of GOLD stage III patients, and 75% of GOLD stage IV patients. Consequently, vertebral fractures are also prevalent among patients with COPD [5]. At least 41% of both male and female COPD patients have been shown to have at least one vertebral fracture and the prevalence increases with COPD severity in men. An increase in COPD severity also correlates with an increase in multiple vertebral fractures.

Risk Factors and Pathophysiology

There are several risk factors in COPD patients that predispose them to become osteoporotic or osteopenic. Smoking, low vitamin D level, low body mass index (BMI), immobility, hypogonadism, and steroid use have been identified as risk factors [6]. Genetic factors, chronic inflammation, and decreased levels of insulin-like growth factor (IGF-1) have also been identified. Smoking has been identified as an independent risk factor for osteoporosis in males. Bone mineral density is lower among men who are smokers. Furthermore, it has been found that smokers with more than 20 pack years have a 12% lower bone mineral density [7]. Subsequently, vertebral and hip fractures are increased among smokers. However, no clear pathophysiologic mechanism has been identified yet to link smoking and bone loss. It has been suggested that peak bone mass may also be decreased among early smokers and when combined with other risk factors such as corticosteroid use in COPD, the result is a greater risk for osteoporosis [8]. Alcohol use in conjunction with smoking increases the rate of bone loss and the prevalence of vertebral and hip fractures.

Vitamin D deficiency also plays a role in the development of osteoporosis in COPD. Vitamin D is essential in the maintenance of mineralization of the bone matrix. Low vitamin D levels have been demonstrated among COPD patients and are most likely due to the patients' poor functional status resulting in poor nutrition and inadequate sun exposure [6].

BMI correlates with bone mineral density such that a higher bone mineral density has been observed in persons with a higher BMI. The explanation is felt to be a greater weight-bearing load on the bones and also higher estrogen levels among obese persons. Conversely, a low BMI predisposes to having a low bone mineral density and persons with COPD have a lower BMI owing to their decreased nutritional intake and increase in energy requirements [9]. A BMI less than 22 kg/m^2 in patients with COPD has actually proven to be the strongest predictor of osteoporosis [10].

Hypogonadism leads to osteoporosis and can be caused by chronic illnesses or corticosteroid use, both of which are present in COPD patients. The mechanism may be due to gonadotropin suppression by corticosteroids at the level of the pituitary gland leading to low estrogen, testosterone, and luteinizing hormones [6]. Increasing age is also related to hypogonadism.

Physical activity is important in relation to bone mineral density and the lower end of the spectrum of physical activity, i.e., paralysis, has been shown to increase bone turnover. Patients with COPD have a very poor functional status owing to dyspnea and deconditioning which leads to poor physical activity and mobility. In addition, decreased activity and strength lead to an increased risk for hip fractures secondary to falls [6].

Chronic oral steroid use has been widely accepted as a risk factor for the development of osteopenia and osteoporosis which occurs in a dose-dependent fashion. Long-term inhaled corticosteroid therapy has been widely studied also and has been shown to affect bone health when used in higher doses. At lower doses, inhaled corticosteroids generally have no or a much lesser risk for osteopenia and osteoporosis.

Inhaled corticosteroids affect bone health in terms of bone mineral density, biomarkers of bone turnover, and fracture risk and this risk differs between inhaled corticosteroid preparations and doses. The more frequently used inhaled corticosteroids include budesonide, beclomethasone, fluticasone, or triamcinolone. At conventional doses, chronic use of inhaled corticosteroids has not been shown to increase fracture risk or affect bone mineral density in randomized controlled trials [11]. However, markers of bone turnover have been noted to be higher when using very high doses of inhaled corticosteroids [11]. Among the different inhaled corticosteroids, inhaled triamcinolone imposes a higher risk for lower BMD levels and increased biomarkers of bone turnover. Data have shown that doses above 750 mcg/day of fluticasone, 800 mcg/day of budesonide, 1,000 mcg/day of flunisolide, and 1,000 mcg/day of beclomethasone may have significant effects on bone loss.

Chronic oral steroid treatment is widely used in asthma patients and its effects on bone mineral density and osteoporosis has been demonstrated in this population. Similarly, COPD patients are also at increased risk for osteoporosis when steroid therapy is instituted. Although continuous oral steroid therapy is used less in this population, they are exposed to oral or systemic steroids during exacerbations. Systemic steroid therapy affects bone mineral density and fracture risk in a dose-dependent manner. Six milligrams per day for more than 6 months has been suggested to be related to an increase in osteoporosis and fracture risk. The osteoporotic effects are much severe during the first 6 months of treatment where there is a 5% decrease in bone mineral density during this period. The rate of bone loss then slows down to about 1–2% per year. In terms of dosing regimens, alternate day regimens are just as detrimental as daily dosing.

Glucocorticoid-induced bone loss is brought about by several processes: (1) Stimulating osteoclasts resulting in an increase in bone resorption while osteoblasts are suppressed hence reducing bone formation; (2) inhibiting formation of type I collagen by osteoblasts thereby altering bone matrix formation; (3) affecting calcium metabolism such that calcium loss is promoted via a secondary hyperparathyroidism pattern; (4) decreasing intestinal absorption of calcium and phosphate and at the same time increasing urinary calcium excretion; and (5) affecting adrenal and gonadal hormone release leading to a loss of the anabolic effects of these hormones. Several studies have shown that COPD is also associated with a systemic inflammatory state as well as to local inflammation in the lungs. Systemic inflammatory markers, CRP, IL-6, IL-8, and TNF, are elevated in patients with severely reduced lung function. Patients with a low BMI and low creatinine–height ratio (which is a measure of muscle mass) or low BMI alone have higher levels of IL-6 and TNF-alpha [12]. Therefore, systemic inflammation is postulated to result in loss of lean body mass in these patients. These inflammatory markers especially IL-1, IL-6, and TNF-alpha stimulate the proliferation and activation of osteoclasts in turn leading to increased bone turnover and loss of bone mineral density.

Diagnostic Studies

Screening

Often, the severity of the pulmonary disease diverts attention away from other important comorbidities, including the presence of osteopenia and osteoporosis. The early detection of decreased bone density allows for aggressive treatment of osteoporosis as well as strategies to prevent progression, with subsequent decrease

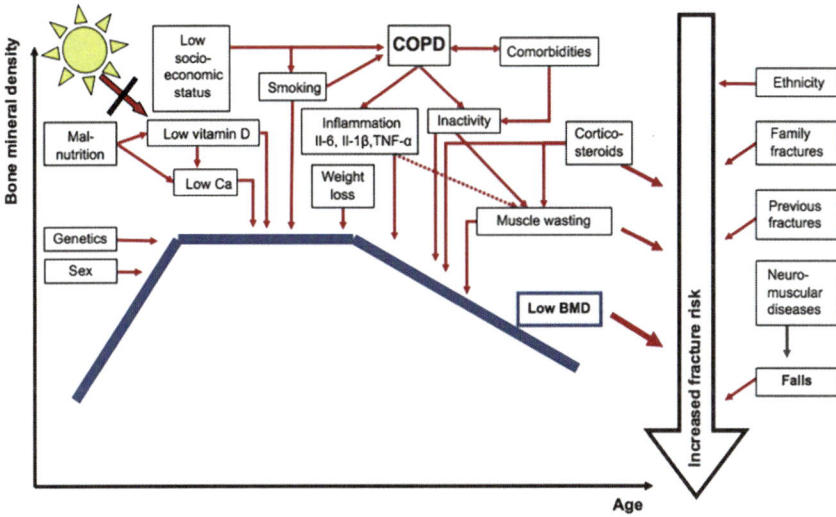

Fig. 5.1 The development of bone mineral density (BMD) throughout life, factors of importance for level of BMD (genetics, sex), COPD-related factors lowering (BMD), and important factors influencing fracture risk in addition to level of BMD. Modified from Langhammer et al. [11]

in morbidity. The wrists, hips, and vertebrae are the most often fractured bones in the osteoporotic patient. Vertebral fractures are often visualized in the lateral views of chest X-rays, images that are frequently obtained for diagnostic purposes at the time of a symptomatic COPD presentation. Their presence may be the first clinical sign of bone fragility. These vertebral compressions are a known predictor of future fractures and an important clue to perform further studies [12].

Unfortunately, visually searching for vertebral fractures in radiographs is inadequate. Quantitative morphometric analysis of these fractures can be performed but it is tedious and, furthermore, may not significantly improve their recognition [13]. Bone mass density (BMD) and bone mineral content (BMC) as determined by dual energy X-ray absorptiometry (DEXA) are considered the standards for diagnosis of osteopenia and osteoporosis. Results are reported as T and Z-scores. T is a calculation of the number of standard deviations from the mean peak bone mass of the same gender, normal individuals; Z is the standard deviation from same gender and age control population. T-scores are more frequently used in clinical practice, with scores between −1.0 and −2.5 defining osteopenia; scores lower than −2.5 defining the presence of osteoporosis. Every standard deviation can increase the risk of fractures threefold [14, 15].

The timing of screening patients for osteoporosis, including COPD patients, has not been firmly established. Studies do correlate the severity of COPD with the presence of osteoporosis, with patients at the highest GOLD (Global Initiative for Obstructive Lung Disease) stage having the highest incidence of bone disease (Fig. 5.1). These patients often have multiple risk factors for osteoporosis, therefore

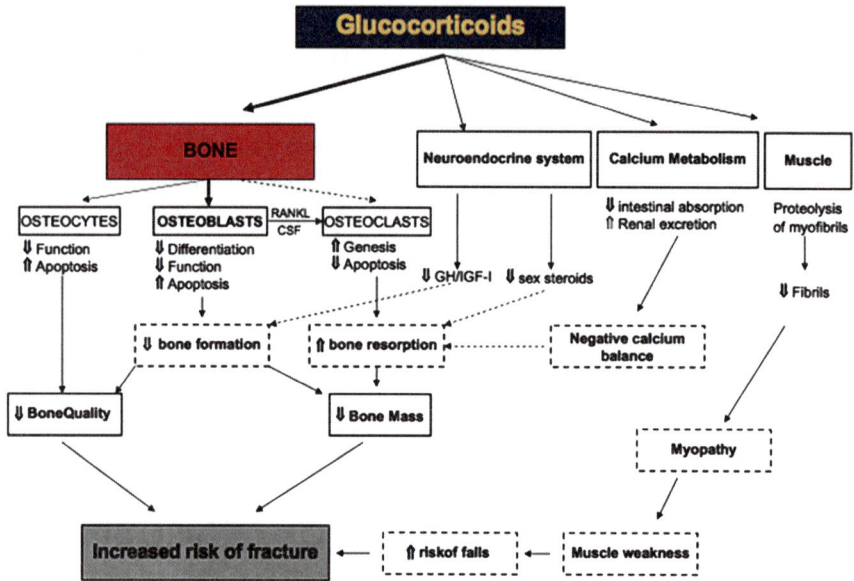

Fig. 5.2 Diagram showing the direct and indirect effects of glucocorticoids on bone leading to glucocorticoid-induced osteoporosis and fractures. Modified from Canalis et al. [25]

yearly DEXA scans are recommended. This group of patients should derive the most benefit from early diagnosis and a DEXA screening scan. All patients with a vertebral compression fracture or with a prior low impact fracture of other bones should also have a bone density evaluation (Fig. 5.2). Recommendations for follow-up scans vary from annually to bi-annually. However, yearly scans seem prudent once osteopenia or osteoporosis has been diagnosed [3].

Prevention

Every attempt should be made to decrease the known risk factors for osteoporosis in COPD patients. Smoking cessation is one of the biggest challenges in those patients who use tobacco. Every visit should be viewed as an opportunity to tell the patient the importance of quitting and ask if they are ready to quit. For certain patients, individual or group therapy may be useful. Some patients may benefit from nicotine substitutes such as nicotine chewing gum and nicotine patches, in particular those with a high level of physical addiction. The use of varenicline and bupropion, together with a patient support program, can significantly increase the success rate by decreasing the nicotine cravings.

Besides decreasing bone mineralization, Vitamin D deficiency may negatively affect muscle strength, and increase heart disease and cancer [16]. Vitamin D levels should be measured in all patients with COPD and corrected if low. Rapid and safe correction can be achieved with the administration of 50,000 IU of ergocalciferol three times a week for 4 weeks. Daily supplement of 800–1,000 IU of Vitamin D is recommended by most experts. It is often very difficult for patients to achieve adequate dietary calcium intake in their diets, especially the elderly, as lactose intolerance increases with age. To insure appropriate calcium intake, calcium supplementation is advised for all patients at 1,200–1,500 mg a day [6].

Low levels of testosterone in men and estrogen in women could lead to osteoporosis. Because of the high incidence of hypogonadism in COPD, men as well as postmenopausal women should be carefully followed and monitored for its development [6]. If there are no contraindications, hormone replacement should be carried out to achieve the appropriate levels [17, 18].

The progressive decrease in physical activity with eventual immobility increases the risk for osteoporosis in the COPD patients [19]. Decreased levels of activity have also been correlated to an increase risk of falls and fractures [20, 21]. Maintaining strength and mobility is a challenge that needs to be approached early and aggressively. Strength and weight-bearing exercises, included as part of pulmonary rehabilitation, could slow the progression of osteopenia.

Pharmacologic Treatment

There are no clear guidelines for the pharmacological treatment of osteoporosis in COPD. The GOLD summary from 2007 does not specifically address this issue [22]. Treatment guidelines for the general population recommend calcium and Vitamin D for patients with osteopenia and the use of biphosphonates in those who have T-scores of −2.5 standard deviations or lower as determined by a DEXA scan [23, 24].

References

1. WHO Study Group on Assessment of fracture risk and its application to screening for postmenopausal osteoporosis. Assessment of fracture risk and its application to screening for postmenopausal osteoprorosis: A Report of a WHO Study Group. Geneva 1994.
2. Cazzola M, Bettoncelli G, Sessa E, Cricelli C, Biscione G. Prevalence of comorbidities in patients with chronic obstructive pulmonary disease. Respiration. 2010;80(2):112–9.
3. Jørgensen NR, Schwarz P, Holme I, Henriksen BM, Petersen LJ, Backer V. The prevalence of osteoporosis in patients with chronic obstructive pulmonary disease: a cross sectional study. Respir Med. 2007;101(1):177–85.
4. Vrieze A et al. Low bone mineral density in COPD patients related to worse lung function, low weight and decreased fat = free mass. Osteoporos Int. 2007;18:1197–202.
5. Nuti R, Siviero P, Maggi S, Guglielmi G, Caffarelli C, Crepaldi G, et al. Vertebral fractures in patients with chronic obstructive pulmonary disease: the EOLO Study. Osteoporos Int. 2009;20(6):989–98.
6. Biskobing DM. COPD and osteoporosis. Chest. 2002;121(2):609–20.
7. Selemenda CW et al. Long term bone loss in men: effects of genetic and environmental factors. Ann Intern Med. 1992;117:286–91.

8. Ionescu AA, Schoon E. Osteoporosis in Chronic obstructive pulmonary disease. Eur Respir J. 2003;22 Suppl 46:64s–75.
9. Schols AM, Wouters EF. Nutritional abnormalities and supplementation in chronic obstructive pulmonary disease. Clin Chest Med. 2000;21:753–62.
10. Incalzi RA, Caradonna P, Ranieri P, et al. Correlates of osteoporosis in chronic obstructive pulmonary disease. Respir Med. 2000;94:1079–84.
11. Langhammer A, Forsmo S, Syversen U. Long-term therapy in COPD: any evidence of adverse effect on bone? Int J COPD. 2009;4:365–80.
12. Ross PD, Davis JW, Epstein RS, Wasnich RD. Pre-existing fractures and bone mass predict vertebral fracture incidence in women. Ann Intern Med. 1991;114:919–23.
13. Carter JD, Patel S, Sultan FL, Thompson ZJ, Margaux H, Sterrett A, et al. The recognition and treatment of vertebral fractures in males with chronic obstructive pulmonary disease. Respir Med. 2008;102:1165–72.
14. Marshall D, Johnell O, Wedel H. Meta-analyses of how well measures of bone mineral density predict the occurrence of osteoporotic fractures. BMJ. 1996;312:1254–9.
15. Kanis JA, Melton III LJ, Christiansen C, Johnston CC, Khaltaev N. The diagnosis of osteoporosis. J Bone Miner Res. 1994;9:1137–41.
16. Janssens W, Lehouck A, Carremans C, Bouillon R, Mathieu C, Decramer M. Vitamin D beyond bones in chronic obstructive pulmonary disease time to act. Am J Respir Crit Care Med. 2009;179:630–6.
17. Adachi JD. Corticosteroid-induced osteoporosis. Am J Med Sci. 1997;313:41–9.
18. Doerr P, Pirke KM. Cortisol-induced suppression of plasma testosterone in normal adult males. J Clin Endocrinol Metab. 1976;43:622–8.
19. Bourjeily G, Rochester CL. Exercise training in chronic obstructive pulmonary disease. Clin Chest Med. 2000;21:763–81.
20. Cooper C, Barker DJ, Wickham C. Physical activity, muscle strength and calcium intake in fractures of the proximal femur in Britain. BMJ. 1988;297:1443–6.
21. Gregg EW, Cauley JA, Seeley DG, et al. Physical activity and osteoporotic fracture risk in older women. Ann Intern Med. 1998;129:81–8.
22. Rabe KF, Hurd S, Anzueto A, et al. Global strategy for the diagnosis, management, and prevention of chronic obstructive pulmonary disease: GOLD executive summary. Am J Respir Crit Care Med. 2007;176:532–55.
23. National Osteoporosis Foundation. NOF physician's guidelines; September 2005. Pharmacologic options. http://www.nof.org/professionals/clinical.htm. Accessed 20 June 2007.
24. US Preventive Services Task Force. Screening for osteoporosis in postmenopausal women: recommendations and rationale. Ann Intern Med. 2002;137:526–8.
25. Canalis E, Mazziotti G, Giustina A, Bilezikian JP. Glucocorticoid-induced osteoporosis: pathophysiology and therapy. Osteoporos Int. 2007;18(10):1319–28.

Chapter 6
Thoracic Malignancies

Matthew D. Jankowich

Abstract Lung cancer is the leading cause of cancer death in the U.S. and in the world. Individuals with chronic obstructive pulmonary disease (COPD) are dispro-portionately affected by lung cancer, even after adjustment for smoking history and other factors. In the Lung Health Study, lung cancer was the leading overall cause of death in follow-up of individuals with mild to moderate COPD. The presence of COPD and lung function impairment may significantly affect treatment options and outcomes after the diagnosis of lung cancer. Thus, lung cancer is a significant comorbidity of COPD. The relation between COPD and lung cancer has also pro-voked interest in common genetic susceptibilities and pathogenetic mechanisms with hopes of gaining insight into these two common diseases. This chapter will examine the epidemiology of lung cancer in COPD, the relationship between emphysema and lung cancer, what is currently known about the genetics and pathophysiology of lung cancer in COPD, and aspects of lung cancer management and outcomes in relation to the presence of COPD.

Keywords Thorax • Malignancy • Cancer • Lung • COPD • Genetic • Pathogen • Epidemiology • Emphysema • Pathophysiology

Introduction

Lung cancer is the leading cause of cancer death in the U.S. and in the world. Individuals with chronic obstructive pulmonary disease (COPD) are disproportion-ately affected by lung cancer, even after adjustment for smoking history and other

M.D. Jankowich (✉)
Division of Pulmonary Medicine, Department of Medicine, Providence VA Medical Center, Providence, RI, USA
e-mail: Matthew_Jankowich@brown.edu

L. Nici and R. ZuWallack (eds.), *Chronic Obstructive Pulmonary Disease: Co-Morbidities and Systemic Consequences*, Respiratory Medicine, DOI 10.1007/978-1-60761-673-3_6,
© Springer Science+Business Media, LLC 2012

factors. In the Lung Health Study, lung cancer was the leading overall cause of death in follow-up of individuals with mild to moderate COPD [1]. The presence of COPD and lung function impairment may significantly affect treatment options and outcomes after the diagnosis of lung cancer. Thus, lung cancer is a significant comorbidity of COPD. The relation between COPD and lung cancer has also provoked interest in common genetic susceptibilities and pathogenetic mechanisms with hopes of gaining insight into these two common diseases. This chapter will examine the epidemiology of lung cancer in COPD, the relationship between emphysema and lung cancer, what is currently known about the genetics and pathophysiology of lung cancer in COPD, and aspects of lung cancer management and outcomes in relation to the presence of COPD.

Epidemiology

COPD as a Risk Factor for Lung Cancer

Numerous studies have established that individuals with COPD have a higher risk of lung cancer than individuals with normal lung function. In a seminal prospective case-control study by Skillrud et al., 113 individuals with airflow limitation (FEV1 <70% predicted) were matched by age, occupation, and smoking history with 113 control subjects [2]. In follow-up, nine individuals with airflow limitation developed lung cancer as compared with two control subjects, corresponding to a significant difference in the probability of developing lung cancer ($p = 0.024$). Ten-year mortality from lung cancer was 7.2% for individuals with airflow limitation and 0% for control subjects [2]. In a study published the following year by Tockman et al., based on data from the Intermittent Positive Pressure Breathing Trial and the Johns Hopkins Lung Project, airway obstruction was found to be a stronger predictor of lung cancer development than age or pack years of smoking [3]. In this study, FEV1 (% predicted) was inversely related to the adjusted risk of lung cancer, with higher lung cancer risk in individuals with lower FEV1% (Fig. 6.1) [3].

Subsequent studies have confirmed that COPD confers an increased risk for lung cancer beyond associations with age or smoking history. The increased risk of lung cancer related to COPD is notable. In the Tockman et al. study, the adjusted odds ratio for lung cancer in the setting of airway obstruction was 4.88 [3]. In a study by Young et al., COPD (GOLD stage 2 or higher) was present in 50% of lung cancer cases as compared with 8% of age-, sex-, and smoking history-matched controls, for an odds ratio of 11.6 ($p < 0.0001$) [4]. As this study selected cases from a specialty clinic, a referral bias for sicker cases with more airway obstruction could have been present. However, in a study conducted using a U.K. primary care database, individuals with a clinical diagnosis of COPD and a control cohort without COPD were followed over 5 years; the incidence of lung cancer in the COPD cohort was 7.8/1,000 person years, as compared to 1.4/1,000 person years in the control group [5].

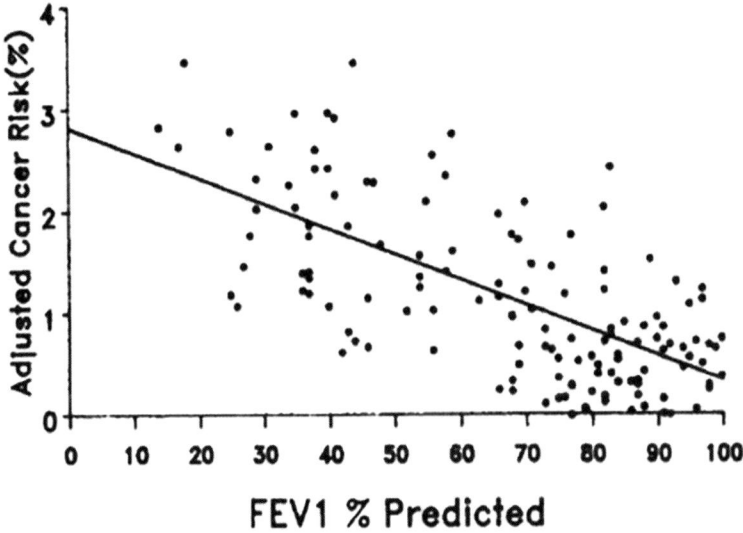

Fig. 6.1 In one study, FEV1 (% predicted) was inversely related to the adjusted risk of lung cancer, with higher lung cancer risk in individuals with lower FEV1% [3]. With permission from the American College of Physicians copyright 1987

The adjusted relative risk of lung cancer in the COPD cohort was 3.33. In a population-based case control study conducted in northern Italy, clinical diagnoses of emphysema, chronic bronchitis, and COPD were associated with increased odds of lung cancer (adjusted odds ratios (OR) of lung cancer: emphysema OR = 1.9 (95% CI 1.4 = 2.8); chronic bronchitis OR = 2.0 (95% CI 1.5–2.5); COPD OR = 2.5 (95% CI 2.0–3.1)) [6]. Confirming that COPD is associated with an increased risk of lung cancer that is unrelated to smoking, a prospective study by Turner et al. in lifelong nonsmokers ($n = 448,600$) showed a significant association between lung cancer mortality and a physician diagnosis of emphysema (hazard ratio 1.66 95% CI 1.06–2.59) [7]. Overall, these studies are consistent in reporting a significant association between COPD and lung cancer that is not explained by smoking or other shared factors.

Interestingly, studies utilizing a clinical diagnosis of COPD as opposed to spirometric diagnosis report lower relative risk of lung cancer, suggesting that a purely clinical diagnosis of airways disease may underestimate the actual risk of lung cancer associated with the presence and degree of airways obstruction. Indeed, lung cancer risk after adjustment for smoking was shown to be highest (relative risk 2.7) in individuals in the lowest quartile of lung function as compared to the highest quartile of lung function in the Tecumseh Community Health Study; a rapid decline in FEV1 also conferred greater risk of lung cancer in current smokers in that study [8]. Kuller et al. found a dose–response relationship between lung function as measured by FEV1 and risk of lung cancer mortality, with individuals in the lowest quintile of FEV1 having a rate of lung cancer death of 3.02/1,000 person-years, as compared to a rate of 0.43/1,000 person years for individuals in the highest quintile of lung function [9]. Purdue et al. also found a dose–response relationship between lung function impairment and lung cancer risk, with a relative risk of lung cancer of 1.5 in individuals with mild COPD, increasing to 2.7 in individuals with severe COPD [10]. Similarly, Mannino et al. found a hazard ratio for incident lung cancer of 1.4 in individuals with mild COPD and 2.8 in individuals with moderate or severe COPD [11]. A meta-analysis of several studies has confirmed the dose–response relationship between lung function as measured by FEV1 and the risk of lung cancer, with even mild decrements in FEV1 being associated with a significantly increased risk of lung cancer [12]. These findings suggest that not only the presence of COPD but also the degree of airflow limitation itself is an important marker of lung cancer risk.

Emphysema, Chronic Bronchitis, and Lung Cancer Risk

Although current definitions of COPD rely on the presence of airway obstruction on spirometry for diagnosis, COPD has traditionally been separated dichotomously on a clinicopathologic basis into chronic bronchitis and emphysema. Some studies have focused on whether underlying chronic bronchitis, a symptom-based diagnosis, or emphysema, a radiologic and pathologic diagnosis, are specific risk factors for lung cancer [13, 14]. An association between chronic bronchitis and lung cancer risk has been suggested. Mucus hypersecretion was found to be an independent risk factor for subsequent lung cancer by Peto et al., with a significant relationship between mucus hypersecretion and lung cancer persisting after adjustment for FEV1 and smoking [15]. After adjustment for smoking, productive cough was also a risk factor for lung cancer in the Tecumseh Community Health Study [8]. In a cohort from the Copenhagen City Heart Study, chronic bronchitis, currently defined as cough and sputum production for more than 3 months for at least 2 consecutive years, was a significant predictor of subsequent mortality from lung cancer (HR 2.0 95% CI 1.4–2.9) after adjustment for age, gender, smoking, FEV1, and other factors [16]. Therefore, the presence of chronic bronchitis symptoms may confer increased risk of lung cancer beyond that related to the presence of impaired FEV1.

Recent studies have focused on the presence of emphysema as a specific risk factor for lung cancer, utilizing computed tomography (CT) to assess for emphysema. In a study by de Torres et al., the presence of emphysema was an independent risk factor for lung cancer after adjustment of factors including age, smoking history, and presence of airway obstruction (relative risk of lung cancer if emphysema: 2.51 95% CI 1.01–6.23) [17]. Interestingly, the presence of both emphysema and airway obstruction was associated with a synergistically increased lung cancer risk [17]. A subsequent study by Wilson et al. demonstrated that even trace quantities of emphysema on CT as assessed visually were associated with a significantly elevated risk of lung cancer [18]. In this study, a synergy between airflow obstruction and emphysema was again noted, with the highest risk of lung cancer seen in individuals with emphysema and moderate or severe airflow obstruction [18]. After adjustment for airflow obstruction and other factors, any emphysema remained a significant independent predictor of lung cancer (RR 3.14 95% CI 1.91–5.15) [18]. A clear dose–response between emphysema severity and lung cancer risk, however, was not seen. By contrast, in a study by Maldonado et al., quantitative analysis of emphysema by CT scan did not show a significant association between percent volume of emphysema and lung cancer, nor even between severe emphysema (emphysema volume >15%) and lung cancer [19]. However, this study did reconfirm the significant association between airflow obstruction and lung cancer [19]. The contradictory results of these studies could relate to differences in diagnosis of emphysema (quantitative versus visual), CT techniques such as slice thickness, or other factors. Further study of emphysema as an independent risk factor for lung cancer is warranted, and may become available from contemporary CT screening studies for lung cancer.

Gender, COPD, and Lung Cancer

Women have been reported to be potentially at greater risk of lung cancer per smoking dose than men. The effects of gender on the relationship between COPD and lung cancer have also been studied. An increased risk of lung cancer is present in women with COPD as compared to women without COPD. A study by Schwartz et al. found increased odds of lung cancer in women with a history of COPD (adjusted OR 1.67 95% CI 1.15–2.41) as compared to controls without COPD after adjustment for multiple confounders [13]. In this study, a prior diagnosis of emphysema was associated with even stronger odds of lung cancer (adjusted OR 3.21 95% CI 1.60–6.45) [13]. In a study by Kiri et al., women represented 40% of all lung cancer patients, but women were slightly less represented (36.8%) among individuals with concomitant lung cancer and COPD [14]. In this study, lung cancer incidence was considerably higher in both men and women with COPD as compared to the general population (lung cancer incidence of 64/10,000 men with COPD as compared to 15/10,000 men in the general population, and 48/10,000 women with COPD as compared to 10/10,000 women in the general population). Mortality rates related to lung cancer were similarly elevated in both men with COPD and women with COPD as compared to all individuals with lung cancer, suggesting gender does not influence the prognosis of lung cancer in individuals with COPD [14]. However, other studies have suggested that impaired lung function may be a greater risk factor for lung cancer in women than in men; in a meta-analysis by Wasswa-Kintu et al., women had higher relative risks for lung cancer than men in every quintile of lung function below the highest quintile (for example, the pooled relative risk for women in the lowest quintile of lung function as compared to the highest was 3.97, vs. a relative risk of 2.23 for men in the lower quintile of lung function) [12].

This suggests potentially important gender influences on lung cancer risk in the setting of impaired lung function.

Asthma, COPD, and Lung Cancer

Is the risk of lung cancer specifically confined to an association with COPD, or does the association extend to individuals with obstructive lung disease from other causes, such as asthma? Some studies have suggested an elevated risk of lung cancer associated with the diagnosis of asthma [20], but others have not [21]. Wu et al. found that a previous diagnosis of asthma was more common in nonsmoking women diagnosed with lung cancer than in controls (adjusted OR 1.67 95% CI 1.1–2.50) [22]. A subsequent meta-analysis of multiple studies has suggested an increased risk of lung cancer even in never smokers with asthma [23]. González-Pérez et al. also found an increased prevalence of lung cancer in individuals with asthma (adjusted OR 1.35 95% CI 1.15–1.59) in a study using the U.K. General Practitioner Research Database; by comparison, in the same study, the adjusted odds ratio for lung cancer in individuals with COPD was 1.86 [24]. Huovinen et al. found an elevated risk of lung cancer in men with asthma after adjustment for smoking, but this association did not remain significant after adjustment for other confounders (hazard ratio 2.36 95% CI 0.88–6.34) [25]. Ramanakumar et al. found no association between lung cancer and asthma in either men or women [21]. Most studies of the relationship between asthma and lung cancer have relied on the clinical diagnosis of asthma, and possible misclassification of COPD as asthma is a limitation of these studies as is the lack of an objective measure for asthma. In a study by Hospers et al., airway hyperresponsiveness, a hallmark of asthma, as measured by response to histamine inhalation, was not associated with an increased risk of lung cancer [26]. In this study, clinical asthma, peripheral eosinophilia, or positive allergen skin tests were also not associated with lung cancer risk [26]. In summary, whether there is an association between lung cancer and asthma is uncertain as study results have been contradictory and misclassification of exposure to asthma versus COPD is a potential problem in some studies, though studies demonstrating an elevated risk of lung cancer in never smokers with asthma are more convincing. Given the significant differences in asthma and COPD pathogenesis, different underlying molecular mechanisms would likely relate these diseases to lung cancer.

COPD and Thoracic Malignancies Aside from Lung Cancer

There is no clear epidemiological data linking COPD to the occurrence of other thoracic malignancies, such as mesothelioma, esophageal cancer, lymphoma, or carcinoid tumors. However, as with lung cancer, COPD may be a frequent comorbidity in smoking-related tumors like esophageal cancer, and may influence the therapeutic options for these cancers, especially with regard to feasibility of surgery.

Pathophysiology of Lung Cancer Related to COPD

While smoking is a shared risk factor for both lung cancer and COPD, the additional risk of lung cancer present in individuals with COPD beyond that related to smoking, as established by epidemiologic studies discussed above, suggests that unique pathophysiologic mechanisms in COPD, not shared by cigarette smokers without obstructive lung disease, directly contribute to lung cancer formation. The additional risk of lung cancer in individuals with COPD may relate to a shared genetic vulnerability to both diseases, and/or to aspects of COPD such as ciliary dysfunction and air trapping resulting in elevated smoke-related carcinogen exposure, local or systemic inflammation, lung tissue remodeling, angiogenesis, or other molecular processes initiated in the COPD lung. At present, the specific pathophysiologic mechanisms that confer an increased risk of lung cancer in individuals with COPD are uncertain. This section will discuss the current state of knowledge of lung cancer pathophysiology as related to COPD.

Genetics and Genomics of Lung Cancer in COPD

The confluence of lung cancer and COPD has suggested the possibility of shared genetic susceptibility. Relatives of patients with COPD or lung cancer have greater rates of impaired pulmonary function than controls, suggesting that familial clustering of pulmonary dysfunction occurs which may lead to one or both diseases [27]. A subset of smokers fails to upregulate detoxification and antioxidant genes in the airway epithelium, suggesting that these individuals may represent a group that is predisposed to subsequent COPD and lung cancer [28]. Despite the relatively limited understanding of the genetics of COPD, there have been a number of studies exploring potential shared genetic causes of lung cancer and COPD.

Alpha-one-antitrypsin deficiency, related to mutations in the $\alpha 1AT$ gene on 14q32.1, is the classic genetic cause of emphysema and chronic obstructive pulmonary disease [29]. A variety of mutant alleles of the $\alpha 1AT$ gene have been described, such as the S allele, Z allele, and other rare alleles like null, with individuals homozygous for the PI*Z allele having abnormally low serum concentrations of alpha-one-antitrypsin protein due to intracellular polymerization of the mutant proteins in the hepatocyte. The consequent deficiency in alpha-one-antitrypsin results in unopposed function of neutrophil elastase, the molecule normally inhibited by alpha-one-antitrypsin, which in turn results in lung parenchymal destruction and panacinar emphysema. Alpha-one-antitrypsin deficiency accounts for approximately 1% of cases of COPD [29]. While heterozygotes for the wild type M allele in combination with a mutant $\alpha 1AT$ allele generally do not develop lung disease, recent evidence suggests that carriers of abnormal $\alpha 1AT$ alleles may be at increased risk for lung cancer. Yang et al. found that 13.7% of lung cancer cases were carriers of at least one $\alpha 1AT$ deficiency allele (S, Z, and other alleles), as compared to 7.8%

of controls [30]. Carriers of a α1AT deficiency allele had 70% higher odds of lung cancer, after adjustment for factors including sex, age, and COPD. In this study, the authors estimated the population attributable risk of lung cancer related to α1AT deficiency allele carriage at 11–12% in their Midwestern U.S. population [30]. Given geographic variance in α1AT allele carriage, this risk estimate may not apply to other geographic distributions. This same group has also reported an association between lung cancer and neutrophil elastase haplotypes, suggesting that protease–antiprotease imbalance may contribute to lung carcinogenesis [31]. This hypothesis and the reported genetic associations need to be tested in other geographically diverse populations.

Aside from alpha-one-antitrypsin deficiency, single-gene mutations are not known to be causes of COPD. A common lung cancer single-gene mutation that accounts for a substantial proportion of lung cancer cases is not known. Therefore, little is presently understood about shared genetic causes of lung cancer and COPD. However, a number of recent studies have begun to examine potential links between lung cancer, COPD, and various genetic loci. The 15q24-25 locus has been linked to lung cancer [32–34]. This region contains nicotinic acetylcholine receptor subunit genes and has also been linked to nicotine dependence [34–36], COPD [37, 38] and emphysema [37, 39]. While the relation between the 15q25 locus and lung cancer remains significant after adjustment for smoking quantity [32, 40, 41] because a factor affecting smoking behavior will clearly confer additional risk for smoking-related diseases such as COPD and lung cancer, this genetic locus may not necessarily explain a smoking-independent lung cancer risk thought to be associated with the presence of COPD. Indeed, an association between the 15q25 locus and lung cancer is not seen in never smokers [32, 41–43], and the association of 15q25 with COPD is weakened by adjustment for smoking quantity as measured by cigarettes per day [35]. Further research will be needed to determine if the 15q25 locus helps to explain a susceptibility to lung cancer in COPD independent of influences on smoking behavior.

Other genes and genetic loci have been investigated as possible determinants of lung cancer and COPD. A genetic locus that has been implicated in lung function in genome-wide association studies is the 4q31 locus near the hedgehog interacting protein [44, 45]. Carriers of the minor allele of the rs13147758 single-nucleotide polymorphism (SNP) have higher values for lung function as measured by the FEV1/FVC ratio [44]. This genetic locus has also been associated with lung cancer in a case-control study [46]. The hedgehog interacting protein is a component of the hedgehog signaling pathway, which has been implicated in tumorigenesis, and may act as a pathway inhibitor; hedgehog interacting protein expression has been reported to be lost in some lung cancers [47]. Larger studies of the 4q31 locus association with lung cancer are needed. The 6p21 locus has also been implicated in both lung cancer [33] and lung function [45]. Polymorphisms in glutathione-s-transferase, an enzyme involved in the detoxification of polycyclic aromatic hydrocarbons in cigarette smokers, resulting in reduced glutathione-s-transferase function may pose an increased risk of lung cancer. The GSTM1 (null) polymorphism has been found to confer an increased risk of lung cancer in analysis of the multiple studies thus far performed (OR 1.22, 95% CI 1.14–1.30) [48]. This risk may be particularly elevated in Asian populations [48, 49]. The GSTM1 (null) polymorphism also seems to confer an elevated risk of COPD, as demonstrated in a recent meta-analysis of a number of studies showing an OR for COPD of 1.45 (95% CI 1.09–1.92) for GSTM1 (null) variants [50]. In summary, genome-wide association studies and case-control genetic studies have identified a number of single nucleotide polymorphisms which have been associated with both lung function/COPD and lung cancer. Further investigation of these loci may shed light on pathogenetic pathways explaining lung cancer risk related to COPD.

Molecular Pathogenesis of Lung Cancer Related to COPD

The pathogenesis of COPD involves a complex molecular response to cigarette smoke within the lung that can be broadly categorized into inflammatory, fibrotic, and proteolytic pathways [51]. The role of inflammation as a central common pathway in the pathogenesis of lung cancer related to COPD has been a subject of interest [52, 53]. The sustained need to repopulate damaged lung tissue in COPD in the setting of chronic inflammation may potentially represent a pro-proliferative impulse in a disease that is otherwise characterized by lung tissue destruction and apoptosis [53]. Inflammation in COPD involves both innate and adaptive immune systems invoking a multicellular immune response, with infiltration and activation of CD[8+] T cells, neutrophils, macrophages; interactions with lung epithelial cells; and activation of a complex cytokine response [51, 54, 55]. How COPD inflammatory pathways may be involved in lung cancer pathogenesis has only begun to be elucidated. However, insights can be gained from certain studies.

The role of local and systemic inflammation in lung cancer pathogenesis in COPD is complex. Increasing levels of c-reactive protein, a marker of systemic inflammation, have been associated with increasing risk for all-cause and cancer-related mortality in COPD [56]. In data from the Lung Health Study, individuals with COPD in the highest quintile of c-reactive protein had a higher proportion of lung cancer deaths (2.9%) than individuals in the lowest quintile of c-reactive protein (1.4%), but the trend was not significant after adjustment for confounders [56]. Given the association between inflammation and cancer, anti-inflammatory medications have been studied as possible agents for lung cancer prevention in COPD. Inhaled corticosteroids prescribed for COPD treatment may be associated with a reduced risk of lung cancer [57, 58]. However, a prospective trial of inhaled steroids in smokers with bronchial dysplasia did not reveal an effect of inhaled steroids on preneoplastic lesion progression or prevention [59]. Studies adequately powered and specifically designed to assess inhaled corticosteroids as chemoprophylactic agents for lung cancer in COPD are needed.

Aspirin and other nonsteroidal anti-inflammatory agents may similarly have a role in lung cancer chemoprophylaxis, presumably through anti-inflammatory mechanisms. Cyclooxygenase is overexpressed in lung tumors, especially adenocarcinomas [60]. Epidemiologic studies have suggested that use of aspirin, a cyclooxygenase inhibitor, may be associated with a reduced risk of lung cancer in population studies [61]. However, a study of the association between lung cancer and NSAID use among individuals with COPD found no reduction in risk of lung cancer in the COPD population [62]. Detection of an effect of aspirin on lung cancer mortality may require long-term follow-up [63]. Interestingly, in a study by Rothwell et al., aspirin reduced lung cancer risk in adenocarcinomas, the type of tumors which appear to most vigorously overexpress cyclooxygenase [63]. Whether risk reduction with aspirin or other nonsteroidals is effective in preventing lung cancer related to COPD will require confirmation with appropriately powered studies with adequate long-term follow-up.

Bacterial colonization and infection is a driver of local inflammation and exacerbations in COPD and may also play a role in lung cancer formation in COPD. Nontypeable (unencapsulated) *Haemophilus influenzae* is an important colonizer of the COPD airway that also commonly contributes to infectious exacerbations of COPD. Nontypeable *H. influenzae* strongly activates nuclear factor kappa-B-mediated inflammation via toll-like receptor-2 signaling in human airway epithelial cells [64]. Exposure of a mouse model of lung cancer (in which a mutant K-ras gene is inserted in the Clara cell secretory protein locus) to nontypeable *H. influenzae* lysates resulted in neutrophilic inflammation and a 3.2-fold increase in lung tumor production [65]. This suggests that inflammation related to bacterial infection may be a specific driver of lung cancer in the setting of COPD. Interestingly, COPD-like inflammation mediated by IL-6 appears to have more of an effect on lung tumorigenesis than allergic inflammation in this mouse model [66]. Further data links the IL-6 inflammatory pathway to lung cancer in COPD. The gene for Stat-3, a signaling molecule downstream from IL-6, is upregulated in lung carcinomas in patients with COPD [67]; matrix metalloproteinase 12 expression may link IL-6 and Stat-3-related inflammation, proteolysis, and lung tumorigenesis in COPD [68]. The compound curcumin has been shown in the mutant K-ras/Clara-cell secretory protein model to inhibit neutrophilic airway inflammation from nontypeable *H. influenzae* with a consequent relative reduction in lung tumor formation [69]. Novel chemoprophylaxis of lung cancer in the high-risk COPD population may involve agents such as antimicrobial agents, IL-6 pathway inhibitors, or inhibitors of neutrophil chemotaxis that will prevent or suppress airway inflammation in response to infection.

Despite the potential role of inflammation in the pathogenesis of both lung cancer and COPD, inhibiting specific inflammatory pathways may produce unpredictable results. In a randomized controlled trial of infliximab, an antitumor necrosis factor-alpha antibody, in individuals with COPD, infliximab therapy resulted in no improvement in health-related quality of life or exercise tolerance [70]. A larger number of cancers, including lung cancers, were diagnosed in the infliximab group as compared to the placebo group [70]. This finding highlights the complex relationship between the immune system, inflammation, and cancer in COPD and suggests that cautious selection and careful testing of anti-inflammatory therapies for COPD and COPD-related lung cancer will be needed.

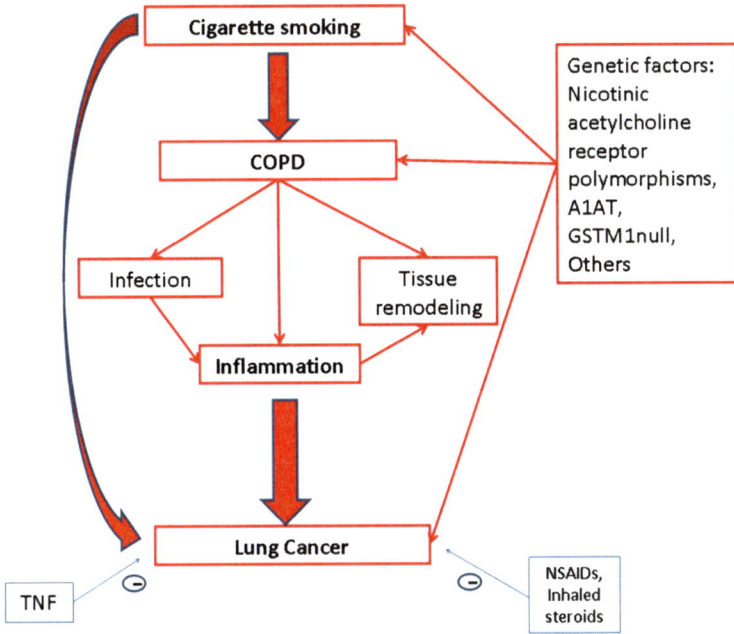

Fig. 6.2 Summary of the current understanding of genetic and molecular pathways in COPD-related lung cancer

Novel Insights into Lung Cancer Pathogenesis in COPD

Genomic, proteomic, and epigenetic studies may allow for specific molecular subtyping of COPD-related lung cancer. In a study by Boelens et al. using laser dissection microscopy to isolate tumor cells, differential gene expression was found in squamous cell lung cancers derived from non-COPD subjects and COPD subjects [71]. Reduced expression of multiple mitochondrial function-related genes was seen in samples from non-COPD tumors compared to COPD tumors, mostly related to increased loss of 5q in the non-COPD patients [71]. A study by Suzuki et al. found that methylation patterns of particular genes distinguished COPD-related lung cancer from non-COPD-related lung cancer; furthermore, HER-2 overexpression was seen more frequently in COPD-related tumors [72]. Future studies will allow further molecular subtyping of COPD-related lung cancer, holding the promise of identifying specific molecular pathways for chemoprevention, early diagnosis, or individualized treatments. Figure 6.2 summarizes currently the understanding of genetic and molecular pathways in COPD-related lung cancer.

Clinical Aspects of Lung Cancer in COPD

At present, the only definitive curative therapy for lung cancer is surgery for early stage disease. However, the presence of impaired lung function, especially with COPD, is a common reason for ineligibility for surgical treatment and for adverse outcomes following surgical resection. Therefore, careful preoperative assessment, staging, and management of COPD following the diagnosis of lung cancer are essential. Minimally invasive techniques that may preserve lung function and preclude the need for surgery, such as radiofrequency ablation and stereotactic radiotherapy, have been developed and may offer therapeutic options for individuals with COPD ineligible for surgery due to reduced lung function. In the setting of progressive lung cancer, end-of-life palliative care is beneficial in addressing symptoms such as dyspnea which are common in the setting of lung cancer and COPD. This section will discuss data on lung cancer clinical management as specifically related to COPD.

Diagnosis of Lung Cancer in COPD

Pulmonary nodules are common in patients with COPD, in one study being present in 35% of subjects with COPD undergoing CT screening [73], and often require serial imaging follow-up or immediate workup for diagnostic purposes depending on the lesion characteristics. In general, the diagnostic workup of suspected lung cancer in the setting of COPD should proceed as for a patient without COPD. Common nonoperative diagnostic procedures to establish a tissue diagnosis include sputum cytology, fiberoptic bronchoscopy, and image-guided transthoracic needle aspiration or biopsy. Sputum cytology examination is noninvasive and is an option for establishing a tissue diagnosis for patients with advanced COPD and suspected lung cancer in whom other procedures are felt to be potentially hazardous [74]. Fiberoptic bronchoscopy is generally a very safe procedure with an associated mortality rate of 0.04% or less in several large studies; however, the presence of severe COPD may increase the risk of complications [75]. Appropriate monitoring of oximetry should be undertaken, and CO_2 retention may be an especial risk in the setting of COPD, conscious sedation, and bronchoscopy. Prebronchoscopy therapy with bronchodilators does not affect the decline in FEV1 that occurs immediately following the procedure, nor does it prevent oxygen desaturation during the procedure [76]. Transthoracic needle aspiration or biopsy, typically performed under CT guidance, is a commonly employed diagnostic procedure, especially for more peripheral lung lesions. Complications including pneumothorax [77], pneumothorax requiring chest tube placement [78, 79], and pulmonary hemorrhage [80] have been reported to be more common in individuals with COPD and/or emphysema. However, lesion depth is generally the strongest risk factor for pneumothorax following CT-guided lung biopsy [79, 80]. Traditional diagnostic techniques for the assessment of possible lung cancer can be utilized in individuals with COPD, though the risks of individual techniques may vary based on lesion and patient characteristics, so an individualized diagnostic approach to lung cancer in a patient with COPD should be undertaken.

Preoperative Assessment

The goal in early stage lung cancer should be curative surgical resection if possible. When early stage, potentially resectable lung cancer is known or suspected, a careful preoperative multidisciplinary assessment should be performed to determine if the patient is a surgical candidate. Pulmonary function tests are a cornerstone of the preoperative assessment in all individuals with lung cancer. A preoperative FEV1 of greater than 1.5 l is associated with low mortality from lobectomy, and a preoperative FEV1 of greater than 2 l, or 80% of predicted is associated with low mortality from pneumonectomy [81]. By contrast, a reduced DLCO is a significant predictor of both mortality and postoperative pulmonary complications [82]. DLCO measurement should be considered in individuals with an FEV1 <80% predicted [81] but could be considered of potential benefit in predicting risk of complications in all patients undergoing lung resection [83]. Substantial reductions in FEV1 and DLCO (values <40% predicted) are associated with high perioperative mortality [81]. However, lung resection surgery can be performed safely even in patients with significantly reduced preoperative FEV1 (<35%). In a study by Linden et al. of 100 patients with an FEV1 <35% predicted undergoing lung resection (wedge resection, lobectomy, and segmentectomy) for suspected lung cancer in a high-volume center, there was only one death in hospital, though 22% of these patients had a prolonged air leak requiring chest tube drainage for greater than 7 days [84]. Thus, there is at present no clear cut-off point for lung function values which precludes surgery in potentially curable patients with COPD and lung cancer.

As many patients with COPD have an abnormal predicted FEV1 or DLCO <80%, further preoperative assessment in such patients should be considered, including formal or informal exercise testing and/or prediction of postoperative lung function. Stair climbing is an inexpensive assessment of exercise capacity prior to lung resection surgery. Individuals able to ascend less than 12 m in height in a stairwell had a mortality of 13% after lung resection, as compared to a mortality of 3.7% in those able to climb 12–22 m, and 1% in those able to climb greater than 22 m [85]. Shuttle walk testing is an alternative form of exercise-tolerance testing, in which a patient walks at gradually increasing pace between two markers set 10 m apart, with the pace of the walk determined by an external signal, until the patient can no longer continue [81]. In a prospective study of 103 patients undergoing lung resection, there was no overall difference in shuttle walk distance between patients having a good surgical outcome (n=69) and those having a major complication (n=34) [86]. However, 8/12 (66%) patients with a shuttle walk distance of less than 250 m had a major complication [86]. Shuttle walk testing has a moderate correlation (r=0.67) with maximal oxygen consumption measures in patients with lung cancer, but may underestimate maximal oxygen consumption in individuals with a low shuttle walk distance of less than 250 m [87]. Formal measurement of maximal oxygen uptake by cardiopulmonary exercise testing (typically cycle-based exercise testing) is another option for preoperative fitness assessment. In a meta-analysis of exercise testing, individuals who did not experience postoperative pulmonary complications had a higher maximal oxygen uptake (20 ml/kg/min) than individuals who experienced complications (16 ml/kg/min) [88]. A maximal oxygen uptake value of less than 10 ml/kg/min denotes high perioperative mortality (on average 26%) [81]. In a recent study of 210 patients with FEV1, <80% who underwent preoperative exercise testing and subsequent lung resection for lung cancer, four perioperative deaths occurred, all in individuals with a maximal oxygen uptake of less than 14 ml/kg/min [89]. However, mortality in the subgroup of 29 patients with a maximal oxygen uptake less than 10 ml/kg/min was 10.3% (3/29) [89], suggesting that even this value does not represent an absolute contraindication to surgery. Exercise testing, either formal or informal, can aid in risk stratification of individuals with COPD contemplating lung resection for lung cancer.

Calculation of predicted postoperative pulmonary function is another tool for predicting risk of lung resection in the patient with impaired lung function and lung cancer. Quantitative perfusion lung scanning is frequently used to help estimate the postoperative percent predicted lung function (FEV1 or DLCO). However, simple counting of lung segments to be removed and application of a predictive equation may also allow a reasonable prediction of postoperative FEV1 comparable to lung scintigraphy [90]. Predictive calculations for postoperative FEV1 may be less accurate (including both under- and overestimation) in the setting of COPD [91]. Predicted postoperative lung function measurements can help determine risk of complications after surgery. For example, for every 10-point increment in postoperative predicted DLCO, there is a reduced risk of pulmonary complications, overall complications, and operative mortality in patients with COPD undergoing lung resection [83]. A reduced postoperative predicted FEV1 or DLCO <40% predicted is associated with increased pulmonary complications [81]. However, as with preoperative measured lung function, there is no absolute cutoff for predicted postoperative values of FEV1 or DLCO that precludes consideration of surgery.

In summary, risk stratification with pulmonary function testing and exercise testing is an important part of the preoperative assessment in individuals with COPD and lung cancer. However, no strict cutoff value for lung function or exercise tolerance absolutely prohibits surgery, and surgical resection of lung cancer can be successfully performed in carefully selected patients at experienced centers even in the setting of severely reduced lung function. The decision to proceed or not to proceed with surgery for lung cancer in an individual with COPD should be made in a multidisciplinary setting after comprehensive evaluation of the patient's overall condition, lung function, exercise tolerance, comorbidities, and individual patient goals and desires.

Perioperative Management of the Patient with COPD and Lung Cancer

Optimal management of COPD in the perioperative period in a patient with lung cancer may impact on postsurgical outcomes [92]. Preoperative smoking cessation in patients with COPD who are current smokers would seem beneficial; however, studies have reported increased complications in recent quitters prior to major non-pulmonary surgery [93, 94]. In a study of 300 patients undergoing thoracotomy for lung tumors, the pulmonary complication was 8% in nonsmokers, 19% in past quitters (>2 months prior to surgery), 23% in recent quitters (quit > 1 week, ≤2 months before surgery), and 23% in ongoing smokers [95]. Pneumonia occurred in 3% of nonsmokers, 10% of past quitters, 15% of recent quitters, and 23% of ongoing smokers in this study. This study would seem to confirm that smoking cessation should be encouraged prior to thoracotomy in ongoing smokers, and even recent smoking cessation may potentially reduce postoperative pneumonia rates but may not affect overall pulmonary complications.

Prescription of appropriate bronchodilator and/or inhaled steroid therapy to the patient with lung cancer and COPD may presumably provide benefit in the perioperative period. However, relatively little data exist in this respect, especially on contemporary therapy with long-acting bronchodilators. In a retrospective study of lung cancer patients with COPD, preoperative treatment with tiotropium, an inhaled long-acting muscarinic antagonist, significantly improved lung function and effectively downstaged severity of COPD in treated patients [96]. In a pilot study of 46 patients with non-small-cell lung cancer and newly diagnosed COPD, subjects were randomized to a regimen of tiotropium, formoterol (a long-acting beta agonist), and budesonide (an inhaled steroid) or a regimen of tiotropium and formoterol alone [97]. The tiotropium/formoterol/budesonide (T/F/B) group had a significantly greater post-treatment improvement in FEV1 compared to the tiotropium/formoterol (T/F) group, with 12/24 patients in the T/F/B group having a ≥10% improvement in FEV1 as compared to 2/22 patients in the T/F group. Of 18 patients in the T/F/B group who underwent surgery, two (11.1%) had postoperative pulmonary complications, as compared to 6/14 in the T/F group [97]. While further data would be beneficial, intensive management of COPD with inhaled medications, especially in previously undiagnosed cases, in the perioperative period would seem to be beneficial in individuals with airway obstruction and lung cancer. Preoperative oral corticosteroids and/or antibiotics are also sometimes utilized in patients with COPD and lung cancer to manage exacerbations, treat postobstructive pneumonia, or optimize lung function, but there are no data to support their routine use.

Strength and exercise training in the perioperative period has also been studied. Inspiratory muscle strength training and incentive spirometry in the pre- and postoperative period is associated with increased inspiratory muscle strength and results in an underestimation of postoperative FEV1 values in subjects with COPD undergoing lung resection [98]. The role of routine preoperative pulmonary rehabilitation in patients with COPD and lung cancer is uncertain. In a pilot study by Bobbio et al., preoperative pulmonary rehabilitation was performed in 12 patients with reduced lung function (mean FEV1 $47 \pm 10\%$) and impaired maximal oxygen uptake (≤ 15 ml/kg/min) in whom lung resection for lung cancer was being contemplated [99]. Patients showed a significant mean improvement in maximal oxygen uptake of 2.8 ml/kg/min. Of the 11 patients who ultimately underwent lobectomy, however, eight had postoperative pulmonary complications. Spruit et al. found a median improvement in a 6-min walk distance of 145 m following a course of inpatient pulmonary rehabilitation in 10 patients with lung cancer [100]. In an eight-patient pilot trial of pulmonary rehabilitation prior to surgery in high-risk patients, significant improvements in forced vital capacity and 6-min walk distance were seen following rehabilitation; all patients subsequently survived their surgery [101]. Further study of the effect of pulmonary rehabilitation on postsurgical outcomes is needed. Intuitively, intensive exercise training and rehabilitation would seem to be beneficial in the preoperative period prior to lung cancer resection in individuals with COPD; however, timing and resource allocation for such programs may limit their applicability in the routine preoperative management of lung cancer in patients with COPD.

Effects of Lung Cancer Surgery on Pulmonary Function in COPD

There is increasing evidence that patients with COPD and lung cancer may experience a relative preservation of or improvement in pulmonary function following lobectomy. In a small study of 32 patients undergoing lobectomy for lung cancer, FEV1 was shown to improve by a mean of 3.7% following surgery in the subgroup of patients with COPD, in contrast to a 15.7% decline in FEV1 in the subgroup without COPD [102]. In a study of 137 patients with and without COPD undergoing lobectomy for lung cancer, FEV1 and FEV1/FVC ratio improved postoperatively in the subgroup of patients with a preoperative FEV1 <65% [103]. By contrast, patients with a preoperative FEV1 $\geq 80\%$ experienced a significant postoperative decline in FEV1 [103]. The relative preservation of FEV1 in patients with impaired preoperative pulmonary function may be due to an incidental "lung volume reduction" effect. In the study by Baldi et al., patients who had baseline air trapping as indicated by a functional residual capacity greater than 115% had no change in FEV1 postsurgery, while in patients with an FRC <115%, FEV1 decreased postoperatively [103].

In a study by Subotic et al. of patients undergoing lobectomy for lung cancer, patients with COPD experienced a smaller decline in FEV1 postsurgery (−11.9%) than patients with normal lung function (−24.6%) [104]. Similar results were found in a retrospective study by Sekine et al. of 521 patients who underwent lung resection surgery for lung cancer and who had pre- and postoperative pulmonary function tests [105]. In the study by Sekine et al., the ratio of actual postoperative FEV1/ predicted postoperative FEV1 was significantly higher in the cohort of 48 patients with COPD as compared to the group of 473 patients without COPD [105]. Interestingly, in this study, resection of the lower or middle lobe was associated with relative FEV1 preservation. By contrast, in a study by Kushibe et al., patients with COPD undergoing lobectomy had on average a 3.7% improvement in FEV1 6-month postright upper lobectomy, and a small decline of 1.9% in FEV1 after left upper lobectomy [106]. These changes were relatively better than in a control group without COPD, in which a 12% decline and a 19% decline in FEV1 occurred following right upper and left upper lobectomy respectively [106]. However, the confidence intervals for the changes in lung function in the COPD group were relatively large, suggesting a number of these patients also experienced significant declines in FEV1. Changes in lung function following lower lobectomy were similar between COPD and non-COPD groups in this study. The relative preservation in pulmonary function following lobectomy in individuals with COPD does not necessarily translate into preserved exercise capacity; in another study by Kushibe et al., maximal oxygen consumption declined by a similar percentage postlobectomy in a group of patients with severe COPD as compared to a group of patients without COPD or a group of patients with mild COPD, despite a significantly smaller decline in pulmonary function values following surgery in the severe COPD group [107]. Bobbio et al. also found that maximal oxygen consumption significantly declined following lung resection in patients with COPD, despite no change in FEV1 and a decline in total lung capacity [108]. Overall, these studies suggest that pulmonary function changes following lobectomy for lung cancer may be less than anticipated in patients with COPD, perhaps due to the effects of incidental lung volume reduction. Therefore, relatively lower thresholds for preoperative pulmonary function may be appropriate in selected patients with COPD and lung cancer. However, postlobectomy exercise capacity may be significantly diminished in patients with COPD despite relative preservation of FEV1 following lung resection, and preoperative determination of exercise capacity may therefore especially complement pulmonary function measurements in determining the appropriateness of surgery for lung cancer in an individual with advanced COPD.

Effect of COPD on Complications and Prognosis After Lung Cancer Surgery

Impaired pulmonary function from COPD is considered to be a risk factor for postoperative complications, especially pulmonary complications, following lung resection. Kearney et al. found that the predicted postoperative FEV1 was the only independent predictor of postoperative medical complications following lung resection [109]. In a study by Licker et al. pulmonary complications following lung cancer surgery occurred in 10% of patients with FEV1 ≥70% predicted, 25% of patients with FEV 50–70%, and 27% of patients with FEV1 <50% [110]. In multivariable regression analysis, an FEV1 <60% predicted was an independent risk factor for pulmonary complications (OR 2.7 95% CI 1.3–6.6) and mortality (OR 1.9 95% CI 1.2–3.9) [110]. Sekine et al. found that 53% of patients with COPD experienced pulmonary complications following lung cancer surgery, including air leaks, pneumothorax, pneumonia, and prolonged mechanical ventilation, as compared to 19.3% of patients without COPD [111]. In a prospective study of 168 patients undergoing major lung resection surgery, COPD was an independent risk factor for postoperative pneumonia [112]. Other specific risks related to COPD include postoperative supraventricular arrhythmias [113] and prolonged air leaks and bronchopleural fistula [114, 115]. These studies and others suggest that COPD is a risk factor for overall and specific cardiopulmonary postoperative complications following lung cancer surgery.

While COPD may prohibit curative surgery in some circumstances, whether the presence of COPD confers a worse prognosis for lung cancer survival following successful surgical resection is uncertain. Sekine et al. found no difference in cancer-related survival following lung resection in a group with COPD compared to a group without COPD; however, the intercurrent survival was significantly lower in the COPD group, due in part to an increased number of deaths from respiratory failure [111]. However, in a subsequent study, this group found a significantly worse overall and disease-free survival in a cohort with early stage surgically resected lung cancer and COPD as compared to a group with early stage resected lung cancer but no COPD [116]. Lopez-Encuentra et al. found no difference between COPD and non-COPD groups in overall 5-year survival in a retrospective analysis of 2,994 surgically treated lung cancer patients [117]. However, conditional survival was lower in the COPD group with early stage disease [117]. In patients older than 70 years of age undergoing lung resection for cancer, chronic obstructive pulmonary disease is a significant risk factor for long-term mortality [118]. While COPD may be a risk factor for a worse prognosis following lung cancer resection, given the poor prognosis of untreated lung cancer, surgery should be considered in all patients with COPD and early stage lung cancer and resection should be performed if feasible.

Nonsurgical Treatment of Lung Cancer in Patients with COPD

Nonsurgical therapies for lung cancer traditionally include chemotherapy and external beam radiotherapy for regionally or systemically advanced lung cancer. However, newer techniques for local disease elimination, such as radiofrequency ablation and stereotactic radiotherapy, have created new options for the treatment of early-stage disease in patients felt to be unable to tolerate surgical therapy. Stereotactic radiotherapy, which applies high doses of radiation via multiple focused beams to a circumscribed area, typically using adjustments for respiratory motion, has shown promise in early-stage disease treatment in inoperable patients. In a study of patients with T1 or T2, N0M0 noncentral lung cancer felt to be inoperable due to respiratory or cardiovascular comorbidities, stereotactic radiation therapy resulted in 3-year local-regional control in 87.2% of patients; 22.1% of patients had disease dissemination by 3 years [119]. Overall survival was 55.8% at 3 years [119]. The majority of adverse events in this study were respiratory or constitutional, with no grade 5 toxicity. This study suggests that patients with early-stage lung cancer who are inoperable due to COPD may benefit from stereotactic radiotherapy for local and regional disease control; however, further study is needed of long-term outcomes and more data are needed comparing stereotactic radiotherapy to limited surgical techniques, e.g., wedge resection. Stereotactic radiotherapy may confer higher risk of toxicity when used to treat central lung tumors, although overall toxicity related to stereotactic radiotherapy was not statistically different when comparing central versus peripheral tumors in a recent study [120]. Radiofrequency ablation involves placement of a probe to deliver thermal energy to a tumor. As an alternative local therapy in inoperable patients, especially for smaller tumors, this technique appears promising. However, complications including pneumothorax, hemorrhage, and hemoptysis do occur and may be fatal [121, 122]. Further data on radiofrequency ablation from prospective, well-designed studies are needed, as is comparative data with other techniques, such as stereotactic radiotherapy and limited surgery.

Patients with COPD and regionally or systemically disseminated disease are generally not candidates for curative local procedures but may require external beam radiation therapy for local-regional disease control or chemotherapy for systemic disease. Chronic obstructive pulmonary disease may pose additional risk in the setting of external beam radiotherapy. Patients with COPD experience a larger decrease in pulmonary function parameters after high-dose radiotherapy for lung cancer than patients without COPD [123]. These patients may also be at increased risk for radiation pneumonitis [124]. This highlights the need for local-regional lung cancer therapies that limit lung function deterioration in patients with COPD.

End-of-Life Care in COPD and Lung Cancer

Limited data are available on end-of-life care in patients with concomitant COPD and lung cancer. Health care utilization in the last 12 months of life in patients with both lung cancer and COPD generally appears to mirror utilization by patients with lung cancer alone as compared to COPD alone [125]. Patients with both lung cancer and COPD were more likely to receive palliative care than patients with COPD alone at the end of life [125]. A study by Au et al. also found that patients with both COPD and lung cancer had health care utilization patterns at the end of life similar to those with lung cancer alone [126]. In this study, patients with lung cancer were more likely to receive palliative medications like opioids and benzodiazepines than patients with COPD, and were less likely to be hospitalized in an ICU [126]. Other studies have also shown that patients with COPD alone are less likely to receive palliative care than patients with lung cancer [127, 128] and were more likely to experience breathlessness [127] and anxiety [128]. These studies highlight differences in end-of-life care for patients with COPD alone and for patients with lung cancer with or without COPD, and suggest that patients with COPD who have received the diagnosis of lung cancer will be more likely to receive appropriate palliative care at the end of life.

Summary

Chronic obstructive pulmonary disease is an important risk factor for lung cancer, with a clear dose–response relationship between impaired lung function and lung cancer risk. We are beginning to identify molecular and genetic differences between lung cancer related to COPD and lung cancer unrelated to COPD, though more work toward personalized approaches to the treatment of lung cancer in COPD is needed. Lung function impairment in COPD may impact on therapeutic options and on the outcomes of lung cancer treatment although we have learned that application of limited surgical techniques may permit curative lung cancer surgery even in individuals with substantial lung function impairment. Newer techniques for local lung cancer control, such as stereotactic radiotherapy, may allow for the potentially curative treatment of inoperable patients with early stage lung cancer and advanced COPD. The future holds the promise of more effective detection, diagnosis, and individualized treatment of lung cancer in individuals with COPD.

References

1. Anthonisen NR, Skeans MA, Wise RA, et al. The effects of a smoking cessation intervention on 14.5 year mortality: a randomized clinical trial. Ann Intern Med. 2005;142:233–9.
2. Skillrud DM, Offord KP, Miller RD. Higher risk of lung cancer in chronic obstructive pulmonary disease: a prospective, matched, controlled study. Ann Intern Med. 1986;105:503–7.
3. Tockman MS, Anthonisen NR, Wright E, et al. Airways obstruction and the risk for lung cancer. Ann Intern Med. 1987;106:512–8.
4. Young RP, Hopkins RJ, Christmas T, et al. COPD prevalence is increased in lung cancer, independent of age, sex, and smoking history. Eur Respir J. 2009;34:380–6.
5. Rodríguez LA, Wallander M-A, Martín-Merino E, et al. Heart failure, myocardial infarction, lung cancer and death in COPD patients: a UK primary care study. Respir Med. 2010;104:1691–9.
6. Koshiol J, Rotunno M, Consonni D, et al. Chronic obstructive pulmonary disease and altered risk of lung cancer in a population-based case-control study. PLoS One. 2009;4:e7380.
7. Turner MC, Chen Y, Krewski D, et al. Chronic obstructive pulmonary disease is associated with lung cancer mortality in a prospective study of never smokers. Am J Respir Crit Care Med. 2007;176:285–90.
8. Islam SS, Schottenfeld D. Declining FEV1 and chronic productive cough in cigarette smokers: a 25-year prospective study of lung cancer incidence in Tecumseh, Michigan. Cancer Epidemiol Biomarkers Prev. 1994;3:289–98.
9. Kuller LH, Ockene J, Meilahn E, et al. Relation of forced expiratory volume in one second (FEV1) to lung cancer mortality in the Multiple Risk Factor Intervention Trial (MRFIT). Am J Epidemiol. 1990;132:265–74.
10. Purdue MP, Gold L, Järvhom B, et al. Impaired lung function and lung cancer incidence in a cohort of Swedish construction workers. Thorax. 2007;62:51–6.
11. Mannino DM, Aguayo SM, Petty TL, et al. Low lung function and incident lung cancer in the United States: data from the First National Health and Nutrition Examination Survey follow-up. Arch Intern Med. 2003;163:1475–80.
12. Wasswa-Kintu S, Gan WQ, Man SF, et al. Relationship between reduced forced expiratory volume in one second and the risk of lung cancer: a systematic review and meta-analysis. Thorax. 2005;60:570–5.

13. Schwartz AG, Cote ML, Wenzlaff AS, et al. Chronic obstructive lung diseases and risk of non-small cell lung cancer in women. J Thorac Oncol. 2009;4:291–9.
14. Kiri VA, Soriano JB, Visick G, et al. Recent trends in lung cancer and its association with COPD: an analysis using the UK GP Research Database. Prim Care Resp J. 2010;19:57–61.
15. Peto R, Speizer FE, Cochrane AL, et al. The relevance in adults of air-flow obstruction, but not of mucus hypersecretion, to mortality from chronic lung disease: results from 20 years of prospective observation. Am Rev Respir Dis. 1983;128:491–500.
16. Lange P, Parner J, Prescott E, et al. Chronic bronchitis in an elderly population. Age Ageing. 2003;32:636–42.
17. de Torres JP, Bastarrika G, Wisnivesky JP, et al. Assessing the relationship between lung cancer risk and emphysema detected on low-dose CT of the chest. Chest. 2007;132:1932–8.
18. Wilson DO, Weissfeld JL, Balkan A, et al. Association of radiographic emphysema and airflow obstruction with lung cancer. Am J Respir Crit Care Med. 2008;178:738–44.
19. Maldonado F, Bartholmai BJ, Swensen SJ, et al. Are airflow obstruction and radiographic evidence of emphysema risk factors for lung cancer? A nested case-control study using quantitative emphysema analysis. Chest. 2010;138:1295–302.
20. Brown DW, Young KE, Anda RF, et al. Asthma and risk of death from lung cancer: NHANES II Mortality Study. J Asthma. 2005;42:597–600.
21. Ramanakumar AV, Parent M-E, Menzies D, et al. Risk of lung cancer following nonmalignant respiratory conditions: evidence from two case-control studies in Montreal, Canada. Lung Cancer. 2006;53:5–12.
22. Wu AH, Fontham ET, Reynolds P, et al. Previous lung disease and risk of lung cancer among lifetime nonsmoking women in the United States. Am J Epidemiol. 1995;141:1023–32.
23. Santillan AA, Camargo CA, Colditz GA. A meta-analysis of asthma and risk of lung cancer (United States). Cancer Causes Control. 2003;14:327–34.
24. González-Pérez A, Fernández-Vidaurre C, Rueda A, et al. Cancer incidence in a general population of asthma patients. Pharmacoepidemiol Drug Safety. 2006;15:131–8.
25. Huovinen E, Kaprio J, Vesterinen E, et al. Mortality of adults with asthma: a prospective cohort study. Thorax. 1997;52:49–54.
26. Hospers JJ, Postma DS, Rijcken B, et al. Histamine airway hyper-responsiveness and mortality from chronic obstructive pulmonary disease: a cohort study. Lancet. 2000;356:1313–7.
27. Cohen BH, Diamond EL, Graves CG, et al. A common familial component in lung cancer and chronic obstructive pulmonary disease. Lancet. 1977;2:523–6.
28. Spira A, Beane J, Shah V, et al. Effects of cigarette smoke on the human airway epithelial cell transcriptome. PNAS. 2004;101:10143–8.
29. ATS/ERS Task Force. American Thoracic Society/European Respiratory Society Statement: standards for the diagnosis and management of individuals with alpha-1 antitrypsin deficiency. Am J Respir Crit Care Med. 2003;168:818–900.
30. Yang P, Sun Z, Krowka MJ, et al. Alpha1-antitrypsin deficiency carriers, tobacco smoke, chronic obstructive pulmonary disease, and lung cancer risk. Arch Intern Med. 2008;168:1097–103.
31. Yang P, Bamlet WR, Sun Z, et al. α1-Antitrypsin and neutrophil elastase imbalance and lung cancer risk. Chest. 2005;128:445–52.
32. Amos CI, Wu X, Broderick P, et al. Genome-wide association scan of tag SNPs identifies a susceptibility locus for lung cancer at 15q25.1. Nat Genet. 2008;40:616–22.
33. Hung RJ, McKay JD, Gaborieau V, et al. A susceptibility locus for lung cancer maps to nicotinic acetylcholine receptor subunit genes on 15q25. Nature. 2008;452:633–7.
34. Thorgeirsson TE, Geller F, Sulem P, et al. A variant associated with nicotine dependence, lung cancer and peripheral arterial disease. Nature. 2008;452:638–41.
35. Saccone NL, Culverhouse RC, Schwantes-An T-H, et al. Multiple independent loci at chromosome 15q25.1 affect smoking quantity: a meta-analysis and comparison with lung cancer and COPD. PLoS Genet. 2010;6:e1001053.
36. Thorgeirsson TE, Gudbjartsson DF, Surakka I, et al. Sequence variants at CHRNB3-CHRNA6 and CYP2A6 affect smoking behavior. Nat Genet. 2010;42:448–53.

37. Pillai SG, Kong X, Edwards LD, et al. Loci identified by genome-wide association studies influence different disease-related phenotypes in chronic obstructive pulmonary disease. Am J Respir Crit Care Med. 2010;182:1498–505.
38. Pillai SG, Ge D, Zhu G, et al. A genome-wide association study in chronic obstructive pulmonary disease (COPD): identification of two major susceptibility loci. PLoS Genet. 2009;5: e1000421.
39. Lambrechts D, Buysschaert I, Zanen P, et al. The 15q24/25 susceptibility variant for lung cancer and chronic obstructive pulmonary disease is associated with emphysema. Am J Respir Crit Care Med. 2010;181:486–93.
40. Lips EH, Gaborieau V, McKay JD, et al. Association between a 15q25 gene variant, smoking quantity and tobacco-related cancers among 17,000 individuals. Int J Epidemiol. 2010;39: 563–77.
41. Wang J, Spitz MR, Amos CI, et al. Mediating effects of smoking and chronic obstructive pulmonary disease on the relation between the CHRNA5-A3 genetic locus and lung cancer risk. Cancer. 2010;116:3458–62.
42. Truong T, Hung RJ, Amos CI, et al. Replication of lung cancer susceptibility loci at chromosomes 15q25, 5p15, and 6p21: a pooled analysis from the International Lung Cancer Consortium. J Natl Cancer Inst. 2010;102:959–71.
43. Galvan A, Dragani TA. Nicotine dependence may link the 15q25 locus to lung cancer risk. Carcinogenesis. 2010;31:331–3.
44. Wilk JB, Chen T-H, Gottlieb DJ, et al. A genome-wide association study of pulmonary function measures in the Framingham Heart Study. PLoS Genet. 2009;5:e1000429.
45. Repapi E, Sayers I, Wain LV, et al. Genome-wide association study identifies five loci associated with lung function. Nat Genet. 2010;42:36–44.
46. Young RP, Whittington CF, Hopkins RJ, et al. Chromosome 4q31 locus in COPD is also associated with lung cancer. Eur Respir J. 2010;36:1375–82.
47. Huang S, Yang L, An Y, et al. Expression of hedgehog signaling molecules in lung cancer. Acta Histochemica 2010; doi:10.1016/j.acthis.2010.06.003.
48. Carlsten C, Sagoo GS, Frodsham AJ, et al. Glutathione s-transferase M1 (GSTM1) polymorphisms and lung cancer: a literature-based systematic HuGE review and meta-analysis. Am J Epidemiol. 2008;167:759–74.
49. Shi X, Zhou S, Wang Z, et al. CYP1A1 and GSTM1 polymorphisms and lung cancer risk in Chinese populations: a meta-analysis. Lung Cancer. 2008;59:155–63.
50. Castaldi PJ, Cho MH, Cohn M, et al. The COPD genetic association compendium: a comprehensive online database of COPD genetic associations. Hum Mol Genet. 2010;19:526–34.
51. Hansel TT, Barnes PJ. New drugs for exacerbations of chronic obstructive pulmonary disease. Lancet. 2009;374:744–55.
52. Brody JS, Spira A. Chronic obstructive pulmonary disease, inflammation, and lung cancer. Proc Am Thorac Soc. 2006;3:535–8.
53. Houghton AM, Mouded M, Shapiro SD. Common origins of lung cancer and COPD. Nat Med. 2008;14:1023–4.
54. Yoshida T, Tuder RM. Pathobiology of cigarette-smoke-induced chronic obstructive pulmonary disease. Physiol Rev. 2007;87:1047–82.
55. Barnes PJ. The cytokine network in chronic obstructive pulmonary disease. Am J Respir Cell Mol Biol. 2009;41:631–8.
56. Man SF, Connett JE, Anthonisen NR, et al. C-reactive protein and mortality in mild to moderate chronic obstructive pulmonary disease. Thorax. 2006;61:849–53.
57. Parimon T, Chien JW, Bryson CL, et al. Inhaled corticosteroids and risk of lung cancer among patients with chronic obstructive pulmonary disease. Am J Respir Crit Care Med. 2007;175: 712–9.
58. Kiri VA, Fabbri LM, Davis KJ, et al. Inhaled corticosteroids and risk of lung cancer among COPD patients who quit smoking. Respir Med. 2009;103:85–90.
59. Lam S, leRiche JC, McWilliams A. A randomized phase IIb trial of Pulmicort Turbuhaler (budesonide) in people with dysplasia of the bronchial epithelium. Clin Cancer Res. 2004;10:6502–11.

60. Wolff H, Saukkonen K, Anttila S, et al. Expression of cyclooxygenase-2 in human lung carcinoma. Cancer Res. 1998;58:4997–5001.
61. Cuzick J, Otto F, Baron JA, et al. Aspirin and non-steroidal anti-inflammatory drugs for cancer prevention: an international consensus statement. Lancet Oncol. 2009;10:501–7.
62. Skriver MV, Nørgaard M, Poulsen AH, et al. Use of nonaspirin NSAIDs and risk of lung cancer. Int J Cancer. 2005;117:873–6.
63. Rothwell PM, Fowkes FG, Belch JF, et al. Effect of daily aspirin on long-term risk of death due to cancer: analysis of individual patient data from randomised trials. Lancet. 2011;377:31–41.
64. Shuto T, Xu H, Wang B, et al. Activation of NF- B by nontypeable Hemophilus influenza is mediated by toll-like receptor 2-TAK1-dependent NIK-IKKα/β-I βα and MKK3/6-p38 MAP kinase signaling pathways in epithelial cells. PNAS. 2001;98:8774–9.
65. Moghaddam SJ, Li H, Cho S-N, et al. Promotion of lung carcinogenesis by chronic obstructive pulmonary disease-like airway inflammation in a K-ras-induced mouse model. Am J Respir Cell Mol Biol. 2009;40:443–53.
66. Ochoa CE, Mirabolfathinejad SG, Venado AR, et al. Interleukin 6, but not T helper cytokines, promotes lung carcinogenesis. Cancer Prev Res. 2011;4:51–64.
67. Qu P, Roberts J, Li Y, et al. Stat3 downstream genes serve as biomarkers in human lung carcinomas and chronic obstructive pulmonary disease. Lung Cancer. 2009;63:341–7.
68. Qu P, Du H, Wang X, et al. Matrix-metalloproteinase 12 overexpression in lung epithelial cells plays a key role in emphysema to lung bronchioalveolar adenocarcinoma transition. Cancer Res. 2009;69:7252–61.
69. Moghaddam SJ, Barta P, Mirabolfathinejad SG, et al. Curcumin inhibits COPD-like airway inflammation and lung cancer progression in mice. Carcinogenesis. 2009;30:1949–56.
70. Rennard SI, Fogarty C, Kelsen S, et al. The safety and efficacy of infliximab in moderate to severe chronic obstructive pulmonary disease. Am J Respir Crit Care Med. 2007;175:926–34.
71. Boelens MC, Gustafson AM, Postma DS, et al. A chronic obstructive pulmonary disease related signature in squamous cell lung cancer. Lung Cancer 2010; doi:10.1016/j.lungcan.2010.08.014.
72. Suzuki M, Wada H, Yoshino M, et al. Molecular characterization of chronic obstructive pulmonary disease-related non-small cell lung cancer through aberrant methylation and alterations of EGFR signaling. Ann Surg Oncol. 2010;17:878–88.
73. Cilli A, Ozkaynak C, Onur R, et al. Lung cancer detection with low-dose spiral computed tomography in chronic obstructive pulmonary disease patients. Acta Radiologica. 2007;48:405–11.
74. Rivera MP, Mehta AC. Initial diagnosis of lung cancer: ACCP evidence-based clinical practice guidelines (2nd edition). Chest. 2007;132:131S–48.
75. British Thoracic Society Bronchoscopy Guidelines Committee, a Subcommittee of the Standards of Care Committee of the British Thoracic Society. British Thoracic Society guidelines on diagnostic flexible bronchoscopy. Thorax. 2001;56(Suppl I):i1–21.
76. Stolz D, Pollak V, Chhajed PN, et al. A randomized, placebo-controlled trial of bronchodilators for bronchoscopy in patients with COPD. Chest. 2007;131:765–72.
77. Oikonomou A, Matzinger FR, Seely JM, et al. Ultrathin needle (25 G) aspiration lung biopsy: diagnostic accuracy and complication rates. Eur Radiol. 2004;14:375–82.
78. Laurent F, Michel P, Latrabe V, et al. Pneumothoraces and chest tube placement after CT-guided transthoracic lung biopsy using a coaxial technique: incidence and risk factors. AJR. 1999;172:1049–53.
79. Kazerooni EA, Lim FT, Mikhail A, et al. Risk of pneumothorax in CT-guided transthoracic needle aspiration biopsy of the lung. Radiology. 1996;198:371–5.
80. Heyer CM, Reichelt S, Peters SA, et al. Computed tomography-navigated transthoracic core biopsy of pulmonary lesions: which factors affect diagnostic yield and complication rates? Acad Radiol. 2008;15:1017–26.
81. Colice GL, Shafazand S, Griffin JP, et al. Physiologic evaluation of the patient with lung cancer being considered for resectional surgery: ACCP evidenced-based clinical practice guidelines (2nd edition). Chest. 2007;132:161S–77.

82. Ferguson MK, Little L, Rizzo L, et al. Diffusing capacity predicts morbidity and mortality after pulmonary resection. J Thorac Cardiovasc Surg. 1988;96:894–900.
83. Ferguson MK, Vigneswaran WT. Diffusing capacity predicts morbidity after lung resection in patients without obstructive lung disease. Ann Thorac Surg. 2008;85:1158–65.
84. Linden PA, Bueno R, Colson YL, et al. Lung resection in patients with preoperative FEV1 <35% predicted. Chest. 2005;127:1984–90.
85. Brunelli A, Refai M, Xiumé F, et al. Performance at symptom-limited stair-climbing test is associated with increased cardiopulmonary complications, mortality, and costs after major lung resection. Ann Thorac Surg. 2008;86:240–8.
86. Win T, Jackson A, Groves AM, et al. Relationship of shuttle walk test and lung cancer surgical outcome. Eur J Cardiothorac Surg. 2004;26:1216–9.
87. Win T, Jackson A, Groves AM, et al. Comparison of shuttle walk with measured peak oxygen consumption in patients with operable lung cancer. Thorax. 2006;61:57–60.
88. Benzo R, Kelley GA, Recchi L, et al. Complications of lung resection and exercise capacity: a meta-analysis. Respir Med. 2007;101:1790–7.
89. Licker M, Schnyder J-M, Frey J-G, et al. Impact of aerobic exercise capacity and procedure-related factors in lung cancer surgery. ERJ Express 2010; doi:10.1183/09031936.00069910.
90. Win T, Laroche CM, Groves AM, et al. Use of quantitative lung scintigraphy to predict post-operative pulmonary function in lung cancer patients undergoing lobectomy. Ann Thorac Surg. 2004;78:1215–8.
91. Wang T, Tagayun A, Bogardus A, et al. How accurately can we predict forced expiratory volume in one second after major pulmonary resection. Am Surgeon. 2007;73:1047–51.
92. Stein M, Cassara EL. Preoperative pulmonary evaluation and therapy for surgery patients. JAMA. 1970;211:787–90.
93. Warner MA, Offord KP, Warner ME, et al. Role of preoperative cessation of smoking and other factors in postoperative complications: a blinded prospective study of coronary artery bypass patients. Mayo Clin Proc. 1989;64:609–16.
94. Bluman LG, Mosca L, Newman N, et al. Preoperative smoking habits and postoperative pulmonary complications. Chest. 1998;113:883–9.
95. Barrera R, Shi W, Amar D, et al. Smoking and timing of cessation: impact on pulmonary complications after thoracotomy. Chest. 2005;127:1977–83.
96. Kobayashi S, Suzuki S, Niikawa H, Sugawara T, Yanai M. Preoperative use of inhaled tiotropium in lung cancer patients with untreated COPD. Respirology 2009;14:675–9.
97. Bölükbas S, Eberlein M, Eckhoff J, et al. Short-term effects of inhalative tiotropium/formoterol/budesonide versus tiotropium/formoterol in patients with newly diagnosed chronic obstructive pulmonary disease requiring surgery for lung cancer. Eur J Cardiothorac Surg 2010; doi:10.1016/j.ejcts.2010.09.025.
98. Weiner P, Man A, Weiner M, et al. The effect of incentive spirometry and inspiratory muscle training on pulmonary function after lung resection. J Thorac Cardiovasc Surg. 1997;113:552–7.
99. Bobbio A, Chetta A, Ampollini L, et al. Preoperative pulmonary rehabilitation in patients undergoing lung resection for non-small cell lung cancer. Eur J Cardiothorac Surg. 2008;33:95–8.
100. Spruit MA, Janssen PP, Willemsen SC, et al. Exercise capacity before and after an 8-week multidisciplinary inpatient rehabilitation program in lung cancer patients: a pilot study. Lung Cancer. 2006;52:257–60.
101. Cesario A, Ferri L, Galetta D, et al. Pre-operative pulmonary rehabilitation and surgery for lung cancer. Lung Cancer. 2007;57:118–9.
102. Korst RJ, Ginsberg RJ, Ailawadi M, et al. Lobectomy improves ventilator function in selected patients with severe COPD. Ann Thorac Surg. 1998;66:898–902.
103. Baldi S, Ruffini E, Harari S, et al. Does lobectomy for lung cancer in patients with chronic obstructive pulmonary disease affect lung function? A multicenter national study. J Thorac Cardiovasc Surg. 2005;130:1616–22.

104. Subotic DR, Mandaric DV, Eminovic RM, et al. Influence of chronic obstructive pulmonary disease on postoperative lung function and complications in patients undergoing operations for primary non-small cell lung cancer. J Thorac Cardiovasc Surg. 2007;134:1292–9.

105. Sekine Y, Iwata T, Chiyo M, et al. Minimal alteration of pulmonary function after lobectomy in lung cancer patients with chronic obstructive pulmonary disease. Ann Thorac Surg. 2003;76:356–62.

106. Kushibe K, Kawaguchi T, Kimura M, et al. Influence of the site of lobectomy and chronic obstructive pulmonary disease on pulmonary function: a follow-up analysis. Interact Cardiovasc Thorac Surg. 2009;8:529–33.

107. Kushibe K, Kawaguchi T, Kimura M, et al. Exercise capacity after lobectomy in patients with chronic obstructive pulmonary disease. Interact Cardiovasc Thorac Surg. 2008;7:398–401.

108. Bobbio A, Chetta A, Carbognani P, et al. Changes in pulmonary function test and cardio-pulmonary exercise capacity in COPD patients after lobar pulmonary resection. Eur J Cardiothorac Surg. 2005;28:754–8.

109. Kearney DJ, Lee TH, Reilly JJ, et al. Assessment of operative risk in patients undergoing lung resection. Importance of predicted pulmonary function. Chest. 1994;105:753–9.

110. Licker MJ, Widikker I, Robert J, et al. Operative mortality and respiratory complications after lung resection for cancer: impact of chronic obstructive pulmonary disease and time trends. Ann Thorac Surg. 2006;81:1830–8.

111. Sekine Y, Behnia M, Fujisawa T. Impact of COPD on pulmonary complications and on long-term survival of patients undergoing surgery for NSCLC. Lung Cancer. 2002;37:95–101.

112. Schussler O, Alifano M, Dermine H, et al. Postoperative pneumonia after major lung resection. Am J Respir Crit Care Med. 2006;173:1161–9.

113. Sekine Y, Kesler KA, Behnia M, et al. COPD may increase the incidence of refractory supraventricular arrhythmias following pulmonary resection for non-small cell lung cancer. Chest. 2001;120:1783–90.

114. Stolz AJ, Schützner J, Lischke R, et al. Predictors of prolonged air leak following pulmonary lobectomy. Eur J Cardiothorac Surg. 2005;27:334–6.

115. Algar FJ, Alvarez A, Aranda JL, et al. Prediction of early bronchopleural fistula after pneumonectomy: a multivariate analysis. Ann Thorac Surg. 2001;72:1662–7.

116. Sekine Y, Yamada Y, Chiyo M, et al. Association of chronic obstructive pulmonary disease and tumor recurrence in patients with stage IA lung cancer after complete resection. Ann Thorac Surg. 2007;84:946–51.

117. López-Encuentra A, Astudillo J, Cerezal J, et al. Prognostic value of chronic obstructive pulmonary disease in 2994 cases of lung cancer. Eur J Cardiothorac Surg. 2005;27:8–13.

118. Birim Ö, Zuydendorp HM, Maat AP, et al. Lung resection for non-small-cell lung cancer in patients older than 70: mortality, morbidity, and late survival compared with the general population. Ann Thorac Surg. 2003;76:1796–801.

119. Timmerman R, Paulus R, Galvin J, et al. Stereotactic body radiation therapy for inoperable early stage lung cancer. JAMA. 2010;303:1070–6.

120. Fakiris AJ, McGarry RC, Yiannoutsos CT, et al. Stereotactic body radiation therapy for early-stage non-small-cell lung carcinoma: four-year results of a prospective phase II study. Int J Radiation Oncol Biol Phys. 2009;75:677–82.

121. Powell JW, Dexter E, Scalzetti EM, et al. Treatment advances for medically inoperable non-small-cell lung cancer: emphasis on prospective trials. Lancet Oncol. 2009;10:885–94.

122. Huang L, Han Y, Zhao J, et al. Is radiofrequency thermal ablation a safe and effective procedure in the treatment of pulmonary malignancies? Eur J Cardiothorac Surg. 2011;39: 348–51.

123. Borst GR, De Jaeger K, Belderbos JS, et al. Pulmonary function changes after radiotherapy in non-small-cell lung cancer patients with long-term disease-free survival. Int J Radiat Oncol Biol Phys. 2005;62:639–44.

124. Moreno M, Aristu J, Ramos LI, et al. Predictive factors for radiation-induced pulmonary toxicity after three-dimensional conformal chemoradiation in locally advanced non-small-cell lung cancer. Clin Transl Oncol. 2007;9:596–602.

125. Goodridge D, Lawson J, Duggleby W, et al. Health care utilization of patients with chronic obstructive pulmonary disease and lung cancer in the last 12 months of life. Respir Med. 2008;102:885–91.
126. Au DH, Udris EM, Fihn SD, et al. Differences in health care utilization at the end of life among patients with chronic obstructive pulmonary disease and patients with lung cancer. Arch Intern Med. 2006;166:326–31.
127. Edmonds P, Karlsen S, Khan S, et al. A comparison of the palliative care needs of patients dying from chronic respiratory diseases and lung cancer. Palliative Med. 2001;15:287–95.
128. Gore JM, Brophy CJ, Greenstone MA. How well do we care for patients with end stage chronic obstructive pulmonary disease (COPD)? A comparison of palliative care and quality of life in COPD and lung cancer. Thorax. 2000;55:1000–6.

Chapter 7
Anxiety and Depression

Vincent S. Fan and Nicholas D. Giardino

Abstract Increasing evidence suggests that depression and anxiety are important comorbidities in COPD, and are associated with a number of adverse outcomes including worse health-related quality of life, an increased risk of exacerbations, and a higher mortality. The burden of depression in COPD is higher than in the general population, and many patients remain undiagnosed. Although treatment of depression and anxiety may include medications or pharmacotherapy, many patients with depressive symptoms do not receive treatment.

Keywords Depression • Anxiety • COPD • Comorbidity • Quality of life • Exacerbation • Mortality • Diagnosis • Medication • Pharmacotherapy • Treatment

Introduction

Increasing evidence suggests that depression and anxiety are important comorbidities in COPD, and are associated with a number of adverse outcomes including worse health-related quality of life, an increased risk of exacerbations, and a higher mortality. The burden of depression in COPD is higher than in the general population, and many patients remain undiagnosed. Although treatment of depression and anxiety may include medications or pharmacotherapy, many patients with depressive symptoms do not receive treatment.

V.S. Fan (✉)
Department of Medicine, VA Puget Sound Health Care System,
University of Washington School of Medicine, Seattle, WA, USA
e-mail: Vincent.Fan@va.gov

N.D. Giardino
Department of Psychiatry, VA Ann Arbor Healthcare System, University of Michigan,
Ann Arbor, MI, USA
e-mail: ngiardin@med.umich.edu

L. Nici and R. ZuWallack (eds.), *Chronic Obstructive Pulmonary Disease: Co-Morbidities and Systemic Consequences*, Respiratory Medicine, DOI 10.1007/978-1-60761-673-3_7,
© Springer Science+Business Media, LLC 2012

Prevalence of Depression and Anxiety in COPD

Depression

The prevalence of depressive symptoms among patients with COPD range from 7 to 75% [1–3], although most studies suggest that the range is between 25 and 50% [4–7]. These estimates vary in part due to the use of different instruments to measure depression, differences in severity of COPD across studies [8], and studies with small sample sizes or in select populations of patients such as those participating in clinical trials.

A diagnosis of depression or anxiety requires an assessment by a psychologist or psychiatrist using DSM-IVR criteria; however, this is not practical in most study settings. Since it is difficult to assess whether patients have a diagnosis of depression, a number of different instruments have been used to measure depressive or anxiety symptoms in COPD (see Table 7.1). These instruments generally have an established cutoff score that is suggestive of moderate-to-severe symptoms. Many of these instruments were developed for adults who did not have a chronic medical condition such as COPD, and therefore evaluating depressive symptoms in COPD may be more difficult because symptoms of depression such as fatigue may overlap with those of COPD. Measures of psychological distress have therefore been developed for use in patients with chronic illness such as COPD, and include the Hospital Anxiety and Depression (HAD) Scale [9] or the Geriatric Depression Scale (GDS) [10].

To examine the prevalence of depressive symptoms in the United States population aged >50, a large epidemiologic study using the Centers for Epidemiology Survey-Depression (CES-D8) found that 40.4% of COPD patients had significant depressive symptoms [11]. The rate of depression in COPD in this study was significantly higher than in other chronic illnesses such as stroke, diabetes, coronary artery disease, arthritis, cancer, or hypertension. The only other medical condition with a similar prevalence of depression was congestive heart failure, another disease with chronic exertional dyspnea as a primary symptom. Another study also found that the prevalence of depression in COPD was higher than in other disabling diseases such as Parkinson's disease, arthritis, stroke, and amputation [12].

Studies have also found that the prevalence of psychological symptoms is higher in COPD than in the general population [7, 12, 13]. Compared to age-matched controls, the risk of depression appears greatest for patients with severe COPD (FEV_1% predicted <50%), who are 2.5 times more likely to have depressive symptoms [14]. In another study, Beck Depression Inventory (BDI) scores were worse among patients with the most severe COPD, further supporting the concept that depression is worse among patients with severe COPD [15]. However, the association between depression and worsening COPD severity is not consistent [7, 13, 16]. For example, the prevalence of depression was not elevated among patients with COPD and long-term home oxygen use compared to those without [17].

Although the prevalence of depression in COPD and heart failure was found to be similar [11], there may be differences in factors associated with depression

Table 7.1 Measures of depressive and anxiety symptoms

Measure	Abbreviation	Range	Depression	Anxiety	Cut-off
Beck Depression Inventory [128, 129]	BDI	0–63	Yes	No	10–18 mild to moderate 19–29 moderate to severe 30–63 severe
Beck Anxiety Inventory [130]	BAI	0–63	No	Yes	8–15 mild 16–25 moderate 26–63 severe
Brief Assessment Schedule Depression Cards [131]	BASDEC	0–21	Yes	No	≥7
Centers for Epidemiology Survey – Depression [132]	CES-D	0–60	Yes	No	≥16
CES-D 10 Item Questionnaire [133]	CES-D 10	0–30	Yes	No	≥10
CES-D 8 Item Questionnaire	CES-D 8	0–24	Yes	No	≥3
Geriatric Depression Scale [10]	GDS	0–30	Yes	No	11–19 mild ≥20 moderate to severe
Geriatric Depression Scale Short Form [134]	GDS-SF, GDS-15	0–15	Yes	No	6–10 depression ≥11 severe
Geriatric Mental State Schedule [67, 135]	GMS	0–5	Yes	Yes	≥3 depression ≥3 anxiety
Hamilton Depression Rating Scale [136–138]	HAM-D	0–53	Yes	No	8–12 mild 13–17 mild to moderate ≥18 moderate to severe
Hospital Anxiety and Depression [139]	HAD-D HAD-A	0–21 0–21	Yes	Yes	≥8 mild ≥11 moderate to severe
Montgomery Asberg Depression Rating Scale [140, 141]	MADRS	0–60	Yes	No	7–19 mild 20–34 moderate ≥35 severe
State-Trait Anxiety Index [142, 143]	STAI	20–80	No	Yes	≥55
Symptom-Checklist-90-Revised [117, 144]	SCL-90-R		Yes	Yes	Symptom-Checklist-90-Revised

between the two diseases. Although both diseases are characterized by chronic exertional dyspnea, patients with COPD and major depression have a greater history of past psychiatric illness, less medical comorbidity, and more severe dyspnea than patients with heart failure [18]. These results suggest that causes of depression in COPD may be different from other chronic illnesses, that depression in COPD may be more difficult to treat, and that different approaches may be needed to address depression in COPD. Smoking is a key risk factor for the development of COPD and a health behavior known to be associated with depression, and therefore may be on the causative pathway between depression and COPD.

Depression in COPD may differ from depression in other chronic diseases in several ways. First, COPD patients experience persistent and worsening shortness of breath, a very distressing symptom [11] that is often more difficult to treat than the symptoms of other chronic diseases. Medications improve but do not eliminate the symptom of dyspnea, which leads to worsening disability that further contributes to depressive symptoms [19]. Second, COPD patients often report anxiety and panic symptoms resulting from their dyspnea. Anxiety may be worsened by COPD treatments such as beta-agonist inhalers, corticosteroids, and the stigma attached to home oxygen therapy [20]. The coexistence of anxiety may make the depression more refractory to treatment [2]. Third, most COPD is related to cigarette smoking, which in turn is associated with alcohol abuse [21]. These two behaviors are associated with both depression and nonadherence to treatment recommendations.

In addition to the high prevalence of depression in COPD, increasing evidence suggests that patients with COPD are at risk for developing a new episode of depression. Patients with COPD without depression were at increased risk of incident depression in the first 2 years following the diagnosis of COPD compared to those without COPD (Hazard Ratio (HR) 2.2, 95% CI 1.6–3.0) [22]. Similar findings were obtained in a study from the United Kingdom, with increasing risk of new depression in COPD compared to those without COPD, and the risk increasing with COPD disease severity [23]. Compared to patients with diabetes, those with COPD also had an increased risk of new depression (HR 1.8, 1.2–2.8) [24]. Given the high prevalence of depression in COPD, and increased risk of new depression episodes, further attention to screening for psychological symptoms should be considered.

Anxiety

The prevalence of anxiety is estimated between 6% and 74% [25]. The wide range is due, in part, to different instruments used to measure anxiety symptoms as well as differences in the study population. Anxiety often overlaps with depression in COPD [16], therefore making it more difficult to examine the independent effect of anxiety on outcomes. Using the HAD questionnaire, there were no differences in the proportion of patients with significant anxiety between those with COPD on home oxygen, and those without [17]. The prevalence of anxiety is not clearly higher among those with more severe COPD measured with FEV_1 alone [16, 26], although disease severity measured with the multicomponent BODE index was associated with increased risk of significant anxiety symptoms [26].

Association Between Depression/Anxiety and Outcomes in COPD

Effect of Depression and Anxiety on COPD Symptoms and Quality of Life

The relationship between psychological distress and symptoms and quality of life in COPD is complex, since the increasing dyspnea and functional impairments associated with COPD can often lead to social isolation and worsening depression. Depression and anxiety can in turn lead to further deconditioning and worsening symptoms and quality of life [27]. Anxiety may also impact quality of life by contributing to tachypnea, which may worsen hyperinflation, leading to worsening dyspnea, limitations in activity, and worse quality of life (Fig. 7.1) [28].

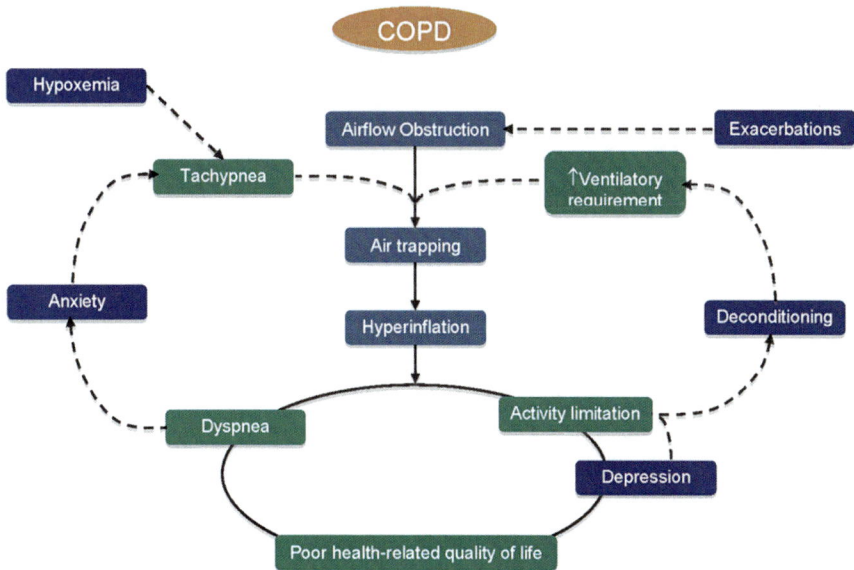

Fig. 7.1 Cycle of anxiety and dyspnea. The connection between chronic obstructive pulmonary disease symptoms and hyperinflation and its impact on exercise and function [28]. Reprinted with permission from Elsevier, copyright 2006

To better understand the relationship between psychological symptoms and COPD symptoms, several cross-sectional studies have looked at different populations of COPD patients. A large epidemiologic study suggests that dyspnea and difficulty walking are strongly associated with depression in COPD patients [11]. In smaller studies of well-characterized patients with COPD, depressive symptoms are associated with dyspnea measured with both the Borg [29, 30] and Medical Research Council (MRC) [13, 29, 31] dyspnea scales. For example, increasing dyspnea on the MRC dyspnea index was associated with an OR 1.8 (95% CI, 1.1–2.9) for depression defined as a BDI score >10 [31].

Depression is also associated with self-reported health-related quality of life (HRQOL), measured with both general and disease-specific HRQOL measures. Poor health status measured among outpatients with the St. George's Respiratory Questionnaire (SGRQ) is associated with depression and anxiety [4, 13], and explains 31% of the variation in health status after adjusting for BODE score, smoking, dyspnea, and fatigue [29]. Worse depression and somatization measured with the Symptom Checklist-90-Revised (SCL-90-R) are also associated with the worse total SGRQ score after adjusting for disease severity [32]. Depression measured with the Brief Assessment Schedule Depression Cards (BASDEC) instrument is also associated with total Chronic Respiratory Questionnaire (CRQ) score after adjusting for disease severity [33].

Some investigators have assessed the impact of both depression and anxiety on HRQOL. For example, both depression and anxiety (measured with the BDI and BAI) were associated with the worse scores on the CRQ Emotion and Mastery Scales, but only the anxiety was associated with the CRQ dyspnea scale [34]. Both depression and anxiety are associated with decreased scores on general measures of health status measured with the SF-36 [34–36]. Depression is also associated with other COPD-related HRQOL measures such as the Seattle Obstructive Lung Disease Questionnaire (SOLDQ) [35] and the Airways Questionnaire 20 (AQ20-R) [37].

Effect of Psychological Symptoms On Functional Outcomes

In addition to symptoms and HRQOL, functional outcomes are an important patient-centered outcome in COPD. A majority of the evidence linking depressive symptoms and impaired functioning in COPD are based on small-to-moderate sized cross-sectional studies that measure physical activity by self-report [4, 38, 39].

Depression is associated with worse performance on the 6-min walk test (6-MWT) in unadjusted analyses [29]. Among patients participating in a pulmonary rehabilitation program, increasing depression on the HAD instrument was associated with less improvement in exercise performance measured with cycle ergometery [40] and 6-MWT [41]. When depression and functional outcomes are measured at the same time, one cannot determine whether, for instance, physical activity is the cause or result of depression. In fact, the association is likely bidirectional and mutually reinforcing because depression leads to physical inactivity and inactivity worsens depression [42–44].

A recent study of German COPD patients found that depression was not associated with total physical activity measured by accelerometry after adjustment for systemic inflammation and other covariates including cardiovascular and COPD disease severity, metabolic status, muscle strength, and anemia [15]. Measurement of physical activity by accelerometry enables the assessment of the actual activity performed by the patient at home outside of the clinical setting, and does not rely on self-report. Since preliminary data in other patient populations suggest that depressed patients appear to underestimate their functional ability [45], it is important that studies perform objective assessments of functional capacity and performance over time in order to accurately model these relationships.

The limited experimental literature offers some insight into the relationship between depression and functional outcomes in patients with COPD. An early study by Borson et al. [46] testing the effect of nortriptyline in 30 patients with moderate to severe COPD showed that despite large improvements in depression and psychosocial functioning after 3 months of treatment, there were no changes in distance walked on a 12-min walk test. In contrast, a recent uncontrolled study of 28 COPD patients showed that unblinded treatment with a serotonin-selective-reuptake inhibitor (SSRI) for 3 months resulted in significant reductions in depression scores and a 58-m increase in 6-min walk distance [47]. These latter findings are consistent with several randomized controlled studies testing the effects of antidepressants and exercise training for medically healthy individuals with major depressive disorders; concurrent improvements in depressive symptoms and functional capacity were reported, at least in adults with major depression and no other significant medical comorbidities [42, 43].

Data from patients with severe emphysema in the National Emphysema Treatment Trial (NETT) assessed the relationship between baseline depressive or anxiety symptoms and functional capacity (6-MWT and cycle ergometry). In this analysis of 1,828 patients screened for the NETT study, both depression and anxiety were independently associated with decreased 6-MWT and workload on cycle ergometry, after adjusting for demographic factors and disease severity. In a separate study, anxiety measured with the HADS was also associated with reduced 6-MWT [26].

Mortality

Depression has been associated with an increased risk of mortality in chronic disease such as ischemic heart disease [48] or diabetes [49], and several studies have investigated the relationship between depression and risk of mortality for COPD patients. Severe COPD is associated with increased depressive symptoms as well as adverse clinical outcomes, therefore adequately adjusting for the severity of COPD is essential in measuring the independent effect of depression on clinical outcomes [50].

An early study investigating the relationship between depression and mortality in COPD found that among patients followed for a median of 838 days after a hospitalization for COPD, depression measured with the Geriatric Depression Scale Short Form was associated with an hazard ratio of 3.6 (95% CI 1.5–8.7) for mortality after adjusting for FEV_1 and other measures of disease severity [51]. Mortality was also increased after a COPD hospitalization with depression measured with the HAD survey among 376 patients in Singapore, with a HR 1.9 (1.0–3.6), after adjustment for disease severity measures including FEV_1, hypoxemia, and dyspnea [4].

The finding that depression is associated with mortality has also been seen in the outpatient setting. In a study of outpatients admitted to a pulmonary rehabilitation center, depression was measured with the BDI and patients were followed for a median of 8.5 years [52]. A BDI ≥ 19 was associated with an increased risk of death (HR 1.9, 95% CI 1.1–3.3) after adjusting for gender, age, and maximal workload on cycle ergometry. Among 610 outpatients with severe emphysema participating in the NETT randomized to medical therapy, 3-year mortality was 34.5% among those with a BDI ≥ 10 versus 23% for those with a BDI < 10 [53]. After extensive adjustment for measures of COPD disease severity including a modified BODE index, hemoglobin level, residual volume, diffusion capacity of carbon monoxide, maximal cardiopulmonary exercise test workload, difference in percentage emphysema by CT, perfusion ratio by perfusion scan, and comorbidity, the risk of 3-year mortality was OR 1.8 (1.0–3.8) for BDI 11–14 and OR 2.7 (1.4–5.3) for a BDI of ≥15 compared to a BDI < 5.

The association between anxiety and mortality has not been extensively studied, but among outpatients enrolled in the NETT trial, anxiety measured with the State-Trait Anxiety Index was not associated with either 1- or 3-year mortality [53]. Anxiety measured with the HADS questionnaire was also not statistically associated with mortality among 491 outpatients with COPD in China [54].

Although not all studies have confirmed the independent effect of depression on mortality [55, 56], these studies indicate that depression is likely associated with a significantly increased risk of mortality for patients with COPD both after an acute hospitalization, and also in the outpatient setting. The mechanism between depression and mortality is not well understood but may include biologic effects of depression such as increased activity of the hypothalamic–pituitary–adrenal axis [57] or increased inflammation [58] that contribute to worse outcomes. Depression also may affect important self-care behaviors such as medication adherence, smoking or alcohol use, physical activity, or interaction with the health care team. Continued smoking is correlated with depressive symptoms [52], suggesting that this is a potential factor on the causal pathway. Data from a cohort of patients with stable coronary heart disease found that the effect of depression on adverse cardiovascular events was explained in large part by behavioral factors, particularly physical activity [59], suggesting that these behavioral factors may play a similar role in COPD. Worse depression and anxiety were predictive of patients not completing pulmonary rehabilitation, supporting the suggestion that psychological factors are associated with health care behaviors in COPD [60]. Additional studies will be needed to better understand the mechanism between depression and adverse outcomes in COPD.

Exacerbations/Hospitalizations

During the course of the disease, patients with COPD frequently experience exacerbations characterized by increasing dyspnea, cough, and sputum production. Several studies have identified risk factors for exacerbations including disease severity such as worsening lung function (FEV1), muscle weakness [61], pulmonary hypertension, hypercapnea [62], impaired quality of life [63], prior COPD exacerbations, and comorbidity [64, 65]. In addition to these factors, depression and anxiety may also contribute to the risk of COPD exacerbations.

Among outpatients with stable COPD, depression measured with the HADS ≥ 11 was associated with symptoms-based exacerbations [incidence rate ratio (IRR) 1.5, 1.0–2.2], those that required treatment with steroids or antibiotics (IRR 1.56, 1.0–2.4), or hospitalization (IRR 1.72, 1.0–2.9) [54]. These analyses were adjusted for disease severity including the components of the BODE index, comorbidity, and medication use. Similarly, the risk of exacerbations in the 1-year period after pulmonary rehabilitation was increased (OR 2.8, 1.1–7.3) among those with significant depressive symptoms measured with the BDI (≥19) [66].

Initial studies suggested that anxiety, measured with the Geriatric Mental State Schedule (GMS), was associated with the frequency of hospitalizations in the past year for patients with COPD after adjusting for depression [67]. In prospective studies, anxiety measured with the HAD questionnaire was found to predict exacerbations, although only among those with worse HRQOL [68]. Another study of stable outpatients also found that the HAD anxiety score was associated with COPD exacerbations with a HR 1.4 (1.0–1.9) [26]. Anxiety may be related to exacerbations since the symptom of dyspnea, which is the cardinal symptom of a COPD exacerbation, is associated with anxiety [26]. Also, medications such as beta agonists and methylxanthines used to treat COPD contribute to symptoms of anxiety. Although several studies have found that anxiety is associated with exacerbations, other studies have not confirmed this relationship measuring anxiety with either the HAD score [54] or the STAI [53].

In addition to exacerbations, patients hospitalized with COPD and with symptoms of depression measured with the HADS had an increased length of stay (6.1 days versus 4.9 days, $p=0.02$), although they were not at increased risk for being readmitted (OR 0.9, 0.7–1.3) [4]. The relationship between depressive symptoms and exacerbations has not been consistent, however, with several studies showing no association [53, 68, 69] with depressive or anxiety symptoms.

Among COPD patients who underwent a structured psychiatric interview, a psychiatric diagnosis (46% anxiety, 17% mood, and 4% dysthymia) was associated with an increased risk of first outpatient exacerbation (RR 1.7, 1.1–2.6) [70]. Psychological symptoms may therefore contribute to an increased risk of COPD exacerbations, although the results may reflect differences in the severity of COPD between studies, the type of measures used to assess depression and anxiety, and the degree to which the studies adjusted for disease severity.

Impact of Depression on Self-care in COPD

Decreased Participation in Pulmonary Rehabilitation

Depression has been shown to adversely affect adherence to self-care regimens, with higher rates of smoking and sedentary lifestyle among depressed patients [71]. In patients with diabetes and heart disease, depression is associated with nonadherence to medications [72, 73]. It is likely, therefore, that depression is associated with decreased self-care behaviors in patients with COPD.

Pulmonary rehabilitation is a guideline-recommended treatment for moderate-to-severe COPD, and a study of patients enrolled in the NETT trial examined whether baseline anxiety or depression were associated with adherence to pulmonary rehabilitation [60]. Participants in the trial were required to complete 8–9 weeks of rehabilitation, however 27% did not complete all 10 required sessions. Patients with a BDI score ≥ 5 were significantly less likely to complete rehabilitation (OR 0.6 95% CI 0.3–0.9). Similarly, after adjusting for depression, anxiety was also independently associated with not completing pulmonary rehabilitation.

These suggest that psychological symptoms in COPD are associated with lack of adherence to an exercise program in COPD. In addition, for patients enrolled in COPD-related self-management programs, depression may moderate the response to these interventions. Patients at high risk for depression (CESD > 15) who received 24 supervised exercise sessions in addition to an independent walking exercise program over 12 months had greater reduction in dyspnea with activities of daily living compared to depressed patients who received only four supervised exercise sessions or no exercise sessions [74].

One of the principal factors for changing patient behavior is to change patient self-confidence, or self-efficacy, to manage their illness. For patients enrolled in a self-management program for chronic illness that includes COPD, only patients with significant depression had an improvement in their self-efficacy to manage their disease [75]. These findings suggest that patients with COPD with greater depressive symptoms may require more intensive interventions in order to achieve a similar improvement in symptoms. As a result, it may be necessary to tailor intervention intensity depending on depression status in order to achieve optimal symptom relief.

Anxiety and Dyspnea

Individual personality differences may also contribute to increased risk for anxiety symptoms in COPD. From a cognitive-behavioral perspective, emotional sensitivity to somatic sensations may lead to greater anxiety when these bodily cues are encountered. The disposition toward this type of heightened reaction has been termed anxiety sensitivity. Patients with high anxiety sensitivity may become vigilant to somatic sensations and react to these sensations with anxiety, and further physiological arousal. In addition, longitudinal experience with exacerbations of respiratory disease may generate fearful or catastrophic beliefs about respiratory symptoms, which, in turn, provoke panic attacks.

Support for this theory is found in a number of studies including one that investigated the relationship between pulmonary function, catastrophic thoughts about anxiety, and panic attacks in patients with COPD [76]. In this study, COPD patients with panic attacks did not differ from those without panic attacks on demographic variables, pulmonary function tests, or general activity levels; but they did have more agoraphobic thoughts and greater fear of bodily sensations. However, this study did not examine panic disorder (PD) per se, and may have limited relevance to this disorder, since 36% of the general population has experienced panic attacks, while only 2–3% develops PD. In another study, women with COPD scored twice as high on the Anxiety Sensitivity Index than men and were three times more likely to have PD [77].

COPD can be associated with near-death episodes, need for ventilatory support, and other illness experiences, which could also influence the development of these frightening thoughts. Livermore and colleagues examined the perception of dyspnea to a series of increasing inspiratory resistive loads in patients with PD or panic attacks and COPD [78]. Participants with COPD and panic reported greater dyspnea during all resistive loads than participants with COPD alone and healthy controls. It should be noted, though, that less than half of the subjects in the "COPD with panic" group actually had PD. Furthermore, this study only measured dyspnea intensity ratings to resistive loads but did not test for differences in the detection of loads. More recently, Giardino et al. attempted to test these findings with patients having COPD and panic disorder and also examine whether group differences in sensitivity to respiratory loads existed between groups [79].

Participants with COPD and panic disorder and COPD without panic disorder first completed a task to determine their detection threshold for inspiratory resistive loads and then a second task in which they rated dyspnea to a series of resistive load similar to those used in the Livermore study above. As in others studies, participants with COPD and PD reported greater dyspnea during loaded breathing, but no group differences in detection thresholds for resistive loads were found. Furthermore, anxiety sensitivity accounted for a significant proportion of the group differences in dyspnea magnitude ratings. Thus, it appears that higher anxiety sensitivity, leading to greater distress in response to uncomfortable respiratory sensations, and not greater interoceptive sensitivity, may account for higher dyspnea scores reported in patients with COPD and panic disorder.

Increased rates of anxiety and depression in patients with COPD may not be primarily explained as a consequence of COPD, however. In many patients with COPD, the onset of anxiety and depression precedes the onset of COPD. Cigarette smoking rates are higher among those with anxiety and depression. Thus, premorbid anxiety problems may be overrepresented in COPD. It is still unclear, though, whether common factors influence the development of anxiety, depression, and smoking; whether anxiety and depression lead to smoking; or whether the reverse is true. More complex mechanisms include the possibility that anxiety and depression, in the presence of smoking, may increase risk for developing COPD. Finally, preexisting vulnerabilities may also lead to the expression of anxiety and depression in the presence of the consequent physiological and psychological stress of COPD.

Causative Mechanisms for the Development of Depression

Role of Depression and Inflammation in COPD

While the biological basis for depression remains incompletely understood, there is accumulating evidence of an interaction between the brain and immune system [80, 81]. Observations that acute depressive episodes frequently occur in patients undergoing cytokine therapy for the treatment of hepatitis C or cancer suggest the possible role of inflammation in the pathophysiology of depression [82, 83]. Interferon-alpha potently stimulates the release of endogenous pro-inflammatory cytokines such as IL-6 [84] and frequently induces major depression [85]. Cytokines have been shown to alter serotonin metabolism by either degrading tryptophan dehydrogenase or by enhancing the activity of indoleamine 2,3-dioxygenase, resulting in reduced availability of tryptophan and consequently provoking depressive symptoms [86]. Another link between inflammation and depression is through activation of the hypothalamo–pituitary–adrenal axis (HPA-axis). Cytokines the size of IL-6 can cross the blood-brain barrier and through corticotrophin-releasing hormone (CRH) modulate the HPA-axis and neurotransmission. Hyperactivity of the HPA-axis is known to be associated with major depression [87].

Experimental studies show that SSRIs, commonly used to treat depression, may decrease systemic cytokine production [88–90]. Patients with depression who were treated with 8 weeks of Sertraline had significant reductions in IL-2, IL-4, IL-12, TNF-α, TGF-B1, and MCP1 levels [89]. Interestingly, two studies by O'Brien et al. [88, 91] reported that SSRIs reduced CRP levels in patients with major depression independent of their impact on depression symptoms and patients with SSRI-resistant depression had significantly higher production of IL-6 and TNF-α compared to normal controls. SSRIs also reduce the secretion of TNF-α from lymphocytes [90], further suggesting that this class of antidepressants have an immunomodulatory effect.

The high prevalence of depression among chronically ill patients raises the possibility that chronic inflammation may increase the risk of depression [80]. The relationship between depression and systemic inflammation has mostly been studied using cross-sectional epidemiologic designs with mixed findings across healthy [92–94] and clinical populations, particularly, patients with cardiovascular diseases [95–98]. Lesperance et al. [95] found an interaction between CRP levels and statin therapy with risk of depression, although no association was seen with IL-6. Similarly, Miller et al. [96] showed that depression severity was associated with higher CRP levels but not with IL-6 or TNF-α in patients with stable heart disease;

yet these results have not been consistent [97]. Although most studies have used cross-sectional designs, one prospective study of middle-age workers found that baseline CRP and IL-6 were predictive of depression 12 years later but not the converse, suggesting that inflammation may precede the development of depression [99].

Only two studies have assessed the relationship between depression and inflammation in COPD with conflicting findings. A recent cross-sectional study of 142 patients with COPD found no relationship between CRP or IL-6 with depressive symptoms as measured by the CES-D [100], whereas a small study that used the HAD Scale found a significant association between TNF-α and depression ($r = 0.42$) [101].

Role of Hypoxemia on Cognitive Function and Psychological Symptoms

Hypoxemia secondary to pulmonary pathophysiology may also play a role in the development of depression and anxiety in patients with COPD. Chronic hypoxia may lead to structural brain changes that cause neuro-cognitive deficits and impairment in emotion regulation. Even mild hypoxia may produce alterations in neurotransmitter systems essential to cognitive-emotional functioning. These impairments in brain function may result directly in psychiatric symptoms, but also may impair the individual's ability to adapt and cope with challenge, including the stress associated with managing a chronic illness. In a longitudinal study of hypoxemic COPD patients on continuous oxygen therapy, lower baseline FVC and FEV$_1$ were associated with decline in cognitive function at 1- and 2-year follow-up [102]. Furthermore, 2-year changes in cognitive function were inversely associated with change in depression scores. However, in another study of nonhypoxemic patients with mild-moderate COPD, no differences in cognitive performance were found when compared to control subjects with chronic nonrespiratory diseases [103].

Repeated experiences with hypoxia may also sensitize the brain circuitry involved in fear responses to become hyperresponsive to subsequent episodes of hypoxia, as well as other respiratory sensations that have been previously associated with hypoxia, including the many sensations related to the experience of dyspnea. Patients may become more vigilant to respiratory sensations and react to these sensations with increased anxiety and physiological arousal. This may lead to an escalating cycle of increasing anxiety that leads to a panic attack. Panic attacks are common in patients with COPD; approximately one-third of COPD patients report having panic attack [76, 104], and approximately 8% will meet full psychiatric criteria for panic disorder (PD) [105]. Fearful thoughts and beliefs about respiratory symptoms can increase risk for anxiety and panic attacks. Given the fearfulness of air hunger, as well as patients' direct or indirect experience with near-death episodes, need for ventilatory support, and other illness experiences, the common development of these frightening thoughts is understandable.

Treatment of Depression and Anxiety in COPD

Pharmacotherapy

Studies in non-COPD populations with other chronic diseases such as ischemic heart disease have demonstrated the effectiveness of sertraline [106], citalopram [107], and cognitive behavioral therapy (CBT) [108] in treating comorbid depression. There is little data regarding the effectiveness of pharmacological treatment of anxiety and depression for patients with COPD. One study showed that 12 weeks of nortriptyline versus placebo significantly improved depressed mood and anxiety, but showed little improvement in dyspnea or physiologic function [46]. This study did find that symptoms of physical distress and quality of life improved, suggesting that nortriptyline may improve the somatic experience of physical symptoms. A 6-week randomized controlled trial (RCT) in 28 depressed COPD patients used an SSRI, paroxetine, followed by a 3-month open-labeled treatment [47]. The authors found that there was no significant improvement in depression or functional outcomes during the 6-week RCT phase, but improvements were observed in depression scores, quality of life, and exercise tolerance after 3 months of treatment in pre–post analysis. In a small 2-week randomized controlled trial, Argyropoulou et al. found that the anxiolytic buspirone produced significant reductions in anxiety and dyspnea, as well as improvements in exercise tolerance, in patients with COPD [109].

Psychotherapy

Nonpharmacologic interventions may also be effective for anxiety and depression treatment in COPD. In a small randomized controlled study, de Godoy and de Godoy reported that addition of psychotherapy to a 12-week pulmonary rehabilitation produced significant reductions in anxiety and depression symptoms not found in rehabilitation alone [110]. A randomized controlled trial of CBT compared to COPD education found that both significantly improved depressive symptoms, but that the effectiveness of CBT and the education program did not differ [111]. In a recent study, CBT was compared with enhanced standard care for patients with COPD and clinically significant anxiety and depression symptoms [112]. In this small randomized controlled trial, CBT, but not the control condition, produced significant improvements in anxiety and depression that were maintained at an 8-month follow-up. As discussed earlier, panic disorder is the most common anxiety disorder diagnosed in patients with COPD. In an interesting application of CBT, Livermore and colleagues tested the efficacy of CBT in *preventing* the development or worsening of panic attacks in patients with COPD [113]. They found that, compared to those in the control condition, patients randomized to the four-session CBT intervention were significantly less likely at 18 months to have experienced a panic attack in the previous 6 months (17% versus 60%). A significant limitation of nearly all of the published studies of psychotherapy in COPD is that study subjects were not selected for participation based on the presence of an anxiety or depressive disorder diagnosis, but rather only for the presence of anxiety or depression symptoms. CBT and related treatments were developed and validated for the treatment of specific anxiety disorders (e.g., panic disorder, generalized anxiety disorder) and major depressive disorder. Thus, their application and efficacy, when targeted at those with symptoms, but not necessarily a clinical disorder, may be questioned. Thus, despite guideline recommendations, these data and a recent review of the limited literature [114] suggest that psychotherapy has not yet been demonstrated to be an effective component of care for depression and anxiety disorders; however, COPD-specific self-management or other psychosocial interventions may be helpful in symptom relief. Research is needed to test the efficacy of psychological interventions for specific anxiety and mood disorders diagnoses in patients with COPD.

Pulmonary Rehabilitation

Addressing the underlying symptoms of dyspnea and decreasing disability may improve psychological symptoms for patients with COPD. Pulmonary rehabilitation is recommended by the COPD GOLD guidelines for patients with moderate-to-severe (stages II–IV) COPD. In addition to exercise training, the American Thoracic Society/European Respiratory Society guidelines on pulmonary rehabilitation also recommends assessing patients for anxiety and depression, and referring patients with significant psychiatric disease to appropriate specialists, and promotion of an adequate patient support system [115]. Pulmonary rehabilitation also generally includes self-management education that may include education on coping with chronic lung disease, managing anxiety, relaxation techniques, and stress management.

A small randomized controlled trial of 30 patients enrolled in a 12-week outpatient pulmonary rehabilitation demonstrated that patients who received pulmonary rehabilitation combined with weekly psychotherapy had significant reduction in both anxiety and depression measured with the BAI and BDI [110]. A 3-arm randomized trial comparing exercise and stress management education to stress management to control found improved scores on the STAI and SCL-anxiety score for patients in the exercise group compared to both the stress management group and the control group [116]. Another study of a 4-month pulmonary rehabilitation program found that among patients who completed the study (35/40), depression and anxiety measured with the SCL-90-R improved following the program [117]. A randomized controlled trial of 24 patients of an 8-week pulmonary rehabilitation program found that rehabilitation was associated with improvement in depression severity measured with the BDI, and anxiety measured with the STAI-trait index [118]. A large study of 200 patients randomized to a 6-week pulmonary rehabilitation program found a significant reduction in depressive symptoms measured with the HAD at 1 year (difference -1.3, $p=0.004$) [119]. A meta-analysis of six randomized controlled trials of comprehensive pulmonary rehabilitation found that pulmonary rehabilitation significantly improved anxiety [SMD −0.33 (−0.57, −0.09) and depression (SMD −0.58 (−0.93, −0.23)] [120]. These studies suggest that pulmonary rehabilitation likely improves psychological symptoms for COPD.

Summary of Treatment

There are surprisingly few studies of treatment of either depression or anxiety in patients with COPD. Those that have been published generally include small numbers of subjects and focus on the reduction of anxiety and depression symptoms, rather than diagnosed psychiatric disorders. This may reflect patient preference not to be treated for psychiatric symptoms and disorders, and there is evidence that patient acceptance of antidepressant medications is poor [121]. This may make it difficult to recruit patients for clinical trials of depression or anxiety treatment. Further research is needed to determine how best to incorporate treatment of anxiety and depression in the care of patients with COPD.

Inadequacy of Treatment of Depression in COPD

Guidelines

Several guidelines have been developed that provide recommendations for treatment of depression in the general populations [122]. Most guidelines recognize the important role played by chronic medical illness when treating depression, and the risk of relapse of depression for elderly patients with coexisting chronic disease [123]. The guidelines also recommend taking into account chronic medical illness when selecting an antidepressant.

Recently, the National Institute for Health and Clinical Excellence (NICE) in England has released guidelines regarding the treatment of depression in adults, and differentiate treatment between those with and without a chronic physical health problem [124]. These guidelines emphasize the role of psychosocial interventions, peer support, and psychotherapy for patients with depression and chronic illness, reserving antidepressant use for those with resistant depression or severe depressive symptoms. The NICE guidelines are the first to recommend that treatment algorithms for depression in the setting of a chronic medical condition may need to be addressed differently.

Adherence to Guidelines

In the United States, a commonly used measure of appropriate depression treatment is the Health Plan Employer Data and Information Set (HEDIS). The HEDIS measure focuses primarily on pharmacologic treatment of depression and whether patients received adequate medication coverage and three or more follow-up appointments in the first 84 days after treatment was initiated.

There is evidence that depressed COPD patients are less likely to get adequate antidepressant therapy compared to patients with heart disease, diabetes, and osteoarthritis [125] .Only 10% of COPD patients receive adequate antidepressants and follow-up [126], with significant geographic variation in care [127]. Overall, these findings suggest that compared to other chronic conditions, patients with COPD are more likely to be depressed, may prefer not to be treated [121], and are less likely to receive guideline-concordant care. These patients may therefore benefit from improved access to mental health care and targeted interventions that improve depressive symptoms such as COPD self-management or psychotherapy that require deployment of additional resources.

Summary

There is a high prevalence of psychological symptoms among patients with COPD. Depression appears to be more common in COPD than in many other chronic medical conditions and is associated with worse clinical outcomes including mortality, COPD exacerbations, and impaired functional status. Although inflammation and hypoxemia may contribute to the development of depressive and anxiety symptoms, the mechanism for the development of psychological symptoms is poorly understood. There are few studies of treatment of either depression or anxiety in patients with COPD, although medications, psychotherapy, and pulmonary rehabilitation may be effective.

References

1. Engstrom CP, Persson LO, Larsson S, Ryden A, Sullivan M. Functional status and well being in chronic obstructive pulmonary disease with regard to clinical parameters and smoking: a descriptive and comparative study. Thorax. 1996;51(8):825–30.
2. Kunik ME, Roundy K, Veazey C, et al. Surprisingly high prevalence of anxiety and depression in chronic breathing disorders. Chest. 2005;127(4):1205–11.
3. Lacasse Y, Rousseau L, Maltais F. Prevalence of depressive symptoms and depression in patients with severe oxygen-dependent chronic obstructive pulmonary disease. J Cardiopulm Rehabil. 2001;21(2):80–6.
4. Ng TP, Niti M, Tan WC, Cao Z, Ong KC, Eng P. Depressive symptoms and chronic obstructive pulmonary disease: effect on mortality, hospital readmission, symptom burden, functional status, and quality of life. Arch Intern Med. 2007;167(1):60–7.
5. Norwood R. Prevalence and impact of depression in chronic obstructive pulmonary disease patients. Curr Opin Pulm Med. 2006;12(2):113–7.
6. van Ede L, Yzermans CJ, Brouwer HJ. Prevalence of depression in patients with chronic obstructive pulmonary disease: a systematic review. Thorax. 1999;54(8):688–92.
7. Wagena EJ, Arrindell WA, Wouters EF, van Schayck CP. Are patients with COPD psychologically distressed? Eur Respir J. 2005;26(2):242–8.

8. Maurer J, Rebbapragada V, Borson S, et al. Anxiety and depression in COPD: current understanding, unanswered questions, and research needs. Chest. 2008;134(4 Suppl):43S–S56.
9. Mykletun A, Stordal E, Dahl AA. Hospital Anxiety and Depression (HAD) scale: factor structure, item analyses and internal consistency in a large population. Br J Psychiatry. 2001;179:540–4.
10. Yesavage JA, Brink TL, Rose TL, et al. Development and validation of a geriatric depression screening scale: a preliminary report. J Psychiatr Res. 1982;17(1):37–49.
11. Schane RE, Walter LC, Dinno A, Covinsky KE, Woodruff PG. Prevalence and risk factors for depressive symptoms in persons with chronic obstructive pulmonary disease. J Gen Intern Med. 2008;23(11):1757–62.
12. Yohannes AM, Roomi J, Baldwin RC, Connolly MJ. Depression in elderly outpatients with disabling chronic obstructive pulmonary disease. Age Ageing. 1998;27(2):155–60.
13. Di Marco F, Verga M, Reggente M, et al. Anxiety and depression in COPD patients: the roles of gender and disease severity. Respir Med. 2006;100(10):1767–74.
14. van Manen JG, Bindels PJ, Dekker FW, IJzermans CJ, van der Zee JS, Schade E. Risk of depression in patients with chronic obstructive pulmonary disease and its determinants. Thorax. 2002;57(5):412–6.
15. Watz H, Waschki B, Boehme C, Claussen M, Meyer T, Magnussen H. Extrapulmonary effects of chronic obstructive pulmonary disease on physical activity: a cross-sectional study. Am J Respir Crit Care Med. 2008;177(7):743–51.
16. Gudmundsson G, Gislason T, Janson C, et al. Depression, anxiety and health status after hospitalisation for COPD: a multicentre study in the Nordic countries. Respir Med. 2006;100(1):87–93.
17. Lewis KE, Annandale JA, Sykes RN, Hurlin C, Owen C, Harrison NK. Prevalence of anxiety and depression in patients with severe COPD: similar high levels with and without LTOT. COPD. 2007;4(4):305–12.
18. Koenig HG. Differences between depressed patients with heart failure and those with pulmonary disease. Am J Geriat Psychiatry. 2006;14(3):211–9.
19. Katz P, Julian L, Omachi TA, et al. The impact of disability on depression among individuals with COPD. Chest. 2009;137(4):838–45.
20. Cullen DL, Stiffler D. Long-term oxygen therapy: review from the patients' perspective. Chron Respir Dis. 2009;6(3):141–7.
21. Daeppen JB, Smith TL, Danko GP, et al. Clinical correlates of cigarette smoking and nicotine dependence in alcohol-dependent men and women. The Collaborative Study Group on the Genetics of Alcoholism. Alcohol Alcohol. 2000;35(2):171–5.
22. Polsky D, Doshi JA, Marcus S, et al. Long-term risk for depressive symptoms after a medical diagnosis. Arch Intern Med. 2005;165(11):1260–6.
23. Schneider C, Jick SS, Bothner U, Meier CR. COPD and the risk of depression. Chest. 2010;137(2):341–7.
24. van den Bemt L, Schermer T, Bor H, et al. The risk for depression comorbidity in patients with COPD. Chest. 2009;135(1):108–14.
25. Yohannes AM, Willgoss TG, Baldwin RC, Connolly MJ. Depression and anxiety in chronic heart failure and chronic obstructive pulmonary disease: prevalence, relevance, clinical implications and management principles. Int J Geriat Psychiatry. 2009;25(12):1209–21.
26. Eisner MD, Blanc PD, Yelin EH, et al. Influence of anxiety on health outcomes in COPD. Thorax. 2010;65(3):229–34.
27. Rabe KF, Hurd S, Anzueto A, et al. Global strategy for the diagnosis, management, and prevention of chronic obstructive pulmonary disease: GOLD executive summary. Am J Respir Crit Care Med. 2007;176(6):532–55.
28. Cooper CB. The connection between chronic obstructive pulmonary disease symptoms and hyperinflation and its impact on exercise and function. Am J Med. 2006;119(10 Suppl 1):21–31.
29. Al-shair K, Dockry R, Mallia-Milanes B, Kolsum U, Singh D, Vestbo J. Depression and its relationship with poor exercise capacity, BODE index and muscle wasting in COPD. Respir Med. 2009;103(10):1572–9.

30. Giardino ND, Curtis JL, Andrei AC, et al. Anxiety is associated with diminished exercise performance and quality of life in severe emphysema: a cross-sectional study. Respir Res. 2010;11:29.
31. Chavannes NH, Huibers MJ, Schermer TR, et al. Associations of depressive symptoms with gender, body mass index and dyspnea in primary care COPD patients. Fam Pract. 2005;22(6):604–7.
32. Kuhl K, Schurmann W, Rief W. Mental disorders and quality of life in COPD patients and their spouses. Int J Chron Obstruct Pulmon Dis. 2008;3(4):727–36.
33. Yohannes AM, Roomi J, Waters K, Connolly MJ. Quality of life in elderly patients with COPD: measurement and predictive factors. Respir Med. 1998;92(10):1231–6.
34. Cully JA, Graham DP, Stanley MA, et al. Quality of life in patients with chronic obstructive pulmonary disease and comorbid anxiety or depression. Psychosomatics. 2006;47(4):312–9.
35. Felker B, Katon W, Hedrick SC, et al. The association between depressive symptoms and health status in patients with chronic pulmonary disease. Gen Hosp Psychiatry. 2001;23(2):56–61.
36. Kim HF, Kunik ME, Molinari VA, et al. Functional impairment in COPD patients: the impact of anxiety and depression. Psychosomatics. 2000;41(6):465–71.
37. Omachi TA, Katz PP, Yelin EH, et al. Depression and health-related quality of life in chronic obstructive pulmonary disease. Am J Med. 2009;122(8):778.
38. Wall MP. Predictors of functional performance in community-dwelling people with COPD. J Nurs Scholarsh. 2007;39(3):222–8.
39. Weaver TE, Narsavage GL. Physiological and psychological variables related to functional status in chronic obstructive pulmonary disease. Nurs Res. 1992;41(5):286–91.
40. Trappenburg JC, Troosters T, Spruit MA, Vandebrouck N, Decramer M, Gosselink R. Psychosocial conditions do not affect short-term outcome of multidisciplinary rehabilitation in chronic obstructive pulmonary disease. Arch Phys Med Rehabil. 2005;86(9):1788–92.
41. Yeh ML, Chen HH, Liao YC, Liao WY. Testing the functional status model in patients with chronic obstructive pulmonary disease. J Adv Nurs. 2004;48(4):342–50.
42. Blumenthal JA, Babyak MA, Doraiswamy PM, et al. Exercise and pharmacotherapy in the treatment of major depressive disorder. Psychosom Med. 2007;69(7):587–96.
43. Blumenthal JA, Babyak MA, Moore KA, et al. Effects of exercise training on older patients with major depression. Arch Intern Med. 1999;159(19):2349–56.
44. Penninx BW, Deeg DJ, van Eijk JT, Beekman AT, Guralnik JM. Changes in depression and physical decline in older adults: a longitudinal perspective. J Affect Disord. 2000;61(1–2):1–12.
45. Skotzko CE, Krichten C, Zietowski G, et al. Depression is common and precludes accurate assessment of functional status in elderly patients with congestive heart failure. J Card Fail. 2000;6(4):300–5.
46. Borson S, McDonald GJ, Gayle T, Deffebach M, Lakshminarayan S, VanTuinen C. Improvement in mood, physical symptoms, and function with nortriptyline for depression in patients with chronic obstructive pulmonary disease. Psychosomatics. 1992;33(2):190–201.
47. Eiser N, Harte R, Spiros K, Phillips C, Isaac MT. Effect of treating depression on quality-of-life and exercise tolerance in severe COPD. COPD. 2005;2(2):233–41.
48. Grace SL, Abbey SE, Kapral MK, Fang J, Nolan RP, Stewart DE. Effect of depression on five-year mortality after an acute coronary syndrome. Am J Cardiol. 2005;96(9):1179–85.
49. Lin EH, Heckbert SR, Rutter CM, et al. Depression and increased mortality in diabetes: unexpected causes of death. Ann Fam Med. 2009;7(5):414–21.
50. Mendes de Leon CF. Depression and social support in recovery from myocardial infarction: confounding and confusion. Psychosom Med. 1999;61(6):738–9.
51. Almagro P, Calbo E, Ochoa de Echaguen A, et al. Mortality after hospitalization for COPD. Chest. 2002;121(5):1441–8.
52. de Voogd JN, Wempe JB, Koeter GH, et al. Depressive symptoms as predictors of mortality in patients with COPD. Chest. 2009;135(3):619–25.

53. Fan VS, Ramsey SD, Giardino ND, et al. Sex, depression, and risk of hospitalization and mortality in chronic obstructive pulmonary disease. Arch Intern Med. 2007;167(21):2345–53.
54. Xu W, Collet JP, Shapiro S, et al. Independent effect of depression and anxiety on chronic obstructive pulmonary disease exacerbations and hospitalizations. Am J Respir Crit Care Med. 2008;178(9):913–20.
55. Yohannes AM. Depression and COPD in older people: a review and discussion. Br J Community Nurs. 2005;10(1):42–6.
56. Yohannes AM, Baldwin RC, Connolly M. Mortality predictors in disabling chronic obstructive pulmonary disease in old age. Age Ageing. 2002;31(2):137–40.
57. Ehlert U, Gaab J, Heinrichs M. Psychoneuroendocrinological contributions to the etiology of depression, posttraumatic stress disorder, and stress-related bodily disorders: the role of the hypothalamus-pituitary-adrenal axis. Biol Psychol. 2001;57(1–3):141–52.
58. Anisman H, Merali Z, Poulter MO, Hayley S. Cytokines as a precipitant of depressive illness: animal and human studies. Curr Pharm Des. 2005;11(8):963–72.
59. Whooley MA, de Jonge P, Vittinghoff E, et al. Depressive symptoms, health behaviors, and risk of cardiovascular events in patients with coronary heart disease. JAMA. 2008;300(20):2379–88.
60. Fan VS, Giardino ND, Blough DK, Kaplan RM, Ramsey SD. Costs of pulmonary rehabilitation and predictors of adherence in the National Emphysema Treatment Trial. COPD. 2008;5(2):105–16.
61. Decramer M, Gosselink R, Troosters T, Verschueren M, Evers G. Muscle weakness is related to utilization of health care resources in COPD patients. Eur Respir J. 1997;10(2):417–23.
62. Kessler R, Faller M, Fourgaut G, Mennecier B, Weitzenblum E. Predictive factors of hospitalization for acute exacerbation in a series of 64 patients with chronic obstructive pulmonary disease. Am J Respir Crit Care Med. 1999;159(1):158–64.
63. Fan VS, Curtis JR, Tu SP, McDonell MB, Fihn SD. Using quality of life to predict hospitalization and mortality in patients with obstructive lung diseases. Chest. 2002;122(2):429–36.
64. Fan VS, Ramsey SD, Make BJ, Martinez FJ. Physiologic variables and functional status independently predict COPD hospitalizations and emergency department visits in patients with severe COPD. COPD. 2007;4(1):29–39.
65. Niewoehner DE, Lokhnygina Y, Rice K, et al. Risk indexes for exacerbations and hospitalizations due to COPD. Chest. 2007;131(1):20–8.
66. Jennings JH, Digiovine B, Obeid D, Frank C. The association between depressive symptoms and acute exacerbations of COPD. Lung. 2009;187(2):128–35.
67. Yohannes AM, Baldwin RC, Connolly MJ. Depression and anxiety in elderly outpatients with chronic obstructive pulmonary disease: prevalence, and validation of the BASDEC screening questionnaire. Int J Geriatr Psychiatry. 2000;15(12):1090–6.
68. Gudmundsson G, Gislason T, Janson C, et al. Risk factors for rehospitalisation in COPD: role of health status, anxiety and depression. Eur Respir J. 2005;26(3):414–9.
69. Cao Z, Ong KC, Eng P, Tan WC, Ng TP. Frequent hospital readmissions for acute exacerbation of COPD and their associated factors. Respirology. 2006;11(2):188–95.
70. Laurin C, Labrecque M, Dupuis G, Bacon SL, Cartier A, Lavoie KL. Chronic obstructive pulmonary disease patients with psychiatric disorders are at greater risk of exacerbations. Psychosom Med. 2009;71(6):667–74.
71. Katon WJ. Clinical and health services relationships between major depression, depressive symptoms, and general medical illness. Biol Psychiatry. 2003;54(3):216–26.
72. Ciechanowski PS, Katon WJ, Russo JE. Depression and diabetes: impact of depressive symptoms on adherence, function, and costs. Arch Intern Med. 2000;160(21):3278–85.
73. Carney RM, Freedland KE, Eisen SA, Rich MW, Jaffe AS. Major depression and medication adherence in elderly patients with coronary artery disease. Health Psychol. 1995;14(1):88–90.
74. Nguyen HQ, Carrieri-Kohlman V. Dyspnea self-management in patients with chronic obstructive pulmonary disease: moderating effects of depressed mood. Psychosomatics. 2005;46(5):402–10.
75. Jerant A, Kravitz R, Moore-Hill M, Franks P. Depressive symptoms moderated the effect of chronic illness self-management training on self-efficacy. Med Care. 2008;46(5):523–31.

76. Porzelius J, Vest M, Nochomovitz M. Respiratory function, cognitions, and panic in chronic obstructive pulmonary patients. Behav Res Ther. 1992;30(1):75–7.
77. Laurin C, Lavoie KL, Bacon SL, et al. Sex differences in the prevalence of psychiatric disorders and psychological distress in patients with COPD. Chest. 2007;132(1):148–55.
78. Livermore N, Butler JE, Sharpe L, McBain RA, Gandevia SC, McKenzie DK. Panic attacks and perception of inspiratory resistive loads in chronic obstructive pulmonary disease. Am J Respir Crit Care Med. 2008;178(1):7–12.
79. Giardino ND, Curtis JL, Abelson JL, et al. The impact of panic disorder on interoception and dyspnea reports in chronic obstructive pulmonary disease. Biol Psychol. 2010;84(1):142–6.
80. Irwin MR, Miller AH. Depressive disorders and immunity: 20 years of progress and discovery. Brain Behav Immun. 2007;21(4):374–83.
81. Miller AH, Maletic V, Raison CL. Inflammation and its discontents: the role of cytokines in the pathophysiology of major depression. Biol Psychiatry. 2009;65(9):732–41.
82. Capuron L, Miller AH. Cytokines and psychopathology: lessons from interferon-alpha. Biol Psychiatry. 2004;56(11):819–24.
83. Dantzer R. Cytokine-induced sickness behaviour: a neuroimmune response to activation of innate immunity. Eur J Pharmacol. 2004;500(1–3):399–411.
84. Taylor JL, Grossberg SE. The effects of interferon-alpha on the production and action of other cytokines. Semin Oncol. 1998;25(1 Suppl 1):23–9.
85. Capuron L, Ravaud A. Prediction of the depressive effects of interferon alfa therapy by the patient's initial affective state. N Engl J Med. 1999;340(17):1370.
86. Booij L, Van der Does W, Benkelfat C, et al. Predictors of mood response to acute tryptophan depletion. A reanalysis. Neuropsychopharmacology. 2002;27(5):852–61.
87. Capuron L, Raison CL, Musselman DL, Lawson DH, Nemeroff CB, Miller AH. Association of exaggerated HPA axis response to the initial injection of interferon-alpha with development of depression during interferon-alpha therapy. Am J Psychiatry. 2003;160(7):1342–5.
88. O'Brien SM, Scott LV, Dinan TG. Antidepressant therapy and C-reactive protein levels. Br J Psychiatry. 2006;188:449–52.
89. Sutcigil L, Oktenli C, Musabak U, et al. Pro- and anti-inflammatory cytokine balance in major depression: effect of sertraline therapy. Clin Dev Immunol. 2007;2007:76396.
90. Taler M, Gil-Ad I, Lomnitski L, et al. Immunomodulatory effect of selective serotonin reuptake inhibitors (SSRIs) on human T lymphocyte function and gene expression. Eur Neuropsychopharmacol. 2007;17(12):774–80.
91. O'Brien SM, Scully P, Fitzgerald P, Scott LV, Dinan TG. Plasma cytokine profiles in depressed patients who fail to respond to selective serotonin reuptake inhibitor therapy. J Psychiatr Res. 2007;41(3–4):326–31.
92. Bremmer MA, Beekman AT, Deeg DJ, et al. Inflammatory markers in late-life depression: results from a population-based study. J Affect Disord. 2008;106(3):249–55.
93. Danner M, Kasl SV, Abramson JL, Vaccarino V. Association between depression and elevated C-reactive protein. Psychosom Med. 2003;65(3):347–56.
94. Ford DE, Erlinger TP. Depression and C-reactive protein in US adults: data from the Third National Health and Nutrition Examination Survey. Arch Intern Med. 2004;164(9):1010–4.
95. Lesperance F, Frasure-Smith N, Theroux P, Irwin M. The association between major depression and levels of soluble intercellular adhesion molecule 1, interleukin-6, and C-reactive protein in patients with recent acute coronary syndromes. Am J Psychiatry. 2004;161(2):271–7.
96. Miller GE, Freedland KE, Carney RM. Depressive symptoms and the regulation of proinflammatory cytokine expression in patients with coronary heart disease. J Psychosom Res. 2005;59(4):231–6.
97. Whooley MA, Caska CM, Hendrickson BE, Rourke MA, Ho J, Ali S. Depression and inflammation in patients with coronary heart disease: findings from the Heart and Soul Study. Biol Psychiatry. 2007;62(4):314–20.
98. Arbelaez JJ, Ariyo AA, Crum RM, Fried LP, Ford DE. Depressive symptoms, inflammation, and ischemic stroke in older adults: a prospective analysis in the cardiovascular health study. J Am Geriatr Soc. 2007;55(11):1825–30.

99. Gimeno D, Kivimaki M, Brunner EJ, et al. Associations of C-reactive protein and interleukin-6 with cognitive symptoms of depression: 12-year follow-up of the Whitehall II study. Psychol Med. 2009;39(3):413–23.

100. Quint JK, Baghai-Ravary R, Donaldson GC, Wedzicha JA. Relationship between depression and exacerbations in COPD. Eur Respir J. 2008;32(1):53–60.

101. Dalar L. Relation between depression and anxiety and inflammatory markers in stable COPD cases. Am J Respir Crit Care Med. 2008;177(Abstracts Issue):A826.

102. Incalzi RA, Chiappini F, Fuso L, Torrice MP, Gemma A, Pistelli R. Predicting cognitive decline in patients with hypoxaemic COPD. Respir Med. 1998;92(3):527–33.

103. Incalzi RA, Bellia V, Maggi S, et al. Mild to moderate chronic airways disease does not carry an excess risk of cognitive dysfunction. Aging Clin Exp Res. 2002;14(5):395–401.

104. Moore MC, Zebb BJ. The catastrophic misinterpretation of physiological distress. Behav Res Ther. 1999;37(11):1105–18.

105. Karajgi B, Rifkin A, Doddi S, Kolli R. The prevalence of anxiety disorders in patients with chronic obstructive pulmonary disease. Am J Psychiatry. 1990;147(2):200–1.

106. Glassman AH, O'Connor CM, Califf RM, et al. Sertraline treatment of major depression in patients with acute MI or unstable angina. JAMA. 2002;288(6):701–9.

107. Lesperance F, Frasure-Smith N, Koszycki D, et al. Effects of citalopram and interpersonal psychotherapy on depression in patients with coronary artery disease: the Canadian Cardiac Randomized Evaluation of Antidepressant and Psychotherapy Efficacy (CREATE) trial. JAMA. 2007;297(4):367–79.

108. Berkman LF, Blumenthal J, Burg M, et al. Effects of treating depression and low perceived social support on clinical events after myocardial infarction: the Enhancing Recovery in Coronary Heart Disease Patients (ENRICHD) Randomized Trial. JAMA. 2003;289(23):3106–16.

109. Argyropoulou P, Patakas D, Koukou A, Vasiliadis P, Georgopoulos D. Buspirone effect on breathlessness and exercise performance in patients with chronic obstructive pulmonary disease. Respiration. 1993;60(4):216–20.

110. de Godoy DV, de Godoy RF. A randomized controlled trial of the effect of psychotherapy on anxiety and depression in chronic obstructive pulmonary disease. Arch Phys Med Rehabil. 2003;84(8):1154–7.

111. Kunik ME, Veazey C, Cully JA, et al. COPD education and cognitive behavioral therapy group treatment for clinically significant symptoms of depression and anxiety in COPD patients: a randomized controlled trial. Psychol Med. 2008;38(3):385–96.

112. Hynninen MJ, Bjerke N, Pallesen S, Bakke PS, Nordhus IH. A randomized controlled trial of cognitive behavioral therapy for anxiety and depression in COPD. Respir Med. 2010;104(7):986–94.

113. Livermore N, Sharpe L, McKenzie D. Prevention of panic attacks and panic disorder in COPD. Eur Respir J. 2010;35(3):557–63.

114. Coventry PA, Gellatly JL. Improving outcomes for COPD patients with mild-to-moderate anxiety and depression: a systematic review of cognitive behavioural therapy. Br J Health Psychol. 2008;13(Pt 3):381–400.

115. Nici L, Donner C, Wouters E, et al. American Thoracic Society/European Respiratory Society statement on pulmonary rehabilitation. Am J Respir Crit Care Med. 2006;173(12):1390–413.

116. Emery CF, Schein RL, Hauck ER, MacIntyre NR. Psychological and cognitive outcomes of a randomized trial of exercise among patients with chronic obstructive pulmonary disease. Health Psychol. 1998;17(3):232–40.

117. Guell R, Resqueti V, Sangenis M, et al. Impact of pulmonary rehabilitation on psychosocial morbidity in patients with severe COPD. Chest. 2006;129(4):899–904.

118. Paz-Diaz H, Montes de Oca M, Lopez JM, Celli BR. Pulmonary rehabilitation improves depression, anxiety, dyspnea and health status in patients with COPD. Am J Phys Med Rehabil. 2007;86(1):30–6.

119. Griffiths TL, Burr ML, Campbell IA, et al. Results at 1 year of outpatient multidisciplinary pulmonary rehabilitation: a randomised controlled trial. Lancet. 2000;355(9201):362–8.
120. Coventry PA, Hind D. Comprehensive pulmonary rehabilitation for anxiety and depression in adults with chronic obstructive pulmonary disease: systematic review and meta-analysis. J Psychosom Res. 2007;63(5):551–65.
121. Yohannes AM, Connolly MJ, Baldwin RC. A feasibility study of antidepressant drug therapy in depressed elderly patients with chronic obstructive pulmonary disease. Int J Geriatr Psychiatry. 2001;16(5):451–4.
122. Davidson JR. Major depressive disorder treatment guidelines in America and Europe. J Clin Psychiatry. 2010;71(Suppl E1):e04.
123. Anderson IM, Ferrier IN, Baldwin RC, et al. Evidence-based guidelines for treating depressive disorders with antidepressants: a revision of the 2000 British Association for Psychopharmacology guidelines. J Psychopharmacol. 2008;22(4):343–96.
124. Pilling S, Anderson I, Goldberg D, Meader N, Taylor C. Depression in adults, including those with a chronic physical health problem: summary of NICE guidance. BMJ. 2009; 339:b4108.
125. Pirraglia PA, Charbonneau A, Kader B, Berlowitz DR. Adequate initial antidepressant treatment among patients with chronic obstructive pulmonary disease in a cohort of depressed veterans. Prim Care Companion J Clin Psychiatry. 2006;8(2):71–6.
126. Jordan N, Lee TA, Valenstein M, Weiss KB. Effect of care setting on evidence-based depression treatment for veterans with COPD and comorbid depression. J Gen Intern Med. 2007;22(10):1447–52.
127. Jordan N, Lee TA, Valenstein M, Pirraglia PA, Weiss KB. Effect of depression care on outcomes in COPD patients with depression. Chest. 2009;135(3):626–32.
128. Beck AT, Ward CH, Mendelson M, Mock J, Erbaugh J. An inventory for measuring depression. Arch Gen Psychiatry. 1961;4:561–71.
129. Beck AT, Steer RA, Garbin M. Psychometric properties of the Beck depression inventory: twenty-five years of evaluation. Clin Psychol Rev. 1988;8:77–100.
130. Beck AT, Steer RA. Beck Anxiety Inventory manual. San Antonio, TX: Psychological Corporation; 1990.
131. Adshead F, Cody DD, Pitt B. BASDEC: a novel screening instrument for depression in elderly medical inpatients. BMJ. 1992;305(6850):397.
132. Radloff L. The CES-D scale: a self-report depression scale for research in the general population. Appl Psychol Meas. 1977;1:385–401.
133. Andresen EM, Malmgren JA, Carter WB, Patrick DL. Screening for depression in well older adults: evaluation of a short form of the CES-D (Center for Epidemiologic Studies Depression Scale). Am J Prev Med. 1994;10(2):77–84.
134. Sheikh JI, Yesavage JA. Geriatric Depression Scale (GDS): recent evidence and development of a shoter version. In: Brink TL, editor. Clinical gerontology: a guide to assessment and intervention. New York: The Haworth Press; 1986. p. 165–73.
135. Copeland JR, Kelleher MJ, Kellett JM, et al. A semi-structured clinical interview for the assessment of diagnosis and mental state in the elderly: the Geriatric Mental State Schedule. I. Development and reliability. Psychol Med. 1976;6(3):439–49.
136. Hamilton M. A rating scale for depression. J Neurol Neurosurg Psychiatry. 1960;23:56–62.
137. Guy W. ECDEU assessment manual of psychopharmacology – revised. Rockville, MD: U.S. Department of Health E, and Welfare; 1976.
138. Kayahan B, Karapolat H, Atyntoprak E, Atasever A, Ozturk O. Psychological outcomes of an outpatient pulmonary rehabilitation program in patients with chronic obstructive pulmonary disease. Respir Med. 2006;100(6):1050–7.
139. Zigmond AS, Snaith RP. The hospital anxiety and depression scale. Acta Psychiatr Scand. 1983;67(6):361–70.
140. Montgomery SA, Asberg M. A new depression scale designed to be sensitive to change. Br J Psychiatry. 1979;134:382–9.

141. Snaith RP, Harrop FM, Newby DA, Teale C. Grade scores of the Montgomery-Asberg Depression and the Clinical Anxiety Scales. Br J Psychiatry. 1986;148:599–601.
142. Spielberger CE, Goruch RL. Manual for the state-trait anxiety inventory. Palo Alto, CA: Consulting Psychologists; 1970.
143. Kvaal K, Ulstein I, Nordhus IH, Engedal K. The Spielberger State-Trait Anxiety Inventory (STAI): the state scale in detecting mental disorders in geriatric patients. Int J Geriatr Psychiatry. 2005;20(7):629–34.
144. Derogatis L. The SCL-90-R manual-I. Baltimore, MD: Clinical Psychometrics Research; 1977.

Chapter 8
Cognitive Function

Paula Meek

Abstract Chronic obstructive pulmonary disease (COPD), as previously discussed in other chapters, is a chronic disease with systemic manifestations affecting individuals impairment in the lungs. The brain and associated cognitive functions are not exempt from the systemic effects of COPD. Cognitive function refers to several cognitive processes that influence an individual's ability to learn, remember, judge, decide, and plan. Deterioration of cognitive processes is known to be associated with age, but has not been as widely appreciated in chronic illnesses such as COPD. Alterations in cognitive function due to COPD are entwined with normal cognitive decline resulting from normal aging. This chapter reviews normal cognitive aging, cognitive function in COPD, common screening techniques used to detect cognitive changes, and treatment approaches.

Keywords COPD • Cognitive function • Systemic effects • Age • Chronic illness • Normal cognitive aging • Screening • Treatment

Introduction

Chronic obstructive pulmonary disease (COPD), as previously discussed in other chapters, is a chronic disease with systemic manifestations affecting individuals beyond the lungs. The brain and the associated cognitive functions are no exception to the systemic effects of COPD. Cognitive function refers to several cognitive processes that influence an individual's ability to learn, remember, judge, decide, and plan. Deterioration of cognitive processes is known to be associated with age, but has not been as widely appreciated in chronic illnesses such as COPD. Alterations in

P. Meek (✉)
Denver College of Nursing, University of Colorado, Aurora, CO, USA
e-mail: paula.meek@ucdenver.edu

L. Nici and R. ZuWallack (eds.), *Chronic Obstructive Pulmonary Disease: Co-Morbidities and Systemic Consequences*, Respiratory Medicine, DOI 10.1007/978-1-60761-673-3_8,
© Springer Science+Business Media, LLC 2012

cognitive function due to COPD are entwined with normal cognitive decline resulting from normal aging. This chapter reviews normal cognitive aging, cognitive function in COPD, common screening techniques used to detect cognitive changes, and treatment approaches.

Cognitive Changes Associated with Aging

In aging, many physiologic changes are seen such as increased atherosclerosis, higher blood pressure, increased risk of cardiovascular disease, increased thickness of the left ventricular wall, increased myocardial stiffness, reduced estrogen (females) and testosterone (males), increased insulin resistance, loss of lung elasticity and capacity, and increasing difficulty oxygenating blood, to name a few. There are many neurological responses to aging including slower reaction time, deterioration in memory, and increased insomnia. Undoubtedly, these changes associated with normal aging are intertwined with changes that may result from COPD itself. Therefore, neither the unique cognitive changes that can be attributed to COPD exclusively nor the exact mechanisms for these changes are known. What is known is that COPD patients may suffer a greater burden in cognitive changes than patients with other chronic diseases (exclusive of those directly affecting the brain, such as Alzheimer's disease). This greater burden may be due to the disproportionate effect of COPD on oxygenation than many other chronic illnesses.

Deterioration in cerebral blood flow, flow velocity, and volume within the intracerebral arteries has been noted with age [1], along with reduced hemodynamic response to brain activity [2, 3]. These changes, when coupled with normal cardiovascular changes, can diminish the ability of the cerebral vessels to react to carbon dioxide and maintain oxygenation. There is, however, minimal neuron loss with normal aging, indicating that changes are not due to actual loss in the basic functional unit, the neuron.

These physiological changes may be important to functional outcomes, but have not been clearly linked to specific cognitive changes. Cognitive alterations are typically evaluated by neuropsychological testing. There are a many common cognitive changes with normal aging that have been identified using these standard neuropsychological tests (Table 8.1). Cognitive domains that can be examined using neuropsychological testing include mental status, attention, executive function, memory, expressive functions (language), and visuospatial functioning. These tests are standardized for age, and education to allow comparisons across individuals.

Neuropsychological testing has demonstrated that general mental status declines with age, but the rate and amount of decline is highly variable across individuals [4]. The ability of an individual to focus their attention is relatively unaffected with age, but selective or divided attention (Table 8.1) along with switching tasks, is decreased in the elderly [4–6]. Language skills, in terms of linguistic rules and semantic knowledge, are unaffected, but word "finding" decreases with age [7]. Visuospatial functioning measured in terms of mental rotation and figure copying or visuospatial construction decline more rapidly than verbal skills and abilities [8].

Table 8.1 Changes in cognitive domains with aging

Domain	Description	Changes seen with aging
Mental status	General cognitive status including memory, attention, and other cognitive functions. Influenced by age, education, and intelligence	Declines, rate, and amount are extremely variable
Attention		
Sustained	Ability to maintain focus and alertness	Relatively unaffected
Selective	Ability to focus on relevant information while inhibiting information irrelevant to the task	Decreased leading to increased disinhibition and distractibility
Divided	Ability to focus on multiple tasks or topics	Elderly particularly susceptible
Task switching	Ability to switch quickly between different tasks or skills	Decreased – complex tasks are worse
Executive function	Higher-order cognitive functions involved in self-management and regulation of behaviors. Influences organization and use of large amounts of information	Decreased – especially with tasks such as assessing, planning, and verbal fluency
Memory		
Working	Not short-term memory, however working memory requires manipulation and processing of information dictating greater use of cognitive resources. A key component of executive function	Decreased – worse with increased complexity of the task (e.g., requires simultaneously remembering and calculating)
Episodic	Recollection of experienced based events	Declines
Semantic	Stored factual information	Increases
Auto-biographical	Stored information about self- and life events	Becomes more semantic and factual
Flash bulb	Specific type of autobiographical memory with vivid recall of a situation that has strong emotional meaning (e.g., recall of the Challenger Space Shuttle explosion)	Unaffected
Implicit (procedural)	Memory where previous incident, situation or episode implicitly affects behavior without deliberate memory recovery or specific awareness of the incident	Unaffected
Prospective	Remembering to carry out future tasks that can be time or event based ("remember to remember")	Declines
Recollection	Effortful retrieval of specific contextual information	Slower processing
Familiarity	A feeling of recognition without appropriate details	Unaffected – but more reliance on this form of memory
False	Recall of an event or specific details of an event that did not occur	More susceptible to false memories

(continued)

Table 8.1 (continued)

Domain	Description	Changes seen with aging
Source	Recall of specifics (social, temporal, and spatial) of how a memory was obtained	Declines
Language	General linguistic rules and semantic knowledge	Unaffected
Word finding	Ability to name or retrieve a specific word	Declines
Visuospatial functioning	Ability to visualize spatial patterns and mentally manipulate them, including mental rotation, visuospatial construction, figure copying	Declines – more rapidly than verbal skills

Most commonly, the cognitive changes associated with aging, center around memory loss, or the stereotype of the "forgetful" older person. However, not all forms of memory naturally decline with age. Recall of events, in terms of semantic, "flash bulb," implicit, and autobiographical memory, are relatively unaffected with age (Table 8.1). In fact, semantic memory, or the storage of factual information, is known to increase with age [4]. Working memory is associated with simultaneously manipulating and processing of information, is known to decrease with aging, particularly in relation to highly complex task that may be associated with intricate medication regimens (e.g., inhaler use). Prospective memory, or the ability to remember to carry out tasks in the future, also declines with age. While familiarity with a situation or event is relatively unaffected, there is more reliance on familiarity, as a form of recall memory and this makes elderly more susceptible to false memories or errors in recollection [9]. Source memory, the ability to recall specifics of how the individual obtained recall of an event or fact, also declines with age. While memory changes are known to occur with aging, these changes/alterations in memory appear to be linked more specifically to the individual's ability to process and manipulate information. As a result, the majority of individuals, as they age, will develop strategies and approaches to deal (often by compensation) with many of these typical cognitive changes. Often these strategies are not detectable to others, but seamlessly allow them to carry out the activities of daily life.

The Brain, Cognitive Function, and COPD

There are specific changes that occur with aging that bear on alterations seen in the individuals with COPD. These changes include brain cortical atrophy [10], alterations in cerebral hemodynamics and cellular metabolism. Brain magnetic resonance imaging studies have found decreased cerebral hemisphere volume, in both the frontal and temporoparietal region area. This chapter does not propose to discuss all possible mechanisms that contribute to cognitive changes in COPD, as studies to date have not been able to delineate the mechanisms for these changes. This is especially the case since cognitive function is not routinely evaluated nor is it

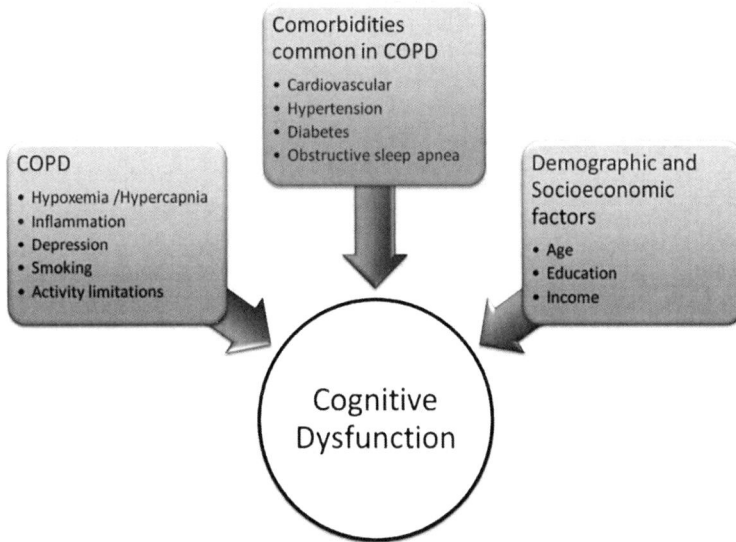

Fig. 8.1 Schema of major factors likely contributing to cognitive dysfunction in COPD patients

reported in studies of COPD. However, a general schematic of the major problems that are believed to contribute to cognitive dysfunction in COPD patients are illustrated in Fig. 8.1. This schema is proposed to summarize the factors that have been raised as contributing to the occurrence of cognitive dysfunction.

In addition to the changes resulting from normal aging, it is important to keep in mind that the systemic impact of COPD can add to or accelerate the cognitive changes that might be seen. No doubt, the most important and common effects on cognition in COPD are related to the changes in oxygen and carbon dioxide levels in the blood. We know that prolonged or sustained changes in both oxygen and carbon dioxide are so critical to life that the body compensates for any changes (e.g., increase ventilation and shunting of blood from hypoxic areas) to maintain homeostasis. It is not clear that the extent to which minor or transient changes in oxygen or carbon dioxide levels affect the brain tissue. Are the changes temporary or do they result in chronic changes, resulting in long-term cognitive dysfunction?

There are recent investigations in oxygenation that provide some evidence of potential long-term issues with hypoxemia impacting the brain. A recent study in rats found that even relatively transient drops in arterial saturation level in the systemic circulation (just below 85% SaO_2) due to a short apneic event, resulted in much more significant drops in the brain tissue oxygen saturation, requiring up to 60 min to fully recover [11]. In a human study, oxygen desaturation with activity provided evidence of brain tissue damage related to "increased frontal choline, which in turn was associated with subcortical white matter attenuation" [12]. The results of these studies suggest that transient drops in oxygenation may cause important acute changes at the tissue level. The clinical significance of these changes, however, has not as yet been determined. Consequently, as research moves forward and we are better able to understand how reductions in oxygenation (or increases in carbon dioxide) affect brain tissue, we will hopefully better understand changes that occur in the cognitive function as a result of COPD. Much work needs to be done on the effects of both hypoxemia and carbon dioxide on brain activity and the subsequent impact of these changes on cognitive function.

Inflammation from the systemic effects of COPD is known to have an impact on cognitive function. Some proteins are, in fact, known to be neurotoxic. Specifically, C-reactive protein has been found to have a direct neurotoxic effect and to contribute to cerebral atherosclerosis [13]. Further, tumor necrosis factor-α, alpha1-antichymotrypsin, as well as interleukin-6 and interleukin-1β have been associated with cognitive dysfunction [12, 14]. It seems fair to say that the presence of chronic inflammation in the COPD patient impacts dysfunction. Precisely how this occurs and what domains of cognition are affected are unclear.

Added to this, individuals with COPD frequently have comorbidities that have been linked to changes in cognitive function. Diabetes, for example, is associated with executive function alterations [15] and vascular risk factors have been associated with general mental status and information processing deficits [16]. At this point in our understanding, it is not possible to totally determine the contribution of comorbidities versus the underling systemic issues associated with COPD. However, it is evident from the literature that hypoxemia, inflammation, vascular disease, and smoking all can lead to damage in neuronal activity and function [16].

The purpose of the next section is to review the occurrence of cognitive dysfunction in COPD, identify what specific cognitive functions have been examined, how they were examined and whether they were found to be different than healthy individuals.

Occurrence of Cognitive Dysfunction in COPD

Some of the first reports of deficits in cognitive function in COPD patients were from the nocturnal oxygen therapy (NOTT) trial [17]. In this trial, neuropsychological testing documented a greater percentage (42%) of moderate cognitive deficits in the COPD group when compared with the controls (14%). In examining these deficits more closely by severity of hypoxemia, it was found that a greater percentage (62%) occurred among those with severe COPD [18]. These numbers remain some of our best estimates of prevalence that we have in the chronically hypoxemic individuals with COPD. However, a recent review reported that even when including individuals with COPD who had mild to no hypoxemia, between 89 and 96% of individuals studied had some degree of cognitive dysfunction [16]. The cognitive dysfunction included 89% verbal or language issues and 96% with attention deficits. From the first reports in the 1980s to the present time, there are clear indications that cognitive dysfunction is an issue in the COPD population, although formal prevalence data do not exist. It is important to note that frequently, cognitive function is not assessed in this population, nor is mentioned in leading respiratory medicine text [19] as a possible complication or associated comorbid condition. Our understanding of cognitive function in the COPD patient is in many ways, in its infancy.

Specific Cognitive Dysfunction

In this section, several important investigations will be reviewed to help provide a detailed look at the specific cognitive dysfunction that has been detected. The findings of the studies that will be reviewed are summarized in Table 8.2. In general, it can be seen that some studies (noted by large, dark diamonds) have consistently demonstrated large improvements in cognitive function than others. These differences can usually be accounted for by more recent studies, using more robust methods of measuring cognition.

As mentioned previously, the first prominent standard neurophysiological testing was done in association with the NOTT [17, 20] studies. In the original study, it is important to note that the inclusion criteria were set so that individuals who participated had to be hypoxemic (mean PaO_2 51 mmHg) compared with healthy controls. The COPD group was found to have important cognitive dysfunction in almost all areas tested, but particularly with what was labeled at the time as abstracting ability, complex perceptual motor skills, and simple motor tasks. When the testing is closely examined, we would say that compared with the healthy controls, that sustained and selective attention, executive function, working memory and recollection as well as verbal memory and visuospatial functioning were all found to be dysfunctional. The next notable study completed at about that same time was the Intermittent Positive Pressure Breathing (IPPB) trial [21]. While the individuals with COPD who participated in this trial were not hypoxemic (mean PaO_2 66 mmHg), they still demonstrated important cognitive dysfunction when compared with matched controls with milder COPD. Particularly, sustained attention measured by digit symbol test used to test divided attention, trail making part B now recognized as a measure of executive function [22], and verbal and nonverbal memory measured by the Wechsler Adult Intelligence Scale (WAIS) were all found to be reduced compared with the normal controls. In a follow-up study that combined the samples of these two investigations, differences remained between control subjects and individuals with even mild hypoxemia on the verbal and nonverbal immediate recall memory and the digit symbol test [20]. In this combined sample, the group with the most severe hypoxemia (PaO_2 44.4±4.1 mmHg) were found to have notable cognitive function decline in 18 (51%) of the 35 neuropsychological tests reported.

An early but small study of 66 stable individuals with COPD, cerebral deficits on several neuropsychological tests were also found [23]. Although the cognitive deficits were present, they were generally small, and considered by the authors to be similar to that of chronic alcoholism in that complex skills (including memory and motor skills) produced the greatest deficits. A multiple regression revealed that divided attention (symbol digit test), motor functioning and processing speed were significantly ($R^2 = 0.63$) related to partial pressure of arterial oxygen. The authors in a follow-up study were able to follow 62 of the individuals with COPD from the original study for 3 years to examine survival. Individuals who survived scored significantly ($p < 0.01$) higher on the neuropsychological tests than those who had died,

Table 8.2 Changes in cognitive domains with COPD identified from the literature reviewed

Domain	References							
	[17, 20]	[23, 30]	[21]	[24, 32–34]	[26, 29, 31]	[25]	[28, 29]	[27]
Mental status	•	•	•	◆	•	◆	◆	◆
Attention								
Sustained	•	•	•			◆	◆	◆ ◆
Selective	•		•		•	◆		
Divided					•	◆	◆	
Task switching								
Executive function	•	•	•	◆	◆	◆		◆
Memory								
Working	•			•	◆	◆	◆	◆
Episodic	•			• •	• ◆	◆ ◆		
Semantic	•	•	•		◆	◆	•	
Auto-biographical								
Flash bulb								
Implicit (procedural)				•				
Prospective								
Recollection	•		•	• •	◆ ◆	•		
Familiarity	•		•	• •	◆	◆		
Verbal memory				◆	•			
				◆	◆	◆		
Language				◆				
Visuospatial functioning	•	•	◆					•

•, small or no differences noted; ◆, larger difference noted; =, not tested

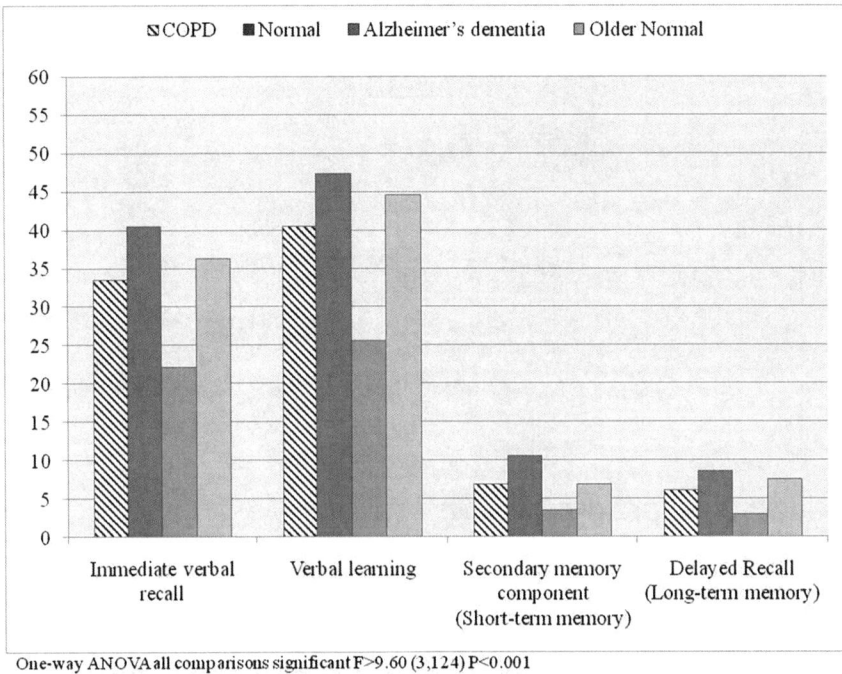

One-way ANOVA all comparisons significant F>9.60 (3,124) P<0.001

Fig. 8.2 Differences in neuropsychological tests in COPD, older normals, Alzheimer's, and elderly normals

with the Benton Visual Motor Retention Test (visual-constructive abilities and processing speed) and the digit symbol test (divided attention and processing speed) of the WAIS, important components of the higher scores on the test battery. The combined evidence from these early investigations supports that it is now anticipated that important cognitive dysfunction could be expected over the course of the disease. Specifically, divided attention and verbal and nonverbal memory deficits consistently were found. Executive function, measured by the trail making test, was also reported as showing impairment and could have important implications for self-care and medication management.

These early studies fueled further research and debate on what cognitive function issues are potentially altered through the course of the disease. Several later studies warrant further discussion. In 1997, Incazli and colleagues [24] closely examined verbal memory using a standardized neuropsychological test battery the Mental Deterioration Battery (MDB) with four known groups. The groups were individuals with stable hypoxic and hypercapnic COPD (age range 62–76), normal age-matched (age range 67–72) individuals, Alzheimer patients (age range 65–76), and older normal (age range 76–79). Verbal memory and learning as well as short- and long-term memory scores were significantly $(F > 9.60 (3,124) P < 0.001)$ worse for individuals with COPD than the age-matched normal individuals, but better than individuals with Alzheimer's dementia (Fig. 8.2). The scores for individuals with

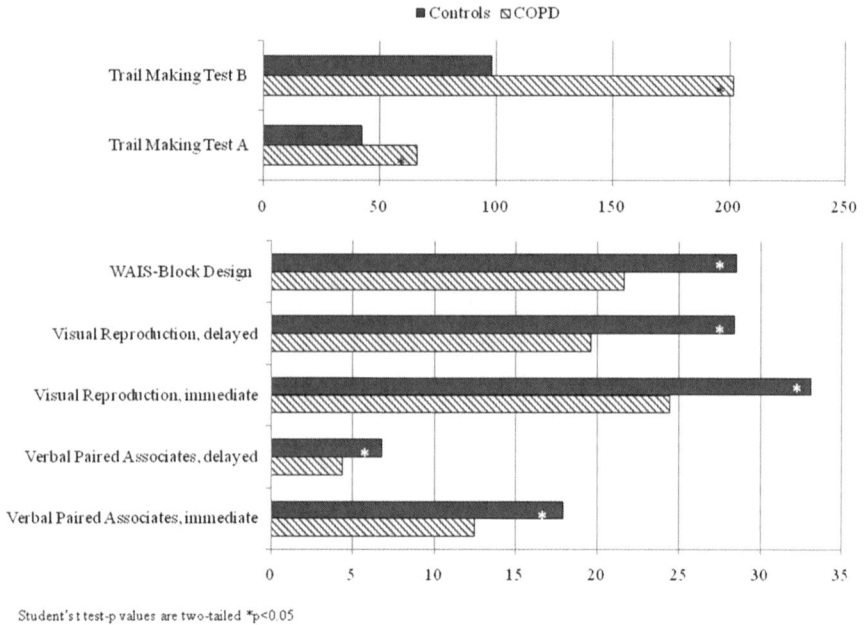

■ Controls ▨ COPD

Student's t test-p values are two-tailed *p<0.05

Fig. 8.3 Differences in scores on tests verbal and visual memory, trail making tests, and WAIS block design

COPD were slightly worse than older normal individuals, but this difference was not significant on post hoc analysis. The important issue again is that when individuals with COPD cognitive function are compared with age-matched controls for verbal and nonverbal memory, they are found to have important deficits. These deficits are similar to normal individuals, 10 years older.

These findings were supported by another small trial ($n = 20$) with the main purpose of determining if improvements could be seen in cognitive function after 3 months of supplemental oxygen [25]. Again a complex battery of neuropsychological test was used including the WAIS, trail making test, simple reaction time (RT), and Complex Choice RT from the California Computerized Assessment Package, immediate recall and 30 min delayed recall subtests from the Wechsler Memory Scale-Revised (WMS-R) and motor functioning: grooved pegboard test. At baseline, the comparison of the hypoxemic ($PaO_2 < 7.3$ kPa) COPD group to age-, gender-, and education-matched healthy controls, demonstrated significantly ($p < 0.05$) lower neuropsychological scores on 10 of the 20 tests. As reported in many of the previous studies, important differences were found on verbal and visual memory tests, trail making test A and B, and WAIS subtest block design (Fig. 8.3). Complex reaction times and motor functioning were also different between controls and COPD individuals, indicating important deficits in processing speed and motor functioning. Despite the small sample, the careful matching and the similar findings from prior work, add to the clear message that there are important cognitive deficits that are seen in individuals with COPD.

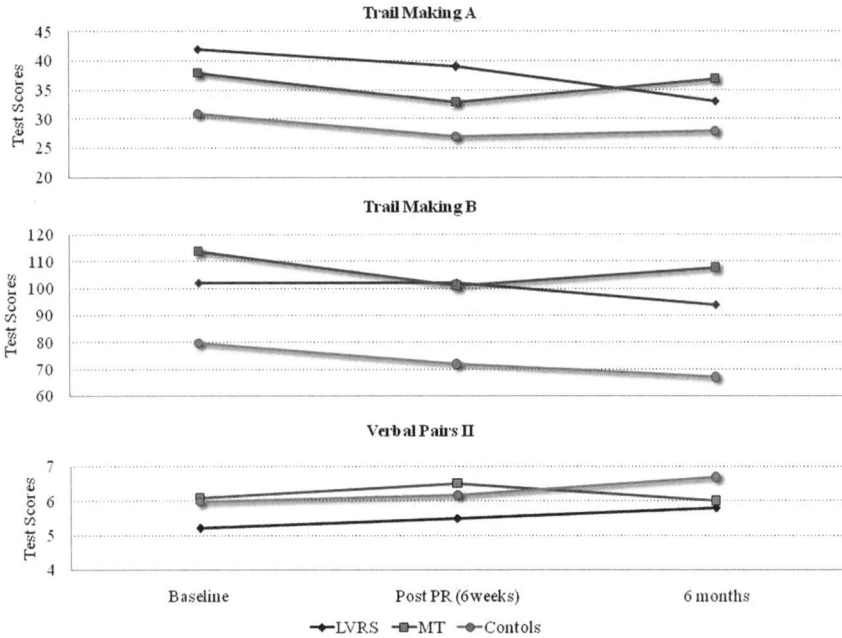

Fig. 8.4 Differences at baseline, 6 weeks, and 6 months on neurospychological tests in the NETT

Another notable documentation of cognitive dysfunction was seen in the National Emphysema Treatment trial (NETT) where age-, gender-, and education-matched COPD patients were compared with healthy individuals [26]. In this study, again an extensive standardized neuropsychological battery (20 tests in total) was used that included the revised WAIS, the Wechsler Memory Scales, trail making test, and the visuospatial clock drawing test, to name a few of the individual test scores obtained. Once COPD individuals had completed a 6-week pulmonary rehabilitation program, they were randomized to lung volume reduction surgery (LVRS) or ongoing medical treatment (MT). Both the LVRS and MT groups were compared with healthy controls to help evaluate the practice effect of repeated neuropsychological testing over the three time periods of baseline, postpulmonary rehabilitation, and 6 months postrandomization. Close examination of both COPD groups at baseline reveals that on many of the neuropsychological tests, cognitive deficits were seen when compared with the healthy controls, although baseline differences were not statistically analyzed. Longitudinal analysis controlling for practice effects revealed significant improvement ($p < 0.05$) in the LVRS group compared with the MT group at 6 months on trail making A test (psychomotor speed) and verbal pairs II (delayed verbal recall) with a trend ($p = 0.053$) toward improved performance on trail making B test (executive function) (Fig. 8.4). The changes seen were in areas that consistently are reported as potential areas where cognitive dysfunction has been reported.

Finally, two recent investigations have also identified important differences in verbal memory and attention. The first of these investigations used newer computerized reaction time task designed, to assess alerting, orienting, and executive functions of attention, along with fluid intelligence measured by standard progressive matrices [27]. Fluid intelligence has been defined as the ability to think and reason abstractly and solve problems and is similar to executive function. In this investigation, individuals with COPD ($n=50$) were compared with age-, gender-, and education-matched healthy controls ($n=50$). All measured neuropsychological tests, with the exception of the test, conflict reaction time, were found to be significantly ($p<0.05$) worse in the COPD group when analyzed using student's t-test. In this analysis, effect sizes were calculated with the largest effect size (−3.4 CI: −3.94 to −2.84) associated with the poor performance of COPD individuals on fluid intelligence.

The second recent investigation was conducted in a very large sample, with a general neuropsychological screening instrument [28]. This investigation used data from the Health and Retirement Study, a national prospective biennial (1996, 1998, 2000, 2002, etc.) survey of Americans over age 50 sponsored by the National Institute on Aging. The cognitive measure used was a 35 item survey with similar questions as the mini-mental state exam (MMSE) that was developed for use in this ongoing national survey [29]. The measure has nine components: immediate and delayed recall, serial 7 s (which requires working memory), identification of dates, counting backward, and various naming of objects and people. This investigation used individuals with 6 years of cognitive testing, and created groups based on self-report of disease severity. Previous work with this cognitive measure has been done that identified a 0.26 drop/year, over a 7-year period, associated with serious declines in independent living such as money and medication management. In this investigation, a drop of 0.90 (95% CI 0.60–1.2, $p<.001$) was associated with individuals with severe COPD, defined as those with oxygen dependence or disease-related activity limitations over the 6 years analyzed. While this decline was not quite at a rate of serious declines in independent living function, it does demonstrate clear declines over time, and the potential implications of problems with self-management.

The investigations reviewed here present a very vibrant picture of the potential for important cognitive dysfunction in individuals with COPD. A potential model of the impact that cognitive dysfunction may have on individuals with COPD in the areas of self-management, health maintenance, and health status and is presented in Fig. 8.5. Deficits with trail making test part B were seen in several studies, along with marked decline in fluid intelligence in a recent investigation. These deficits are associated with declines in higher-order cognitive functions involved in self-management and regulation of behaviors such as medication management. Compounding the self-management issue is the consistent finding of deficits in verbal memory or verbal learning that have been identified. In other words, it can be extremely difficult for individuals with COPD to recall verbal instructions about medication or self-management. Finally, the difficulties in cognitive function have been associated with declines in independent living functions. All of these issues ultimately impact the patient's quality of life and can affect morbidity and mortality.

Fig. 8.5 Potential impact
cascade of cognitive
dysfunction in COPD patients

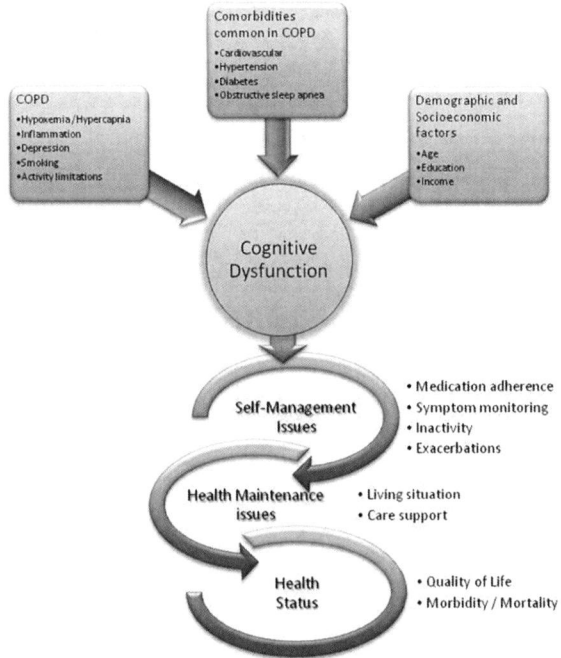

Treatment Approach

The treatment approaches available are quite limited. It is believed that higher levels
of education protect against dementia, a fact that has led to the "reserve hypothesis"
of brain aging [4]. One prediction of the reserve hypothesis is that, among elderly
individuals with similar age-related brain changes, those with more education would
demonstrate less cognitive impairment than those with less education. However,
what is not clear is if ongoing education could also have this impact. Consequently
for the purposes of this chapter, we review only three main treatment options that
have been investigated in individuals with COPD, namely oxygen supplementation,
pulmonary rehabilitation, and cognitive training.

Oxygen

Several early studies suggested a strong correlation between degree of hypoxemia
and cognitive function [23, 30]; however, other studies have not found the same
relationship [17, 31].

In a follow-up study to NOTT, individuals were given either nocturnal or continuous
oxygen supplementation for 6 months with cognitive function measured with the
Halstead-Reitan battery. The Halstead-Reitan battery is a formal neuropsychological

battery that assesses several specific cognitive skills and abilities, such as conceptual and problem-solving skills, attention, verbal and nonverbal learning and memory, visuoconstructional skills, and a variety of sensory-perceptual and motor abilities [22]. The authors did not find important differences in cognitive function between those who were on continuous and nocturnal oxygen supplementation, but there were important differences compared with the untreated normal subjects. Specifically, the amount of change/improvement from baseline in those receiving supplemental oxygenation and healthy normal subjects was significantly different in the trail making test, a measure of attention and problem solving, and the finger-tapping test, a measure of self-directed motor skills. The trail making test has been linked to executive function performance or the ability to execute and modify a plan, while the finger-tapping test is said to be predictive of daily living skills in the elderly [22]. This initial group of investigations was the foundation of our understanding concerning cognitive dysfunction in those individual with COPD who are hypoxemic and potential benefits of oxygen supplementation. To date, this trial has longest follow-up (12 months), but one investigation has reported anecdotal improvement as early as 3-months [25], while others have reported little improvement.

Pulmonary Rehabilitation

Pulmonary rehabilitation has been investigated as treatment that can benefit cognitive function [26, 32, 33]. As mentioned earlier in the chapter, improvements were seen in cognitive function during the NETT trial, although the final end point was LVRS and analysis was not done on the benefits of pulmonary rehabilitation. Reexamination of Fig. 8.4 with a focus on the MT group will show that there was a pattern of improvement in the trail making tests postrehabilitation that unfortunately was not sustained at 6 months. This is consistent with one of the first investigations was an in-depth comprehensive program that required individuals to attend daily for 30 days and also captured important cognitive neuropsychological tests including the trail making test, WAIS digit symbol, and the tapping test [33]. Sixty-four individuals with COPD but unfortunately there was not a control group. In this investigation, improvement in all cognitive tests was seen upon completion of the pulmonary rehabilitation program. A MANOVA was used, with the trail making tests (A and B) along with digit symbol as the multivariate outcome and examining for a gender effect. A significant main effect ($F[3,56] = 34.39$, $p < 0.001$) of the pulmonary rehabilitation was seen as well as a significant gender main effect ($F[3,55] = 2.87$, $p < 0.05$), although no interaction was found. Univariate examination of the gender effect indicated that males improved more on trail making B and digit symbol but that women also improve on these measures. The results of the MANOVA when the tapping test with the dominant hand was analyzed had similar results for improvement by both genders and men preforming better on the test than women. In an additional investigation that followed using a waitlist control group and an intervention without exercise, the majority of the findings were confirmed [34].

The COPD individuals participating in the program improving the other two groups for trail making and WAIS digit symbol tests.

The findings of improvements in cognitive function have been validated in another small controlled trial of pulmonary rehabilitation where 30 individuals with COPD were compared with healthy controls and COPD individuals not undergoing rehabilitation [32]. The report in the literature was a very brief report so some details are missing. However, using ANCOVA and post hoc analysis, significant group differences were found on a sustained visual attention test the digit vigilance test ($p=0.006$), and a verbal test of word fluency ($p=0.04$) scores with those COPD undergoing pulmonary rehabilitation making the greatest improvements.

One other study is worth mentioning in this context [35]. In this investigation while it was not a look at the effect of a comprehensive pulmonary rehabilitation program, the study was designed to determine associations between cognitive performance and aerobic fitness measured by 6 min walk. This cross-sectional study measures were obtained during baseline testing in individuals with COPD who had agreed to participate in an exercise intervention. Not all neuropsychological tests were performed on all individuals to cut down on the measurement burden. Individuals were randomly assigned to a fluid intelligence ($n=60$), processing speed ($n=34$), or working memory span ($n=29$) test. Regression analysis was used to determine the predictors of cognitive tests with education and depression entering the equation first to control for those relationships. The performance on the 6 min walk ($F[1,56]=15.27$) accounted for 17% of the variance in fluid intelligence with age ($F[1,55]=7.52$) another 8% of the variance. On the speed-of-processing task, the 6 min walk ($F[1,30]=8.17$) again contributed an important portion of the explained variance (20%), with maximum voluntary ventilation ($F[1,29]=5.81$) contributing 16%, and age ($F[1,28]=5.26$) another 10%. Forced expiratory volume was the only variable that contributed ($F[1,25]=6.37$) to the explaining the variance (18%) of working memory span. These findings support our understanding that the exercise component is an important piece of the cognitive improvements that may result from pulmonary rehabilitation. It is important to note that more quality research is needed on how pulmonary rehabilitation may improve cognitive function. It is conceivable that improvements in cognitive functions such as executive function might help to improve self-management skills and potentially assist in sustaining the other substantial benefits of pulmonary rehabilitation.

Cognitive Training

There is only one formal investigation of cognitive training as a treatment for cognitive dysfunction in COPD [36]. The aim of the investigation was not to directly improve but to preserve cognitive abilities in individuals with hypoxemic COPD with cognitive training. A total of 105 individuals with COPD who were free from dementia but with at rest or effort induced hypoxemia. The neuropsychological testing was carried out using the MDB at baseline, after 1.5, 4, and 6 months.

The individuals were randomized to multidimensional care with ($n = 53$) or without ($n = 52$) cognitive retraining but included standardization of pharmacological therapy, health education, selection of inhalers according to patient's ability, and comprehensive pulmonary rehabilitation, oxygen therapy, and a control visits. The cognitive training targeted learning, logical-deductive thinking, and stimulating attention. The repeated measures ANOVA showed no statistically significant changes in cognitive performance. It is a disappointing finding that cognitive training seems ineffective in individuals with COPD. It is important to note that in the many of the investigations reviewed that deteriorations in cognitive function was not seen at 6 months and to effectively target preserving function may require extensive longitudinal measurement.

Summary

COPD patients are often older, suffering from the natural declines in cognition from aging. The COPD patient, at an even earlier age than healthy individuals, is also affected by disease-related issues such as hypoxemia, hypercapnea, potential neurotoxic effects of chronic inflammation, and the numerous consequences of smoking from cardiovascular disease and comorbidities. The management of COPD relies on self-management (or at the very least, the ability to understand instructions) for control of symptoms, medication management, and exacerbation prevention and treatment. Cognitive issues complicate the standard approaches to helping these patients manage their disease. We assume all COPD patients understand and retain verbal instructions. This chapter raises many questions in terms of our expectations of these patients to receive and process information we provide.

In terms of identifying the magnitude of cognitive issues and the specific changes induced by hypoxemia, we have only touched "the tip of the iceberg" in our current understanding. Future studies in COPD should address systematically, both in the laboratory and clinical setting, the impact of COPD on patients. Without this information, we will only see the process described in Fig. 8.1 and never understand the important issues described, but still poorly understood in Fig. 8.5, self-management, health maintenance, and maximizing health status.

References

1. Grady CL. Age-related differences in face processing: a meta-analysis of three functional neuroimaging experiments. Can J Exp Psychol. 2002;56(3):208–20.
2. Madden DJ et al. Aging and recognition memory: changes in regional cerebral blood flow associated with components of reaction time distributions. J Cogn Neurosci. 1999;11(5):511–20.
3. Grady CL et al. The effects of age on the neural correlates of episodic encoding. Cereb Cortex. 1999;9(8):805–14.

4. Drag LL, Bieliauskas LA. Contemporary review 2009: cognitive aging. J Geriatr Psychiatry Neurol. 2010;23(2):75–93.
5. Kray J, Lindenberger U. Adult age differences in task switching. Psychol Aging. 2000; 15(1):126–47.
6. Mayr U, Kliegl R. Task-set switching and long-term memory retrieval. J Exp Psychol Learn Mem Cogn. 2000;26(5):1124–40.
7. Mortensen L, Meyer AS, Humphreys GW. Age-related effects on speech production: a review. Lang Cogn Process. 2006;21:238–90.
8. Coffey CE et al. Cognitive correlates of human brain aging: a quantitative magnetic resonance imaging investigation. J Neuropsychiatry Clin Neurosci. 2001;13(4):471–85.
9. Bastin C, Van der Linden M. The contribution of recollection and familiarity to recognition memory: a study of the effects of test format and aging. Neuropsychology. 2003;17(1): 14–24.
10. Grady CL et al. Age-related changes in cortical blood flow activation during visual processing of faces and location. J Neurosci. 1994;14(3 Pt 2):1450–62.
11. Almendros I et al. Changes in oxygen partial pressure of brain tissue in an animal model of obstructive apnea. Respir Res. 2010;11:3.
12. Borson S et al. Modeling the impact of COPD on the brain. Int J Chron Obstruct Pulmon Dis. 2008;3(3):429–34.
13. Duong T, Acton PJ, Johnson RA. The in vitro neuronal toxicity of pentraxins associated with Alzheimer's disease brain lesions. Brain Res. 1998;813(2):303–12.
14. Engelhart MJ et al. Inflammatory proteins in plasma and the risk of dementia: the rotterdam study. Arch Neurol. 2004;61(5):668–72.
15. Kuo HK et al. Effect of blood pressure and diabetes mellitus on cognitive and physical functions in older adults: a longitudinal analysis of the advanced cognitive training for independent and vital elderly cohort. J Am Geriatr Soc. 2005;53(7):1154–61.
16. Dodd JW, Getov SV, Jones PW. Cognitive function in COPD. Eur Respir J. 2010;35(4): 913–22.
17. Grant I et al. Neuropsychologic findings in hypoxemic chronic obstructive pulmonary disease. Arch Intern Med. 1982;142(8):1470–6.
18. Grant I et al. Progressive neuropsychologic impairment and hypoxemia. Relationship in chronic obstructive pulmonary disease. Arch Gen Psychiatry. 1987;44(11):999–1006.
19. Mason RJ et al. Murray and Nadel's textbook of respiratory medicine. 5th ed. Philadelphia: Sanders Elsiver; 2010.
20. Heaton RK et al. Psychologic effects of continuous and nocturnal oxygen therapy in hypoxemic chronic obstructive pulmonary disease. Arch Intern Med. 1983;143(10):1941–7.
21. Prigatano GP et al. Neuropsychological test performance in mildly hypoxemic patients with chronic obstructive pulmonary disease. J Consult Clin Psychol. 1983;51(1):108–16.
22. Strauss E, Sherman EMS, Spreen O. A compedium of neuropsychological test: administration, norms, and commentary. 3rd ed. New York: Oxford University Press; 2006.
23. Fix AJ et al. Neuropsychological deficits among patients with chronic obstructive pulmonary disease. Int J Neurosci. 1982;16(2):99–105.
24. Incalzi RA et al. Verbal memory impairment in COPD: its mechanisms and clinical relevance. Chest. 1997;112(6):1506–13.
25. Hjalmarsen A et al. Effect of long-term oxygen therapy on cognitive and neurological dysfunction in chronic obstructive pulmonary disease. Eur Neurol. 1999;42(1):27–35.
26. Kozora E et al. Improved neurobehavioral functioning in emphysema patients following lung volume reduction surgery compared with medical therapy. Chest. 2005;128(4):2653–63.
27. Klein M et al. Impact of chronic obstructive pulmonary disease (COPD) on attention functions. Respir Med. 2010;104(1):52–60.
28. Hung WW et al. Cognitive decline among patients with chronic obstructive pulmonary disease. Am J Respir Crit Care Med. 2009;180(2):134–7.
29. Herzog AR, Wallace RB. Measures of cognitive functioning in the AHEAD Study. J Gerontol B Psychol Sci Soc Sci. 1997;52:37–48. Spec No.

30. Fix AJ et al. Cognitive functioning and survival among patients with chronic obstructive pulmonary disease. Int J Neurosci. 1985;27(1–2):13–7.
31. Kozora E et al. Cognitive functioning in patients with chronic obstructive pulmonary disease and mild hypoxemia compared with patients with mild Alzheimer disease and normal controls. Neuropsychiatry Neuropsychol Behav Neurol. 1999;12(3):178–83.
32. Antonelli Incalzi R et al. Cognitive impairment in chronic obstructive pulmonary disease – a neuropsychological and spect study. J Neurol. 2003;250(3):325–32.
33. Incalzi RA et al. Chronic obstructive pulmonary disease. An original model of cognitive decline. Am Rev Respir Dis. 1993;148(2):418–24.
34. Antonelli-Incalzi R et al. Correlation between cognitive impairment and dependence in hypoxemic COPD. J Clin Exp Neuropsychol. 2008;30(2):141–50.
35. Etnier J, Johnston R, Dagenbach D et al. The relationships among pulmonary function, aerobic fitness, and cognitive functioning in older COPD patients. Chest. 1999;116:953–60.
36. Incalzi RA, Corsonello A, Trojano L et al. Cognitive training is ineffective in hypoxemic COPD: a six-month randomized controlled trial. Rejuvenation Res. 2008;11:239–50.

Chapter 9
Skeletal Muscle Dysfunction

Marc-André Caron, Marie-Eve Thériault, Richard Debigaré, and François Maltais

Abstract Chronic obstructive pulmonary disease (COPD) is highly prevalent and the burden of this disease is only expected to increase in the coming 15–20 years. Once viewed as a disease limited to the lung, COPD is now recognized as a multisystemic disease with various organ dysfunctions. Skeletal muscle dysfunction is one of the most devastating systemic manifestations of COPD. Skeletal muscle dysfunction is such a reality in COPD that, depending on the clinical situations, 20–35% of the patients refer to leg fatigue as the main cause of exercise cessation, whereas 41% consider it to be at least a major contributor to exercise limitation.

Keywords COPD • Multisystem disease • Skeletal muscle • Systemic manifestations • Leg fatigue • Exercise • Limitation • Respiratory muscles • Mechanisms • Muscle dysfunction

Introduction

Chronic obstructive pulmonary disease (COPD) is highly prevalent and the burden of this disease is only expected to increase in the coming 15–20 years. Once viewed as a disease limited to the lung, COPD is now recognized as a multisystemic disease with various organ dysfunctions. Skeletal muscle dysfunction is one of the most devastating systemic manifestations of COPD [1]. Skeletal muscle dysfunction is such a reality in COPD that, depending on the clinical situation, 20–35% of the patients refer to leg fatigue as the main cause of exercise cessation [2, 3], whereas 41% consider it to be at least a major contributor to exercise limitation [4].

M.-A. Caron (✉) • M.-E. Thériault • R. Debigaré • F. Maltais
Department of Respirology, Institut Universitaire de Cardiologie et de Pneumologie de Québec, Quebec, QC, Canada
e-mail: marc-andre.caron@criucpq.ulaval.ca; marie-eve.theriault.2@ulaval.ca; richard.debigare@rea.ulaval.ca; francois.maltais@med.ulaval.ca

L. Nici and R. ZuWallack (eds.), *Chronic Obstructive Pulmonary Disease: Co-Morbidities and Systemic Consequences*, Respiratory Medicine, DOI 10.1007/978-1-60761-673-3_9, © Springer Science+Business Media, LLC 2012

This chapter, dedicated to skeletal muscle dysfunction in COPD, is divided into four sections. In the first section, the clinical consequences of muscle dysfunction in COPD are presented. A description of the main alterations observed in the lower limb and respiratory muscles is provided in the second section. The third section highlights the probable mechanisms promoting development of muscle dysfunction, while possible treatments are presented in the final section.

Clinical Consequences of Muscle Dysfunction in COPD

Skeletal muscle dysfunction significantly contributes to COPD morbidity. From the COPD patient's point of view, a major restriction is the incapacity to adequately perform daily activities. Upper (*pectoralis major* and *latissimus dorsi*) and lower extremities (*vastus lateralis*) skeletal muscle strength is decreased by 15–25% in patients with COPD when compared to age-matched controls [5]. Furthermore, quadriceps fatigue, defined as a reversible postexercise reduction in muscle strength, can be documented in about 50% of patients with COPD [6]. While not being abnormal in itself, muscle fatigue occurs with greater amplitude and at much lower exercise intensities in these individuals than in sedentary age-matched controls [7, 8]. Consequently, along with impaired lung function, patients with COPD have to deal with weaker and less-enduring muscles to perform their everyday tasks.

Arguably, the most critical consequence of muscle dysfunction is its negative effect on life expectancy. Parameters such as reduced mid-thigh cross-sectional area [9, 10] and lower quadriceps strength [11] are predictors of mortality in subjects with COPD. For clinicians, these findings stress the importance of assessing body composition when evaluating a patient with COPD in daily practice. COPD must be considered a systemic illness and should be treated as such.

Skeletal Muscle Adaptations in COPD

Skeletal muscle dysfunction in COPD encompasses a variety of alterations affecting both locomotor and respiratory muscles. Historically, studies in COPD have focused predominantly on the *vastus lateralis* and the diaphragm as key representatives of their respective muscle group. Accordingly, this section will report the principal abnormalities in these two muscles, while some insights on other muscles will also be provided.

Atrophy

Skeletal muscle atrophy is common in COPD. It is estimated that 15% of the patients with COPD present a low whole body fat-free mass index (FFMI) (<14.62 kg/m^2 for women, <17.05 kg/m^2 for men) [12]. Reduced FFMI can be observed as early as GOLD I stage, though it is more frequent in severe stages of the disease [12]. Patients with COPD directly feel the adverse effects of the decline in FFMI in their everyday life. In the COPD patient, poor muscle mass is associated with a decreased quality of life [13], altered exercise performance [5], and more frequent hospitalizations [14]. It should also be recognized that body mass index (BMI) may be a misleading indicator of the degree of muscle atrophy. In fact, some studies have reported that a substantial proportion of subjects with a normal BMI exhibit lower muscle mass [12, 15]. Accordingly, tools such as dual-energy X-ray absorptiometer and bioelectrical impedance are more accurate than BMI to predict muscle mass in patients with COPD.

Lower limb muscles are particularly affected by the atrophying process in COPD. In two studies, mid-thigh cross-sectional area (CSA) was reduced by 15–20% in patients with moderate COPD when compared to age-matched controls [5, 16]. Studies involving biopsies of *vastus lateralis* reveal that the fiber CSA is lower in patients with COPD and that all fiber types are affected [17] although there is some dispute about this last finding [18]. This observation diverges from what is observed in upper extremity muscles such as deltoids, where muscle fiber CSA is preserved in COPD when compared to healthy controls [19].

Whether the diaphragm also suffers from atrophy in COPD is a difficult question to answer because the size of the human diaphragm cannot be easily quantified. Despite increased work of breathing in this disease [20], the diaphragm fiber CSA is reduced by 40–60% in patients with severe disease when compared to healthy controls [21]. A decrease in diaphragmatic myosin heavy chain content, an indicator of muscle protein degradation, is also observed in mild to moderate patients [22]. The latter implies that the diaphragmatic atrophy process could occur at early stages of COPD. However, one theory postulates that the observed reduction in diaphragmatic muscle fiber CSA and activation of proteolysis could be the reflection of a muscle reorganization process resulting from changes in chest wall configuration and altered muscle fiber length/tension relationship rather than implying a true maladaptive atrophy phenomenon [23].

Fiber-Type Distribution Shifting

A typical feature of COPD is a shift in normal skeletal muscle fiber-type proportions in the quadriceps. In contrast to the decrease in type II fiber proportion typically seen with aging [24], patients suffering from COPD exhibit a reduction in type I fiber proportion in favor of type IIx in the quadriceps [17, 25]. In addition, the degree of fiber-type shifting correlates with disease severity [26] and is not observed in upper extremity muscles such as the deltoid [19]. Type IIx muscle fibers are glycolytic, fast-twitch, and easily fatigable fibers principally required for short exercise in opposition to oxidative, slow-twitch, and enduring type I fibers useful for sustained activities. Consequently, this fiber-type shifting that occurs in the quadriceps of COPD patients likely contributes to the exercise intolerance reported in this disease and the resulting decline in functional capacity. Premature leg fatigue [6, 27, 28], early muscle acidosis [29], and heightened perception of leg fatigue [30] are all examples of how muscle fiber-type shift may contribute to exercise intolerance in COPD.

The diaphragm also exhibits a fiber-type shift in the opposite direction, with an increase in type I fibers. This fiber shift may happen earlier in the disease process than what is seen in the quadriceps [31]. The enhanced-type fiber I proportion is likely due to a chronically increased work of breathing that provides a continuous training stimulus [32].

Contractility

As mentioned in the section "Introduction", patients with COPD commonly have weak quadriceps. An appealing hypothesis to explain this clinical observation is the presence of an inefficient contractile apparatus in the muscle tissue. However, the fact that muscle weakness and atrophy are usually proportional in patients with COPD [5] makes the existence of defective contractile machinery unlikely. Besides, *vastus lateralis* single fibers isolated from patients with COPD and sedentary age-matched controls have similar in vitro twitch contractile properties [33]. This implies that reduction in strength seen in COPD most certainly occurs despite a preserved contractile apparatus. However, a disproportional loss in muscle strength than in muscle mass may occasionally occur, for example, in patients exposed to systemic corticosteroids where a myopathic process may take place [34].

The presence or absence of a contractile defect in the diaphragm is still a matter of debate. On one hand, diaphragmatic strength is preserved in patients with COPD in comparison to normal subjects when lung volumes are taken into account [35]. Moreover, the average and maximal isometric tension of isolated diaphragm fibers are not different between patients with COPD of any GOLD stages and control subjects [31]. Conversely, a diminution of passive tension was reported in diaphragm muscle fibers of patients with COPD, even in mild stages of the disease [36]. It appears that genetic variations in the gene coding for titin, an important protein of the contractile unit, could be responsible for this diminution [36]. Finally, skinned muscle fibers isolated from COPD diaphragms display decreased calcium sensitivity, an important parameter for force generation [22].

Metabolic Alterations

Skeletal muscles of patients with COPD display a number of metabolic adaptations. When analyzing the enzymatic profile of the *vastus lateralis*, a propensity toward glycolytic metabolism is observed. Oxidative enzymes such as 3-hydroxyacyl-CoA dehydrogenase, essential for β-oxidation of the lipids, and citrate synthase, a rate-limiting enzyme of the citric acid cycle, exhibit reduced activity in the quadriceps of patients with moderate to severe COPD [37, 38]. Although less documented, some investigators have reported an increased activity of glycolytic enzymes in the COPD *vastus lateralis* [8, 38, 39]. This strong tendency toward greater reliance on the glycolytic metabolism is well illustrated by the shift of the oxidative/glycolytic enzyme activity ratio in favor of glycolytic metabolism in the quadriceps of patients with COPD. Thus, these patients are likely to use less effective metabolic pathways to produce ATP since Krebs cycle and β-oxidation pathways are downregulated in favor of the glycolytic metabolism in their quadriceps, a situation most certainly contributing to deterioration in exercise performance during endurance tasks [6, 8, 27, 29].

The metabolic portrait of the COPD diaphragm is the mirror image of what is seen in the *vastus lateralis*. Consistent with the fiber-type profile, the diaphragm displays an increased oxidative metabolism in patients with COPD. The activity of succinate dehydrogenase, a mitochondrial enzyme implicated in the Krebs cycle and the electron transport chain, is increased in all diaphragmatic fiber types of patients with severe COPD [40]. Moreover, lactate dehydrogenase, a glycolytic enzyme, has lower activity in the diaphragms of patients with mild-to-moderate COPD [41], suggesting an early effect of the disease.

Capillarization Defect

Adequate muscle oxygen delivery is essential for optimal muscle and exercise performance. The capillary network is responsible for proper blood flow distribution throughout this tissue and allows appropriate oxygen transport to myofibers. In COPD, the absolute number of capillaries is lowered when compared to controls. This probably reflects the reduced muscle fiber CSA since the capillary to muscle fiber CSA ratio is typically normal [17]. Still, there is a tendency toward reduced capillary contacts specifically with oxidative type I and intermediate type IIa quadriceps fibers [17]. The capillary density seems to be a determinant of muscle fatigue in COPD. In one study, a reduced capillary content in all fiber types was associated with the susceptibility to develop contractile fatigue of the quadriceps during cycling exercise [42]. This observation suggests that, although not universal among patients, a defect in capillarization in lower limb muscles may negatively impact on exercise performance.

Unlike the quadriceps, the diaphragmatic capillary network is expanded in COPD. In fact, all fiber types have increased capillary contacts when compared to age-matched controls with normal lung function [41]. This physiological adaptation could be interpreted as a positive adaptation to the increased muscle mitochondrial demand measured in these patients (detailed in the section "Mitochondrial Adaptations and Oxidative Stress Production").

Mitochondrial Adaptations and Oxidative Stress Production

Mitochondria are the energy factories of eukaryotic cells and modulators of exercise performance [43]. The respiratory function of isolated mitochondria from the quadriceps of patients with COPD is preserved when compared to age-matched controls, a statement that is supported by the observation that individual mitochondria produce an equivalent quantity of energy irrespective of the presence of COPD [44]. Nevertheless, as efficient as mitochondria may be in COPD, their total number in a given area of muscle section is reduced in *vastus lateralis* [45]. This situation most certainly contributes to decreasing oxidative capacity of skeletal muscles in COPD and is an important component of muscle dysfunction.

Another essential aspect of mitochondrial function is their role in generating oxidative stress. Oxidative stress is defined as a cellular imbalance between total reactive oxygen and/or nitrogen species (ROS and RNS, respectively) production and antioxidant capacities. Mitochondria, through the respiratory chain, are the main cellular source of ROS [46]. In COPD, an increased mitochondrial ROS generation is measured in quadriceps when compared to age-matched subjects with normal lung function [47]. This oxidative stress could potentially oxidize surrounding proteins and promote their degradation, contributing to development of muscle atrophy and dysfunction. In fact, oxidative stress in the limb muscles of patients with COPD has been associated with premature muscle fatigue [48], muscle weakness [49], and wasting [50].

Once again, the respiratory muscle mitochondrial function is not affected in the same way as the lower limb muscles in COPD. The capacity of the diaphragmatic mitochondrial respiratory chain is higher in patients with moderate to severe COPD than in controls [51, 52]. In addition, mitochondrial concentration is increased in the diaphragm of these patients [53], indicating a higher potential to generate energy from the oxidative metabolism in diseased subjects. However, one potential adverse consequence of having higher mitochondrial density is an exaggerated oxidative stress production. In one study [41], patients with mild-to-moderate COPD had no evidence of enhanced oxidative stress, while enhanced protein carbonylation and superoxide anions were found in patients with advanced disease [54, 55]. The COPD diaphragm attempts to adapt to oxidative bursts by increasing considerably their antioxidant defenses, as demonstrated by the 90% higher catalase activity in these subjects when compared to controls [56]. These results suggest that more oxidant products are generated in diseased diaphragms but that this tissue is capable of counterbalancing this stress by enhancing antioxidant defenses.

Mechanisms of Muscle Dysfunction in Patients with COPD

Although the clinical significance of skeletal muscle dysfunction is well established in COPD, the underlying mechanisms of this dysfunction are not fully elucidated. Several mechanisms have been proposed to explain structural and functional alterations of the lower and upper limb muscles in COPD. We will summarize the possible implication of malnutrition, disuse, hypoxemia, oxidative stress, and systemic inflammation in skeletal muscle adaptations observed in patients with COPD. Even though each mechanism will be reviewed individually, it should be noted that they are interrelated and potentially interacting with each other.

Malnutrition

Malnutrition is the result of an imbalance between energy expenditure and intake, a situation that will favor muscle protein breakdown to provide amino acids to maintain whole body homeostasis. This compensatory phenomenon will eventually compromise the maintenance of muscle mass. Calorie intake may be diminished in patients with COPD, particularly in advanced disease and during episodes of exacerbation [57]. Subsequently, basal and activity-related metabolic rates are often amplified, creating metabolic imbalance [58].

Malnutrition may lead to skeletal muscle dysfunction among healthy individuals and those with a chronic respiratory disease [59]. Malnutrition is associated with muscle weakness of the lower and upper extremities [60] and decreased muscle endurance leading to fatigability [61]. Evidence of malnutrition and its link with muscle atrophy is also present in COPD. Approximately one-third of patients with COPD will show some degree of malnutrition that may be severe in advanced stages of the disease [62]. Recognition that patients with COPD may have reduced fat-free mass even with a normal body weight supports the hypothesis of nutritional depletion as a potential cause of muscle atrophy [15]. Similarly, respiratory muscle strength is reduced in underweight patients with COPD compared to their normal weight counterparts [63]. However, the modest impact of nutritional interventions on skeletal muscle function suggests that nutritional imbalance is not the main mechanism of skeletal muscle dysfunction in COPD.

Disuse

Chronic inactivity leads to deconditioning, a process that initiates muscle structural and functional changes. These changes include a reduction in proportion of type I fiber, in oxidative enzyme capacity, in muscle cross-sectional area, in antioxidant enzyme levels, and in capillarization [64–66].

Chronic inactivity in COPD is intuitively related to pulmonary and functional impairments and the resulting deconditioning [67]. The availability of portable devices capable of monitoring daily activities have confirmed the clinical suspicion that patients with COPD are relatively inactive compared to healthy-matched controls [68, 69]. Importantly, inactivity occurs early in the course of the disease.

Reduced walking time may already be present in patients with GOLD Stage I COPD, although this reduction is more dramatic in advanced disease [70, 71].

The relationship between the level of physical activity and peripheral muscle alterations in COPD is insufficient to explain the range of skeletal muscle abnormalities seen in this disease. For instance, exercise training does not completely restore the histochemical and morphological abnormalities, suggesting that factors other than disuse need to be considered [5, 17]. Furthermore, considering that altered activity is generalized in the COPD population [72], it would be arguable that the prevalence of peripheral muscle atrophy should be higher. Current data demonstrate that 4–35% of patients with COPD have peripheral muscle atrophy [12, 73]. Finally, skeletal muscle alterations, including decreased oxidative capacity, have been demonstrated in emphysematous hamsters in comparison to their healthy counterparts, despite similar activity levels in both groups of animals [74].

Hypoxemia

Hypoxemia and resulting tissue hypoxia may contribute to upper and lower limb adaptive changes. In healthy active individuals, chronic or intermittent hypoxia induces a significant reduction in skeletal muscle strength, endurance, and cross-sectional area [75]. For instance, after 8 weeks of exposure to altitudes higher than 5,000 m, a 10% reduction in muscle mass and maximal muscular power has been reported [75, 76]. In addition, mountaineers have decreased oxidative capacity due to a 25% reduction of muscle mitochondrial volume [76]. Although muscle tissue alterations could be related to hypoxia itself, malnutrition is also present during high-altitude expeditions and is a potential confounder contributing to muscle impairment in high-altitude studies [77].

Approximately 25% of patients with COPD will undergo episodes of hypoxemia during their daily activities [62], sleep [78], and exercise [79]. Hypoxemic patients with COPD demonstrate a reduced proportion of type I fibers in lower limbs when compared to nonhypoxemic patients [80]. A better understanding of the biological events induced by hypoxia and their relationship with peripheral muscle dysfunction in COPD is currently emerging. Hypoxia is a specific and strong inducer of hypoxia-inducible factor-1α (HIF-1α), a subunit of the heterodimeric transcription factor HIF-1. HIF-1 downregulates the expression of oxidative enzymes and upregulates the expression of glycolytic enzymes as well as angiogenic factors. These HIF-1-induced modifications represent an appropriate tissue adaptation to low oxygen levels [81]. The von Hippel-Lindau protein (pVHL), an E3 ligase involved in the proteasomal degradation of HIF-1α, is significantly increased in the *vastus lateralis* of mild-to-moderate patients with COPD [82]. Since HIF-1 is responsible for transcription of VEGF, an angiogenic factor, it can be speculated that a reduction in HIF-1α in peripheral skeletal muscles of patients with COPD could lead to lower angiogenesis and, therefore, to a reduced capillarization. Targeting pVHL may thus represent a potential therapeutic strategy to restore muscle function and its adverse consequences in patients with COPD.

Beyond the effects of compromised muscle oxygenation, chronic hypoxia may also jeopardize skeletal muscle homeostasis through the induction of oxidative stress and an inflammatory response. These responses are believed to contribute to the deterioration of skeletal muscle function (discussed in sections "Metabolic Alterations"and "Capillarization Defect"). Specifically, hypoxia increases the production of ROS by altering the mitochondrial function [83]. Similarly, an inflammatory response is observed during hypoxic events through the activation of inflammatory cells such as monocytes [84]. In agreement with this, lipid peroxydation and oxidized protein levels in *vastus lateralis* muscle are increased after exercise in hypoxemic patients with COPD [85].

Hypoxia may alter muscle regeneration and homeostasis. Following muscle injury, satellite cells are activated in order to produce a sufficient number of myoblasts to repair muscle fiber [86, 87]. Under hypoxic conditions, MyoD, a crucial transcription factor for myoblast growth and differentiation is degraded, thus compromising the muscle regeneration process in this setting [88]. Furthermore, in cultured myotubes, hypoxia decreases protein synthesis while promoting protein degradation. This observation is compatible with the initiation and the development of muscle atrophy observed in COPD [89]. Taken together, hypoxia has the potential to affect muscle tissue homeostasis through several mechanisms in the subset of patients with COPD that experience hypoxemia in the course of their disease.

Oxidative Stress

Oxidative stress may compromise muscle tissue functions in COPD. For example, oxidative stress can damage lipids and contractile proteins, alter mitochondrial respiration, and impair function of sarcoplasmic reticulum and mitochondrial membranes [90]. Oxidative stress may also affect muscle function by inhibiting Na^+/K^+ ATPase pump which, in turn, decreases contractility and endurance while increasing fatigability [91, 92]. Subsequently, N-acetylcysteine, an antioxidant, may circumvent diaphragm fatigue related to oxidative stress produced during repetitive contractions [93].

ROS and RNS are stress molecules normally produced by neutrophils and mitochondria [94]. In addition to physiological conditions, oxidative stress molecules may be produced in response to several factors such as cigarette smoke, hypoxia, and sepsis [95, 96]. As a defense mechanism, antioxidants such as glutathione and others, neutralize oxidants in skeletal muscle to maintain proper contractility [97]. Excessive oxidative stress has been reported in lower limb muscles of patients with COPD at rest, after exercise, and also during acute exacerbation of the disease [48, 98–100]. Additionally, the expected increased antioxidant level observed after exercise in healthy subjects is absent in patients with COPD [48, 101]. In parallel, decreased muscle levels of glutathione has been noted in patients with emphysema [102], indicating that the antioxidant system could be impaired.

Despite direct evidence of increased oxidative stress in plasma, urine, and skeletal muscles [103], a cause–effect role for these molecules on skeletal muscle adaptations still needs to be established. However, as previously stated, indirect evidence supports a potential role for oxidative stress in depressed muscle endurance and contractility in patients with COPD [104]. In addition, cellular models have shown that excessive oxidative burst can trigger protein catabolism [105]. However, the concentration of oxidants that were used to produce muscle protein catabolism was much higher than what has been reported in patients with COPD.

Systemic Inflammation

A state of low-grade systemic inflammation is common in patients with stable COPD [106], a situation that may be worsened during acute exacerbations of the disease. Increased levels of interleukin-1β (IL-1β), IL-6, IL-8, IL-18, tumor necrosis factor α (TNFα), soluble TNF receptors (sTNF-R55 and sTNF-R75), and C-reactive protein (CRP) have been reported in stable patients with COPD [106–109]. This is relevant because pro-inflammatory molecules may induce muscle alterations at the cellular level [110]. A chronic inflammatory state is a likely trigger of muscle loss in a variety of chronic diseases such as chronic heart failure [111], chronic kidney failure [112], cancer [113], and COPD [114]. Systemic inflammation is a risk factor for peripheral muscle weakness and reduced exercise tolerance in COPD [115–117]. Systemic inflammation also correlates with poor contractile performance [118], an observation that could be due to a direct negative effect of pro-inflammatory cytokines on muscle strength and endurance [119]. Mediators of inflammation may also increase energy expenditure, contributing to energy imbalance [109].

The adverse effects of pro-inflammatory cytokines have been confirmed in experimental models of cachexia. Inflammation can impair anabolism by inhibiting IGF-I secretion, an important positive muscle mass modulator [120]. TNFα can adversely influence muscle growth and contractility, induce apoptosis, and enhance protein degradation through the ubiquitin–proteasome pathway [116]. Furthermore, transgenic mice over expressing TNFα exhibit enhanced protein catabolism through NF-κB pathway [121]. TNFα exerts its inhibitory effect on muscle contractility by decreasing myofilament protein sensitivity to Ca^{++} and by enhancing generation of oxidants [122, 123]. Increased plasma levels of TNFα and its soluble receptors are found in COPD, particularly in those suffering from weight loss, providing evidences for involvement of this cytokine in muscle tissue depletion [124].

Despite all scientific data supporting a role for inflammation in skeletal muscle dysfunction in COPD, there are still areas of uncertainties. Increased circulating pro-inflammatory cytokine levels are not universal in patients with COPD [125]. The relative preservation of diaphragm function in patients with COPD suggests that systemic inflammation is not the sole factor explaining skeletal muscle dysfunction in this disease. Although in vitro studies have confirmed that inflammation alone is able to promote muscle atrophy through the ubiquitin–proteasome system and to alter muscle regeneration [126], the level of pro-inflammatory cytokines required to induce cellular and molecular adaptations is far higher than plasma concentrations measured in patients with stable COPD. Conversely, it is possible that acute inflammatory bursts occurring during COPD exacerbations may be sufficient to compromise muscle performance [110]. Further research is needed to clearly establish the role of inflammatory response in altering muscle function in the context of COPD.

Although COPD is clearly associated with systemic inflammation, the source of pro-inflammatory cytokines is still to be defined. One possibility is a spillover of cytokines from the airways and lungs to the systemic circulation [127], although this still needs to be confirmed [128]. Respiratory muscle may also contribute to the inflammatory process by producing several inflammatory cytokines in response to the elevated work of breath [129]. Visceral adiposity can also contribute to worsen systemic inflammation in COPD [130].

Treatments and Prevention

Skeletal muscle dysfunction decreases quality of life and functional capacity in patients with COPD. Since there is currently no cure for this problem, the development of therapies aimed at stopping or slowing the progression of muscle dysfunction is essential. Today, interventions focusing on exercise training, nutritional supplementation, and medication alone, or in combination, have been shown to improve various aspects of muscle function, resulting in better quality of life and enhanced exercise tolerance in COPD [131–137].

Exercise Training

Exercise training is a major component of pulmonary rehabilitation and an essential tool in the clinical management of patients with COPD [138]. In healthy subjects, both endurance and resistance training have been shown to induce structural and functional changes in the muscle tissue [138]. These changes include an increase in the number of mitochondria, muscle capillarization, and muscle oxidative enzyme activity [139]. After intense training, the proportion of type I fibers increases, whereas a shift from type IIb to type IIa fibers may occur [32]. A training program combining aerobic with resistance exercises induces clinically relevant improvement in exercise performance in patients with COPD [140–142]. While the aerobic component of training improves muscle oxidative capacity [140, 141, 143] and reduces susceptibility to fatigue [144], resistance training induces muscle hypertrophy and promotes muscle growth [145]. One interesting feature of resistance training is that it allows a high muscle training stimulus at a low ventilatory cost so that dyspnea is not a limiting factor [146]. Enhanced muscle function in response to exercise is in part attained by an increased expression of myogenic factors [147, 148], a reduced expression of atrogenes [149], and a decreased susceptibility to apoptosis [150]. Exercise training can also be effective in reducing the negative impact of acute COPD exacerbations on muscle function [151].

Interestingly, the response to exercise training may be suboptimal in some patients with COPD. Systemic inflammation [119] and oxidative stress [50, 101] may be worsened by exercise training, particularly in wasted patients. Currently, the clinical significance of these findings is unclear but it will be important to learn how to optimize training responses in individuals with COPD.

Accessibility to training facilities remains problematic for many patients [152]. To circumvent this issue, home-based rehabilitation has been reported as a valuable alternative to institutional-based programs for patients with COPD producing equivalent improvements in exercise tolerance and quality of life while facilitating access to the intervention [153, 154].

Nutrition

COPD symptoms and systemic inflammation may impair dietary intake, particularly in advanced disease. Under such circumstances, nutritional support may be a valuable option to protect against the adverse consequences of nutritional imbalance on muscle tissue. Studies have consistently reported significantly greater mortality rates in underweight COPD than in overweight COPD, an observation arguing in favor of nutritional support therapy [155].

In undernourished patients with COPD, nutritional supplementation can improve body weight and respiratory and peripheral muscle strength, although the magnitude of these changes is relatively modest [62, 156, 157]. One limitation of this intervention, however, is that the gain in body weight is predominantly an increase in fat over muscle tissue [158]. Although quality-of-life indices improved after nutritional therapy in patients with COPD, these results were obtained with a limited number of subjects and further studies with larger sample size are needed. It is also unclear to what extent the improvement in muscle function relates to an increase in muscle mass with nutritional interventions [159]. For instance, after the first few days of repletion, muscle function improves from 10 to 20% without any demonstrable gain in tissue protein [160].

Evidence suggests that, in some nutritionally depleted patients with COPD, weight loss may be related to a systemic catabolic response induced by inflammation [161]. In such patients, nutritional support may not address the underlying problem, and therefore will not be effective. One way to tackle this problem could be to combine nutritional support with exercise or anti-inflammatory therapy (see below), since this could theoretically lead to superior results. The use of appetite-stimulating therapy in underweight patients with COPD has also been tested [162].

Progestogens, administered to stimulate appetite while acting as an antagonist of pro-inflammatory cytokines, have been reported to improve the 6-minute walk test distance and lower inflammatory cytokines [163]. One limitation of this treatment is that it induces gain in fat tissue and does promote muscle growth [164].

Weight loss and loss in fat mass is primarily the result of a negative balance between dietary intake and energy expenditure, while muscle wasting is a consequence of an impaired balance between protein synthesis and protein breakdown. In advanced stages of COPD, both sides of this equation are disturbed. Therefore, nutritional therapy may be more effective in COPD when combined with anabolic stimuli to further enhance contractile protein synthesis [143]. However, the optimal combination of nutritional support and anabolic therapy has yet to be developed.

Medication

Several pharmacological strategies have been explored to promote muscle mass gain in underweight patients with COPD, although none has been translated into clinical practice. Hormonal supplementation, anti-inflammatory molecules, and antioxidants are avenues with some therapeutic potential to address the muscle consequences of COPD. Based on the recent advances in skeletal muscle biology, new therapeutic targets that could block muscle catabolism and/or enhance muscle anabolism are under development since they should attenuate or even reverse muscle tissue loss.

Growth hormone and anabolic steroids have been studied in patients with COPD with the goal of improving muscle mass. Anabolic hormones are important mediators of muscle growth while growth hormone exerts its effects primarily by increasing levels of insulin-like growth factors, a potent inducer of protein synthesis [165]. In growth-hormone-deficient adults, administration of growth hormone increases muscle mass and strength [166], and improves exercise performance [167]. In COPD, growth-hormone-replacement therapy has been tested with inconsistent and disappointing results. For instance, the daily administration of recombinant human growth hormone for 3 weeks increased lean body mass but did not improve muscle strength or exercise tolerance in underweight patients with COPD [168].

Supplementation with testosterone appears to be an effective therapy to treat muscle dysfunction in COPD, as it increases strength and muscle mass [143]. In one study, a 10-week testosterone supplementation program resulted in a significant gain of lean body mass, though better improvements are observed when combined with exercise training [143]. Testosterone supplementations have long-term detrimental effects that may overcome short-term benefits [169]. The use of pharmacological derivates such as Selective Androgen Receptor Modulators, SARM, a molecule designed to mimic testosterone effect without the side effects, is a promising treatment for muscle wasting in this context [170].

Since systemic inflammation may directly affect muscle function and decrease the effectiveness of exercise training [119], nutritional and hormonal supplementation combined with anti-inflammatory drugs such as corticosteroids may be an effective strategy. Corticosteroids are generally prescribed to attenuate bronchial inflammation either during the stable phase of the disease or following an exacerbation, but their long-term use induces muscle protein degradation [171], type II fiber atrophy [172], and could accentuate risk of infection and sepsis [138]. Inhibitors of pro-inflammatory cytokines, such as TNFα, may be a more appealing alternative to corticosteroids [138], although the first studies employing this strategy have been negative [173, 174].

Emerging pharmacological approaches are currently under development. Levosimendan, a calcium sensitizer known to improve muscle contractile protein functions, could be used to increase muscle strength and function. In one study, Levosimendan enhanced the force-generating capacity of diaphragm fibers from patients with and without COPD by increasing calcium muscle cell sensitivity [175]. However, short- and long-term effects of Levosimendan on skeletal muscle need to be documented. Development of potent and selective pharmacological inhibitors of the inflammatory response and the ubiquitin–proteasome proteolytic pathway is also in progress [134].

Summary

In this chapter, we presented an overview of the clinical importance of the changes in muscle structure and function and the contributing factors to this dysfunction in patients with COPD. Muscle atrophy, fiber-type shifting, reduced contractility, metabolic alterations, capillarization defect, and mitochondrial modifications are important adaptations in COPD. A large body of literature has demonstrated that these factors alone, or in combination, impact on muscle function, functional capacity, and even survival of affected subjects.

Future scientific and clinical research is needed to better understand the problem and to design appropriate interventions. Currently, the best therapeutic option to improve muscle function is exercise training. However, poor availability of exercise programs and lack of specific pharmaceutical intervention are barriers to the optimal clinical management of COPD.

References

1. Agusti AG. Systemic effects of chronic obstructive pulmonary disease. Proc Am Thorac Soc. 2005;2:367–70 [discussion 371–2].
2. Maltais F, Hamilton A, Marciniuk D, Hernandez P, Sciurba FC, Richter K, et al. Improvements in symptom-limited exercise performance over 8 h with once-daily tiotropium in patients with COPD. Chest. 2005;128:1168–78.

3. Pepin V, Saey D, Whittom F, LeBlanc P, Maltais F. Walking versus cycling: sensitivity to bronchodilation in chronic obstructive pulmonary disease. Am J Respir Crit Care Med. 2005;172:1517–22.

4. O'Donnell DE, Laveneziana P. Dyspnea and activity limitation in COPD: mechanical factors. COPD. 2007;4:225–36.

5. Bernard S, LeBlanc P, Whittom F, Carrier G, Jobin J, Belleau R, et al. Peripheral muscle weakness in patients with chronic obstructive pulmonary disease. Am J Respir Crit Care Med. 1998;158:629–34.

6. Saey D, Debigaré R, LeBlanc P, Mador MJ, Côté CH, Jobin J, et al. Contractile leg fatigue after cycle exercise: a factor limiting exercise in patients with chronic obstructive pulmonary disease. Am J Respir Crit Care Med. 2003;168:425–30.

7. Mador MJ, Deniz O, Aggarwal A, Kufel TJ. Quadriceps fatigability after single muscle exercise in patients with chronic obstructive pulmonary disease. Am J Respir Crit Care Med. 2003;168:102–8.

8. Saey D, Lemire BB, Gagnon P, Bombardier E, Tupling AR, Debigaré R, et al. Quadriceps metabolism during constant workrate cycling exercise in chronic obstructive pulmonary disease. J Appl Physiol. 2011;110:116–24.

9. Marquis K, Debigaré R, Lacasse Y, LeBlanc P, Jobin J, Carrier G, et al. Midthigh muscle cross-sectional area is a better predictor of mortality than body mass index in patients with chronic obstructive pulmonary disease. Am J Respir Crit Care Med. 2002;166: 809–13.

10. Schols AM, Broekhuizen R, Weling-Scheepers CA, Wouters EF. Body composition and mortality in chronic obstructive pulmonary disease. Am J Clin Nutr. 2005;82:53–9.

11. Swallow EB, Reyes D, Hopkinson NS, Man WD, Porcher R, Cetti EJ, et al. Quadriceps strength predicts mortality in patients with moderate to severe chronic obstructive pulmonary disease. Thorax. 2007;62:115–20.

12. Vestbo J, Prescott E, Almdal T, Dahl M, Nordestgaard BG, Andersen T, et al. Body mass, fat-free body mass, and prognosis in patients with chronic obstructive pulmonary disease from a random population sample: findings from the Copenhagen City Heart Study. Am J Respir Crit Care Med. 2006;173:79–83.

13. Mostert R, Goris A, Weling-Scheepers C, Wouters EF, Schols AM. Tissue depletion and health related quality of life in patients with chronic obstructive pulmonary disease. Respir Med. 2000;94:859–67.

14. Decramer M, Gosselink R, Troosters T, Verschueren M, Evers G. Muscle weakness is related to utilization of health care resources in COPD patients. Eur Respir J. 1997;10:417–23.

15. Schols AM, Soeters PB, Dingemans AM, Mostert R, Frantzen PJ, Wouters EF. Prevalence and characteristics of nutritional depletion in patients with stable COPD eligible for pulmonary rehabilitation. Am Rev Respir Dis. 1993;147:1151–6.

16. Mathur S, Takai KP, Macintyre DL, Reid D. Estimation of thigh muscle mass with magnetic resonance imaging in older adults and people with chronic obstructive pulmonary disease. Phys Ther. 2008;88:219–30.

17. Whittom F, Jobin J, Simard PM, Leblanc P, Simard C, Bernard S, et al. Histochemical and morphological characteristics of the vastus lateralis muscle in patients with chronic obstructive pulmonary disease. Med Sci Sports Exerc. 1998;30:1467–74.

18. Gosker HR, Engelen MP, van Mameren H, van Dijk PJ, van der Vusse GJ, Wouters EF, et al. Muscle fiber type IIX atrophy is involved in the loss of fat-free mass in chronic obstructive pulmonary disease. Am J Clin Nutr. 2002;76:113–9.

19. Gea JG, Pasto M, Carmona MA, Orozco-Levi M, Palomeque J, Broquetas J. Metabolic characteristics of the deltoid muscle in patients with chronic obstructive pulmonary disease. Eur Respir J. 2001;17:939–45.

20. Orozco-Levi M. Structure and function of the respiratory muscles in patients with COPD: impairment or adaptation? Eur Respir J Suppl. 2003;46:41s–51.

21. Levine S, Kaiser L, Leferovich J, Tikunov B. Cellular adaptations in the diaphragm in chronic obstructive pulmonary disease. N Engl J Med. 1997;337:1799–806.

22. Ottenheijm CA, Heunks LM, Sieck GC, Zhan WZ, Jansen SM, Degens H, et al. Diaphragm dysfunction in chronic obstructive pulmonary disease. Am J Respir Crit Care Med. 2005;172:200–5.
23. Caron MA, Debigaré R, Dekhuijzen PN, Maltais F. Comparative assessment of the quadriceps and the diaphragm in patients with COPD. J Appl Physiol. 2009;107:952–61.
24. Larsson L. Histochemical characteristics of human skeletal muscle during aging. Acta Physiol Scand. 1983;117:469–71.
25. Maltais F, Sullivan MJ, LeBlanc P, Duscha BD, Schachat FH, Simard C, et al. Altered expression of myosin heavy chain in the vastus lateralis muscle in patients with COPD. Eur Respir J. 1999;13:850–4.
26. Gosker HR, Zeegers MP, Wouters EF, Schols AM. Muscle fibre type shifting in the vastus lateralis of patients with COPD is associated with disease severity: a systematic review and meta-analysis. Thorax. 2007;62:944–9.
27. Gagnon P, Saey D, Vivodtzev I, Laviolette L, Mainguy V, Milot J, et al. Impact of preinduced quadriceps fatigue on exercise response in chronic obstructive pulmonary disease and healthy subjects. J Appl Physiol. 2009;107:832–40.
28. Amann M, Regan MS, Kobitary M, Eldridge MW, Boutellier U, Pegelow DF, et al. Impact of pulmonary system limitations on locomotor muscle fatigue in patients with COPD. Am J Physiol Regul Integr Comp Physiol. 2010;299:R314–24.
29. Maltais F, Jobin J, Sullivan MJ, Bernard S, Whittom F, Killian KJ, et al. Metabolic and hemodynamic responses of lower limb during exercise in patients with COPD. J Appl Physiol. 1998;84:1573–80.
30. Hamilton AL, Killian KJ, Summers E, Jones NL. Muscle strength, symptom intensity, and exercise capacity in patients with cardiorespiratory disorders. Am J Respir Crit Care Med. 1995;152:2021–31.
31. Stubbings AK, Moore AJ, Dusmet M, Goldstraw P, West TG, Polkey MI, et al. Physiological properties of human diaphragm muscle fibres and the effect of chronic obstructive pulmonary disease. J Physiol. 2008;586:2637–50.
32. Howald H, Hoppeler H, Claassen H, Mathieu O, Straub R. Influences of endurance training on the ultrastructural composition of the different muscle fiber types in humans. Pflugers Arch. 1985;403:369–76.
33. Debigaré R, Côté CH, Hould FS, LeBlanc P, Maltais F. In vitro and in vivo contractile properties of the vastus lateralis muscle in males with COPD. Eur Respir J. 2003;21:273–8.
34. Decramer M, Lacquet LM, Fagard R, Rogiers P. Corticosteroids contribute to muscle weakness in chronic airflow obstruction. Am J Respir Crit Care Med. 1994;150:11–6.
35. Similowski T, Yan S, Gauthier AP, Macklem PT, Bellemare F. Contractile properties of the human diaphragm during chronic hyperinflation. N Engl J Med. 1991;325:917–23.
36. Ottenheijm CA, Heunks LM, Hafmans T, van der Ven PF, Benoist C, Zhou H, et al. Titin and diaphragm dysfunction in chronic obstructive pulmonary disease. Am J Respir Crit Care Med. 2006;173:527–34.
37. Maltais F, LeBlanc P, Whittom F, Simard C, Marquis K, Bélanger M, et al. Oxidative enzyme activities of the vastus lateralis muscle and the functional status in patients with COPD. Thorax. 2000;55:848–53.
38. Green HJ, Bombardier E, Burnett M, Iqbal S, D'Arsigny CL, O'Donnell DE, et al. Organization of metabolic pathways in vastus lateralis of patients with chronic obstructive pulmonary disease. Am J Physiol Regul Integr Comp Physiol. 2008;295:R935–41.
39. Jakobsson P, Jorfeldt L, Henriksson J. Metabolic enzyme activity in the quadriceps femoris muscle in patients with severe chronic obstructive pulmonary disease. Am J Respir Crit Care Med. 1995;151:374–7.
40. Levine S, Gregory C, Nguyen T, Shrager J, Kaiser L, Rubinstein N, et al. Bioenergetic adaptation of individual human diaphragmatic myofibers to severe COPD. J Appl Physiol. 2002;92:1205–13.
41. Doucet M, Debigare R, Joanisse DR, Cote C, Leblanc P, Gregoire J, et al. Adaptation of the diaphragm and the vastus lateralis in mild-to-moderate COPD. Eur Respir J. 2004;24:971–9.

42. Saey D, Michaud A, Couillard A, Cote CH, Mador MJ, LeBlanc P, et al. Contractile fatigue, muscle morphometry, and blood lactate in chronic obstructive pulmonary disease. Am J Respir Crit Care Med. 2005;171:1109–15.

43. Rasmussen UF, Rasmussen HN, Krustrup P, Quistorff B, Saltin B, Bangsbo J. Aerobic metabolism of human quadriceps muscle: in vivo data parallel measurements on isolated mitochondria. Am J Physiol Endocrinol Metab. 2001;280:E301–7.

44. Picard M, Godin R, Sinnreich M, Baril J, Bourbeau J, Perrault H, et al. The mitochondrial phenotype of peripheral muscle in chronic obstructive pulmonary disease: disuse or dysfunction? Am J Respir Crit Care Med. 2008;178:1040–7.

45. Gosker HR, Hesselink MK, Duimel H, Ward KA, Schols AM. Reduced mitochondrial density in the vastus lateralis muscle of patients with COPD. Eur Respir J. 2007;30:73–9.

46. Turrens JF. Mitochondrial formation of reactive oxygen species. J Physiol. 2003;552:335–44.

47. Puente-Maestu L, Perez-Parra J, Godoy R, Moreno N, Tejedor A, Gonzalez-Aragoneses F, et al. Abnormal mitochondrial function in locomotor and respiratory muscles of COPD patients. Eur Respir J. 2009;33:1045–52.

48. Couillard A, Maltais F, Saey D, Debigaré R, Michaud A, Koechlin C, et al. Exercise-induced quadriceps oxidative stress and peripheral muscle dysfunction in patients with chronic obstructive pulmonary disease. Am J Respir Crit Care Med. 2003;167:1664–9.

49. Barreiro E, Peinado VI, Galdiz JB, Ferrer E, Marin-Corral J, Sanchez F, et al. Cigarette smoke-induced oxidative stress: a role in chronic obstructive pulmonary disease skeletal muscle dysfunction. Am J Respir Crit Care Med. 2010;182:477–88.

50. Rabinovich RA, Ardite E, Mayer AM, Polo MF, Vilaro J, Argiles JM, et al. Training depletes muscle glutathione in patients with chronic obstructive pulmonary disease and low body mass index. Respiration. 2006;73:757–61.

51. Wijnhoven JH, Janssen AJ, van Kuppevelt TH, Rodenburg RJ, Dekhuijzen PN. Metabolic capacity of the diaphragm in patients with COPD. Respir Med. 2006;100:1064–71.

52. Ribera F, N'Guessan B, Zoll J, Fortin D, Serrurier B, Mettauer B, et al. Mitochondrial electron transport chain function is enhanced in inspiratory muscles of patients with chronic obstructive pulmonary disease. Am J Respir Crit Care Med. 2003;167:873–9.

53. Orozco-Levi M, Gea J, Lloreta JL, Felez M, Minguella J, Serrano S, et al. Subcellular adaptation of the human diaphragm in chronic obstructive pulmonary disease. Eur Respir J. 1999;13:371–8.

54. Barreiro E, de la Puente B, Minguella J, Corominas JM, Serrano S, Hussain SN, et al. Oxidative stress and respiratory muscle dysfunction in severe chronic obstructive pulmonary disease. Am J Respir Crit Care Med. 2005;171:1116–24.

55. Marin-Corral J, Minguella J, Ramirez-Sarmiento AL, Hussain SN, Gea J, Barreiro E. Oxidized proteins and superoxide anion production in the diaphragm of severe COPD patients. Eur Respir J. 2009;33:1309–19.

56. Wijnhoven HJ, Heunks LM, Geraedts MC, Hafmans T, Vina JR, Dekhuijzen PN. Oxidative and nitrosative stress in the diaphragm of patients with COPD. Int J Chron Obstruct Pulmon Dis. 2006;1:173–9.

57. Schols AM. Nutritional and metabolic modulation in chronic obstructive pulmonary disease management. Eur Respir J Suppl. 2003;46:81s–6.

58. Schols AM, Soeters PB, Mostert R, Saris WH, Wouters EF. Energy balance in chronic obstructive pulmonary disease. Am Rev Respir Dis. 1991;143:1248–52.

59. Pichard C, Jeejeebhoy KN. Muscle dysfunction in malnourished patients. Q J Med. 1988;69:1021–45.

60. Engelen MP, Schols AM, Baken WC, Wesseling GJ, Wouters EF. Nutritional depletion in relation to respiratory and peripheral skeletal muscle function in out-patients with COPD. Eur Respir J. 1994;7:1793–7.

61. Lopes J, Russell DM, Whitwell J, Jeejeebhoy KN. Skeletal muscle function in malnutrition. Am J Clin Nutr. 1982;36:602–10.

62. Ferreira IM, Brooks D, Lacasse Y, Goldstein RS, White J. Nutritional supplementation for stable chronic obstructive pulmonary disease. Cochrane Database Syst Rev. 2005;CD000998.

63. Nishimura Y, Tsutsumi M, Nakata H, Tsunenari T, Maeda H, Yokoyama M. Relationship between respiratory muscle strength and lean body mass in men with COPD. Chest. 1995;107:1232–6.

64. Franssen FM, Wouters EF, Schols AM. The contribution of starvation, deconditioning and ageing to the observed alterations in peripheral skeletal muscle in chronic organ diseases. Clin Nutr. 2002;21:1–14.

65. Lawler JM, Song W, Demaree SR. Hindlimb unloading increases oxidative stress and disrupts antioxidant capacity in skeletal muscle. Free Radic Biol Med. 2003;35:9–16.

66. Remels AH, Schrauwen P, Broekhuizen R, Willems J, Kersten S, Gosker HR, et al. Peroxisome proliferator-activated receptor expression is reduced in skeletal muscle in COPD. Eur Respir J. 2007;30:245–52.

67. Serres I, Gautier V, Varray A, Prefaut C. Impaired skeletal muscle endurance related to physical inactivity and altered lung function in COPD patients. Chest. 1998;113:900–5.

68. Pitta F, Troosters T, Spruit MA, Decramer M, Gosselink R. Activity monitoring for assessment of physical activities in daily life in patients with chronic obstructive pulmonary disease. Arch Phys Med Rehabil. 2005;86:1979–85.

69. Walker PP, Burnett A, Flavahan PW, Calverley PM. Lower limb activity and its determinants in COPD. Thorax. 2008;63:683–9.

70. Pitta F, Troosters T, Spruit MA, Probst VS, Decramer M, Gosselink R. Characteristics of physical activities in daily life in chronic obstructive pulmonary disease. Am J Respir Crit Care Med. 2005;171:972–7.

71. Troosters T, Sciurba F, Battaglia S, Langer D, Valluri SR, Martino L, et al. Physical inactivity in patients with COPD, a controlled multi-center pilot-study. Respir Med. 2010;104:1005–11.

72. Casaburi R. Activity monitoring in assessing activities of daily living. COPD. 2007;4:251–5.

73. Coronell C, Orozco-Levi M, Gea J. COPD and body weight in a Mediterranean population. Clin Nutr. 2002;21:437 [author reply 437–437; author reply 438].

74. Mattson JP, Poole DC. Pulmonary emphysema decreases hamster skeletal muscle oxidative enzyme capacity. J Appl Physiol. 1998;85:210–4.

75. Hoppeler H, Kleinert E, Schlegel C, Claassen H, Howald H, Kayar SR, et al. Morphological adaptations of human skeletal muscle to chronic hypoxia. Int J Sports Med. 1990;11 Suppl 1:S3–9.

76. Ferretti G, Hauser H, di Prampero PE. Maximal muscular power before and after exposure to chronic hypoxia. Int J Sports Med. 1990;11 Suppl 1:S31–4.

77. Westerterp KR, Kayser B. Body mass regulation at altitude. Eur J Gastroenterol Hepatol. 2006;18:1–3.

78. Plywaczewski R, Sliwinski P, Nowinski A, Kaminski D, Zielinski J. Incidence of nocturnal desaturation while breathing oxygen in COPD patients undergoing long-term oxygen therapy. Chest. 2000;117:679–83.

79. Poulain M, Durand F, Palomba B, Ceugniet F, Desplan J, Varray A, et al. 6-Minute walk testing is more sensitive than maximal incremental cycle testing for detecting oxygen desaturation in patients with COPD. Chest. 2003;123:1401–7.

80. Gosker HR, van Mameren H, van Dijk PJ, Engelen MP, van der Vusse GJ, Wouters EF, et al. Skeletal muscle fibre-type shifting and metabolic profile in patients with chronic obstructive pulmonary disease. Eur Respir J. 2002;19:617–25.

81. Hoppeler H, Vogt M, Weibel ER, Fluck M. Response of skeletal muscle mitochondria to hypoxia. Exp Physiol. 2003;88:109–19.

82. Jatta K, Eliason G, Portela-Gomes GM, Grimelius L, Caro O, Nilholm L, et al. Overexpression of von Hippel-Lindau protein in skeletal muscles of patients with chronic obstructive pulmonary disease. J Clin Pathol. 2009;62:70–6.

83. Guzy RD, Schumacker PT. Oxygen sensing by mitochondria at complex III: the paradox of increased reactive oxygen species during hypoxia. Exp Physiol. 2006;91:807–19.

84. Demasi M, Cleland LG, Cook-Johnson RJ, Caughey GE, James MJ. Effects of hypoxia on monocyte inflammatory mediator production: Dissociation between changes in cyclooxygenase-2 expression and eicosanoid synthesis. J Biol Chem. 2003;278:38607–16.

85. Koechlin C, Maltais F, Saey D, Michaud A, LeBlanc P, Hayot M, et al. Hypoxaemia enhances peripheral muscle oxidative stress in chronic obstructive pulmonary disease. Thorax. 2005;60:834–41.
86. Hawke TJ, Garry DJ. Myogenic satellite cells: physiology to molecular biology. J Appl Physiol. 2001;91:534–51.
87. Charge SB, Rudnicki MA. Cellular and molecular regulation of muscle regeneration. Physiol Rev. 2004;84:209–38.
88. Di Carlo A, De Mori R, Martelli F, Pompilio G, Capogrossi MC, Germani A. Hypoxia inhibits myogenic differentiation through accelerated MyoD degradation. J Biol Chem. 2004;279:16332–8.
89. Caron MA, Thériault ME, Paré ME, Maltais F, Debigaré R. Hypoxia alters contractile protein homeostasis in L6 myotubes. FEBS Lett. 2009;583:1528–34.
90. Reid MB. Role of nitric oxide in skeletal muscle: synthesis, distribution and functional importance. Acta Physiol Scand. 1998;162:401–9.
91. Koechlin C, Couillard A, Simar D, Cristol JP, Bellet H, Hayot M, et al. Does oxidative stress alter quadriceps endurance in chronic obstructive pulmonary disease? Am J Respir Crit Care Med. 2004;169:1022–7.
92. Comellas AP, Dada LA, Lecuona E, Pesce LM, Chandel NS, Quesada N, et al. Hypoxia-mediated degradation of Na, K-ATPase via mitochondrial reactive oxygen species and the ubiquitin-conjugating system. Circ Res. 2006;98:1314–22.
93. Barreiro E, Sanchez D, Galdiz JB, Hussain SN, Gea J. N-acetylcysteine increases manganese superoxide dismutase activity in septic rat diaphragms. Eur Respir J. 2005;26:1032–9.
94. Cadenas E, Davies KJ. Mitochondrial free radical generation, oxidative stress, and aging. Free Radic Biol Med. 2000;29:222–30.
95. Heunks LM, Dekhuijzen PN. Respiratory muscle function and free radicals: from cell to COPD. Thorax. 2000;55:704–16.
96. Khawli FA, Reid MB. N-acetylcysteine depresses contractile function and inhibits fatigue of diaphragm in vitro. J Appl Physiol. 1994;77:317–24.
97. Reid MB. Nitric oxide, reactive oxygen species, and skeletal muscle contraction. Med Sci Sports Exerc. 2001;33:371–6.
98. Couillard A, Koechlin C, Cristol JP, Varray A, Préfaut C. Evidence of local exercise-induced systemic oxidative stress in chronic obstructive pulmonary disease patients. Eur Respir J. 2002;20:1123–9.
99. Van Helvoort HA, Heijdra YF, Thijs HM, Vina J, Wanten GJ, Dekhuijzen PN. Exercise-induced systemic effects in muscle-wasted patients with COPD. Med Sci Sports Exerc. 2006;38:1543–52.
100. Rahman I, Skwarska E, MacNee W. Attenuation of oxidant/antioxidant imbalance during treatment of exacerbations of chronic obstructive pulmonary disease. Thorax. 1997;52:565–8.
101. Rabinovich RA, Ardite E, Troosters T, Carbo N, Alonso J, Gonzalez de Suso JM, et al. Reduced muscle redox capacity after endurance training in patients with chronic obstructive pulmonary disease. Am J Respir Crit Care Med. 2001;164:1114–8.
102. Engelen MP, Schols AM, Does JD, Deutz NE, Wouters EF. Altered glutamate metabolism is associated with reduced muscle glutathione levels in patients with emphysema. Am J Respir Crit Care Med. 2000;161:98–103.
103. Mercken EM, Hageman GJ, Schols AM, Akkermans MA, Bast A, Wouters EF. Rehabilitation decreases exercise-induced oxidative stress in chronic obstructive pulmonary disease. Am J Respir Crit Care Med. 2005;172:994–1001.
104. Wouters EF, Creutzberg EC, Schols AM. Systemic effects in COPD. Chest. 2002;121:127S–30.
105. Li YP, Chen Y, Li AS, Reid MB. Hydrogen peroxide stimulates ubiquitin-conjugating activity and expression of genes for specific E2 and E3 proteins in skeletal muscle myotubes. Am J Physiol Cell Physiol. 2003;285:C806–12.
106. Gan WQ, Man SF, Senthilselvan A, Sin DD. Association between chronic obstructive pulmonary disease and systemic inflammation: a systematic review and a meta-analysis. Thorax. 2004;59:574–80.

107. Schols AM, Buurman WA, Staal van den Brekel AJ, Dentener MA, Wouters EF. Evidence for a relation between metabolic derangements and increased levels of inflammatory mediators in a subgroup of patients with chronic obstructive pulmonary disease. Thorax. 1996;51: 819–24.
108. Dentener MA, Creutzberg EC, Schols AM, Mantovani A, Van't Veer C, Buurman WA, et al. Systemic anti-inflammatory mediators in COPD: increase in soluble interleukin 1 receptor II during treatment of exacerbations. Thorax. 2001;56:721–6.
109. Degens H, Alway SE. Control of muscle size during disuse, disease, and aging. Int J Sports Med. 2006;27:94–9.
110. Spruit MA, Gosselink R, Troosters T, Kasran A, Gayan-Ramirez G, Bogaerts P, et al. Muscle force during an acute exacerbation in hospitalised patients with COPD and its relationship with CXCL8 and IGF-I. Thorax. 2003;58:752–6.
111. Anker SD, Swan JW, Volterrani M, Chua TP, Clark AL, Poole-Wilson PA, et al. The influence of muscle mass, strength, fatigability and blood flow on exercise capacity in cachectic and non-cachectic patients with chronic heart failure. Eur Heart J. 1997;18:259–69.
112. Kopple JD. Pathophysiology of protein-energy wasting in chronic renal failure. J Nutr. 1999;129:247S–51.
113. Tisdale MJ. Mechanisms of cancer cachexia. Physiol Rev. 2009;89:381–410.
114. Debigaré R, Côté CH, Maltais F. Peripheral muscle wasting in chronic obstructive pulmonary disease. Clinical relevance and mechanisms. Am J Respir Crit Care Med. 2001;164:1712–7.
115. Broekhuizen R, Wouters EF, Creutzberg EC, Schols AM. Raised CRP levels mark metabolic and functional impairment in advanced COPD. Thorax. 2006;61:17–22.
116. Pinto-Plata VM, Mullerova H, Toso JF, Feudjo-Tepie M, Soriano JB, Vessey RS, et al. C-reactive protein in patients with COPD, control smokers and non-smokers. Thorax. 2006;61:23–8.
117. Yende S, Waterer GW, Tolley EA, Newman AB, Bauer DC, Taaffe DR, et al. Inflammatory markers are associated with ventilatory limitation and muscle dysfunction in obstructive lung disease in well functioning elderly subjects. Thorax. 2006;61:10–6.
118. Agusti AG, Noguera A, Sauleda J, Sala E, Pons J, Busquets X. Systemic effects of chronic obstructive pulmonary disease. Eur Respir J. 2003;21:347–60.
119. Sin DD, Man SF. Skeletal muscle weakness, reduced exercise tolerance, and COPD: is systemic inflammation the missing link? Thorax. 2006;61:1–3.
120. De Benedetti F, Alonzi T, Moretta A, Lazzaro D, Costa P, Poli V, et al. Interleukin 6 causes growth impairment in transgenic mice through a decrease in insulin-like growth factor-I. A model for stunted growth in children with chronic inflammation. J Clin Invest. 1997;99: 643–50.
121. Ladner KJ, Caligiuri MA, Guttridge DC. Tumor necrosis factor-regulated biphasic activation of NF-kappa B is required for cytokine-induced loss of skeletal muscle gene products. J Biol Chem. 2003;278:2294–303.
122. Reid MB, Durham WJ. Generation of reactive oxygen and nitrogen species in contracting skeletal muscle: potential impact on aging. Ann N Y Acad Sci. 2002;959:108–16.
123. Wilcox P, Milliken C, Bressler B. High-dose tumor necrosis factor alpha produces an impairment of hamster diaphragm contractility. Attenuation with a prostaglandin inhibitor. Am J Respir Crit Care Med. 1996;153:1611–5.
124. de Godoy I, Donahoe M, Calhoun WJ, Mancino J, Rogers RM. Elevated TNF-alpha production by peripheral blood monocytes of weight-losing COPD patients. Am J Respir Crit Care Med. 1996;153:633–7.
125. Wouters EF. Chronic obstructive pulmonary disease. 5: systemic effects of COPD. Thorax. 2002;57:1067–70.
126. Langen RC, Van Der Velden JL, Schols AM, Kelders MC, Wouters EF, Janssen-Heininger YM. Tumor necrosis factor-alpha inhibits myogenic differentiation through MyoD protein destabilization. FASEB J. 2004;18:227–37.

127. Vassilakopoulos T, Katsaounou P, Karatza MH, Kollintza A, Zakynthinos S, Roussos C. Strenuous resistive breathing induces plasma cytokines: role of antioxidants and monocytes. Am J Respir Crit Care Med. 2002;166:1572–8.
128. Broekhuizen R, Grimble RF, Howell WM, Shale DJ, Creutzberg EC, Wouters EF, et al. Pulmonary cachexia, systemic inflammatory profile, and the interleukin 1beta −511 single nucleotide polymorphism. Am J Clin Nutr. 2005;82:1059–64.
129. Vassilakopoulos T, Roussos C, Zakynthinos S. The immune response to resistive breathing. Eur Respir J. 2004;24:1033–43.
130. Poulain M, Doucet M, Drapeau V, Fournier G, Tremblay A, Poirier P, et al. Metabolic and inflammatory profile in obese patients with chronic obstructive pulmonary disease. Chron Respir Dis. 2008;5:35–41.
131. Casaburi R. Skeletal muscle function in COPD. Chest. 2000;117:267S–71.
132. Celli BR, MacNee W. Standards for the diagnosis and treatment of patients with COPD: a summary of the ATS/ERS position paper. Eur Respir J. 2004;23:932–46.
133. Mador MJ, Bozkanat E. Skeletal muscle dysfunction in chronic obstructive pulmonary disease. Respir Res. 2001;2:216–24.
134. Gosker HR, Wouters EF, van der Vusse GJ, Schols AM. Skeletal muscle dysfunction in chronic obstructive pulmonary disease and chronic heart failure: underlying mechanisms and therapy perspectives. Am J Clin Nutr. 2000;71:1033–47.
135. Man WD, Kemp P, Moxham J, Polkey MI. Skeletal muscle dysfunction in COPD: clinical and laboratory observations. Clin Sci (Lond). 2009;117:251–64.
136. Decramer M, Rennard S, Troosters T, Mapel DW, Giardino N, Mannino D, et al. COPD as a lung disease with systemic consequences – clinical impact, mechanisms, and potential for early intervention. COPD. 2008;5:235–56.
137. Wagner PD. Skeletal muscles in chronic obstructive pulmonary disease: deconditioning, or myopathy? Respirology. 2006;11:681–6.
138. Hansen MJ, Gualano RC, Bozinovski S, Vlahos R, Anderson GP. Therapeutic prospects to treat skeletal muscle wasting in COPD (chronic obstructive lung disease). Pharmacol Ther. 2006;109:162–72.
139. Holloszy JO, Coyle EF. Adaptations of skeletal muscle to endurance exercise and their metabolic consequences. J Appl Physiol. 1984;56:831–8.
140. Casaburi R, Patessio A, Ioli F, Zanaboni S, Donner CF, Wasserman K. Reductions in exercise lactic acidosis and ventilation as a result of exercise training in patients with obstructive lung disease. Am Rev Respir Dis. 1991;143:9–18.
141. Maltais F, LeBlanc P, Simard C, Jobin J, Berubé C, Bruneau J, et al. Skeletal muscle adaptation to endurance training in patients with chronic obstructive pulmonary disease. Am J Respir Crit Care Med. 1996;154:442–7.
142. Troosters T, Gosselink R, Decramer M. Short- and long-term effects of outpatient rehabilitation in patients with chronic obstructive pulmonary disease: a randomized trial. Am J Med. 2000;109:207–12.
143. Casaburi R, Bhasin S, Cosentino L, Porszasz J, Somfay A, Lewis MI, et al. Effects of testosterone and resistance training in men with chronic obstructive pulmonary disease. Am J Respir Crit Care Med. 2004;170:870–8.
144. Mador MJ, Kufel TJ, Pineda LA, Steinwald A, Aggarwal A, Upadhyay AM, et al. Effect of pulmonary rehabilitation on quadriceps fatiguability during exercise. Am J Respir Crit Care Med. 2001;163:930–5.
145. Bernard S, Whittom F, Leblanc P, Jobin J, Belleau R, Berubé C, et al. Aerobic and strength training in patients with chronic obstructive pulmonary disease. Am J Respir Crit Care Med. 1999;159:896–901.
146. Richardson RS, Sheldon J, Poole DC, Hopkins SR, Ries AL, Wagner PD. Evidence of skeletal muscle metabolic reserve during whole body exercise in patients with chronic obstructive pulmonary disease. Am J Respir Crit Care Med. 1999;159:881–5.

147. Siu PM, Donley DA, Bryner RW, Alway SE. Myogenin and oxidative enzyme gene expression levels are elevated in rat soleus muscles after endurance training. J Appl Physiol. 2004;97:277–85.
148. Vogiatzis I, Stratakos G, Simoes DC, Terzis G, Georgiadou O, Roussos C, et al. Effects of rehabilitative exercise on peripheral muscle TNFalpha, IL-6, IGF-I and MyoD expression in patients with COPD. Thorax. 2007;62:950–6.
149. Siu PM, Bryner RW, Martyn JK, Alway SE. Apoptotic adaptations from exercise training in skeletal and cardiac muscles. FASEB J. 2004;18:1150–2.
150. Léger B, Cartoni R, Praz M, Lamon S, Deriaz O, Crettenand A, et al. Akt signalling through GSK-3beta, mTOR and Foxo1 is involved in human skeletal muscle hypertrophy and atrophy. J Physiol. 2006;576:923–33.
151. Troosters T, Probst VS, Crul T, Pitta F, Gayan-Ramirez G, Decramer M, et al. Resistance training prevents deterioration in quadriceps muscle function during acute exacerbations of chronic obstructive pulmonary disease. Am J Respir Crit Care Med. 2010;181:1072–7.
152. Brooks D, Sottana R, Bell B, Hanna M, Laframboise L, Selvanayagarajah S, et al. Characterization of pulmonary rehabilitation programs in Canada in 2005. Can Respir J. 2007;14:87–92.
153. Maltais F, Bourbeau J, Shapiro S, Lacasse Y, Perrault H, Baltzan M, et al. Effects of home-based pulmonary rehabilitation in patients with chronic obstructive pulmonary disease: a randomized trial. Ann Intern Med. 2008;149:869–78.
154. Vieira DS, Maltais F, Bourbeau J. Home-based pulmonary rehabilitation in chronic obstructive pulmonary disease patients. Curr Opin Pulm Med. 2010;16:134–43.
155. Prescott E, Almdal T, Mikkelsen KL, Tofteng CL, Vestbo J, Lange P. Prognostic value of weight change in chronic obstructive pulmonary disease: results from the Copenhagen City Heart Study. Eur Respir J. 2002;20:539–44.
156. Whittaker JS, Ryan CF, Buckley PA, Road JD. The effects of refeeding on peripheral and respiratory muscle function in malnourished chronic obstructive pulmonary disease patients. Am Rev Respir Dis. 1990;142:283–8.
157. Schols AM. Nutritional modulation as part of the integrated management of chronic obstructive pulmonary disease. Proc Nutr Soc. 2003;62:783–91.
158. Broekhuizen R, Creutzberg EC, Weling-Scheepers CA, Wouters EF, Schols AM. Optimizing oral nutritional drink supplementation in patients with chronic obstructive pulmonary disease. Br J Nutr. 2005;93:965–71.
159. Schols AM, Soeters PB, Mostert R, Pluymers RJ, Wouters EF. Physiologic effects of nutritional support and anabolic steroids in patients with chronic obstructive pulmonary disease. A placebo-controlled randomized trial. Am J Respir Crit Care Med. 1995;152:1268–74.
160. Fiaccadori E, Borghetti A. Pathophysiology of respiratory muscles in course of undernutrition. Ann Ital Med Int. 1991;6:402–7.
161. Di Francia M, Barbier D, Mege JL, Orehek J. Tumor necrosis factor-alpha levels and weight loss in chronic obstructive pulmonary disease. Am J Respir Crit Care Med. 1994;150:1453–5.
162. Fuld JP, Kilduff LP, Neder JA, Pitsiladis Y, Lean ME, Ward SA, et al. Creatine supplementation during pulmonary rehabilitation in chronic obstructive pulmonary disease. Thorax. 2005;60:531–7.
163. Matsuyama W, Mitsuyama H, Watanabe M, Oonakahara K, Higashimoto I, Osame M, et al. Effects of omega-3 polyunsaturated fatty acids on inflammatory markers in COPD. Chest. 2005;128:3817–27.
164. Weisberg J, Wanger J, Olson J, Streit B, Fogarty C, Martin T, et al. Megestrol acetate stimulates weight gain and ventilation in underweight COPD patients. Chest. 2002;121:1070–8.
165. Isgaard J, Nilsson A, Vikman K, Isaksson OG. Growth hormone regulates the level of insulin-like growth factor-I mRNA in rat skeletal muscle. J Endocrinol. 1989;120:107–12.
166. Cuneo RC, Salomon F, Wiles CM, Hesp R, Sonksen PH. Growth hormone treatment in growth hormone-deficient adults. I. Effects on muscle mass and strength. J Appl Physiol. 1991;70:688–94.

167. Cuneo RC, Salomon F, Wiles CM, Hesp R, Sonksen PH. Growth hormone treatment in growth hormone-deficient adults. II. Effects on exercise performance. J Appl Physiol. 1991;70:695–700.
168. Burdet L, de Muralt B, Schutz Y, Pichard C, Fitting JW. Administration of growth hormone to underweight patients with chronic obstructive pulmonary disease. A prospective, randomized, controlled study. Am J Respir Crit Care Med. 1997;156:1800–6.
169. Bhasin S, Calof OM, Storer TW, Lee ML, Mazer NA, Jasuja R, et al. Drug insight: testosterone and selective androgen receptor modulators as anabolic therapies for chronic illness and aging. Nat Clin Pract Endocrinol Metab. 2006;2:146–59.
170. Allan G, Sbriscia T, Linton O, Lai MT, Haynes-Johnson D, Bhattacharjee S, et al. A selective androgen receptor modulator with minimal prostate hypertrophic activity restores lean body mass in aged orchidectomized male rats. J Steroid Biochem Mol Biol. 2008;110:207–13.
171. Tisdale MJ. The ubiquitin-proteasome pathway as a therapeutic target for muscle wasting. J Support Oncol. 2005;3:209–17.
172. Decramer M, de Bock V, Dom R. Functional and histologic picture of steroid-induced myopathy in chronic obstructive pulmonary disease. Am J Respir Crit Care Med. 1996;153:1958–64.
173. Dentener MA, Creutzberg EC, Pennings HJ, Rijkers GT, Mercken E, Wouters EF. Effect of infliximab on local and systemic inflammation in chronic obstructive pulmonary disease: a pilot study. Respiration. 2008;76:275–82.
174. Rennard SI, Fogarty C, Kelsen S, Long W, Ramsdell J, Allison J, et al. The safety and efficacy of infliximab in moderate to severe chronic obstructive pulmonary disease. Am J Respir Crit Care Med. 2007;175:926–34.
175. van Hees HW, Dekhuijzen PN, Heunks LM. Levosimendan enhances force generation of diaphragm muscle from patients with chronic obstructive pulmonary disease. Am J Respir Crit Care Med. 2009;179:41–7.

Chapter 10
Inactivity

Judith Garcia-Aymerich

Abstract Patients with chronic obstructive pulmonary disease (COPD) have reduced levels of physical activity compared to their counterparts. Such inactivity is considered a consequence of several pulmonary and extrapulmonary manifestations of COPD. Evidence in the last decade has shown that reduced levels of activity have deleterious prognostic effects in these patients. This has driven an increasing amount of research aimed at a better understanding of the causes and effects of reduced physical activity in COPD, as well as a search for the best methodological tools and statistical approaches to ascertain physical activity. The current chapter focuses on the determinants, the levels, and the effects of regular physical activity in COPD patients, as well as on interventions to counteract the effects of inactivity. The role of regular physical activity as a protecting factor for developing COPD will not be covered.

Keywords COPD • Pulmonary manifestations • Extrapulmonary manifestations • Activity • Exercise • Inactivity • Physical activity • Physical fitness

Introduction

Patients with chronic obstructive pulmonary disease (COPD) have reduced levels of physical activity compared to their counterparts [1]. Such inactivity is considered a consequence of several pulmonary and extrapulmonary manifestations of COPD [2]. Evidence in the last decade has shown that reduced levels of activity have deleterious prognostic effects in these patients [3]. This has driven an increasing amount of research aimed at a better understanding of the causes and effects of

J. Garcia-Aymerich (✉)
Centre for Research in Environmental Epidemiology (CREAL), Barcelona, Spain
e-mail: jgarcia@creal.cat

L. Nici and R. ZuWallack (eds.), *Chronic Obstructive Pulmonary Disease: Co-Morbidities and Systemic Consequences*, Respiratory Medicine, DOI 10.1007/978-1-60761-673-3_10, © Springer Science+Business Media, LLC 2012

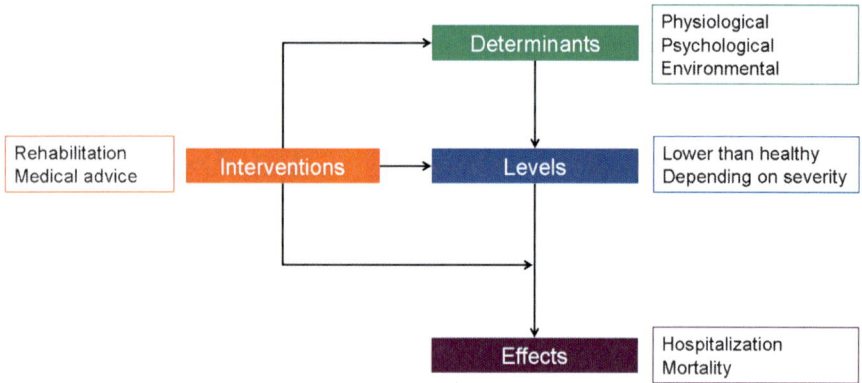

Fig. 10.1 Determinants, levels and effects of regular physical activity in COPD patients

reduced physical activity in COPD, as well as a search for the best methodological tools and statistical approaches to ascertain physical activity. The current chapter focuses on the determinants, the levels, and the effects of regular physical activity in COPD patients, as well as on interventions to counteract the effects of inactivity (Fig. 10.1). The role of regular physical activity as a protecting factor for developing COPD [4] will not be covered.

The Concept of Physical Activity

The terms physical activity, physical fitness, and exercise are often used inter-changeably, despite the fact that they describe different concepts. For the purpose of this chapter, the interpretational framework provided by Caspersen *et al.* in 1985 is used, which relates each of these concepts to health and disease [5]. Physical activity is defined as "any bodily movement produced by skeletal muscles which results in energy expenditure." Physical activity can be categorized in several ways, such as according to intensity (mild, moderate, or high), according to the portions of daily life during which the activities occur (sleeping, at work, or at leisure), or according to the type (conditioning, household, or other). Each method of categorization may be useful for the study of the levels of physical activity as well as the study of its effects in health. Importantly, physical activity is a complex behavior, difficult to assess in itself, and whose determinants are even more difficult to assess. Exercise is defined as "a subset of physical activity that is planned, structured, and repetitive and has as a final or an intermediate objective the improvement or maintenance of physical fitness." Thus, some of the abovementioned physical activities such as sports, or even household activities when they are planned to develop muscular strength or to "burn" calories, may be considered exercise. Finally, physical fitness is defined as "a set of attributes that are either health- or skill-related." Fitness relates to the ability to perform physical activities, and its health-related components include cardio-respiratory endurance, muscle endurance, muscle strength, body composition, and flexibility. The three concepts (physical activity, physical fitness, and exercise) are strongly related among them but need to be distinguished both in clinical practice and in research, and therefore measured with specific tests.

In the context of COPD, physical activity may refer to leisure-time activities such as walking or cycling, or, in nonretired patients, to work-related activities. Physical activity is measured using either direct measures (movement detectors such as accelerometers or pedometers) or indirect measures (questionnaires). In COPD, physical fitness is often labeled as exercise capacity or tolerance, and is regularly measured using field or cardiopulmonary exercise tests. Exercise, as defined above, has been traditionally incorrectly restricted to sports. However, structured activities designed to improve fitness, such as exercise training in the frame of pulmonary rehabilitation programs, should be considered exercise.

Determinants of Physical (In)Activity in COPD

It is generally accepted that respiratory function impairment and symptoms of COPD lead patients to reduce their physical activity. In turn, a sedentary lifestyle deconditions their bodies and reduces the threshold for physical activity-related dyspnea. Progressively, patients enter a stage of reduced physical activity, high symptom burden, reduced health-related quality of life, and even psychological disorders [6]. This situation has been labeled as "the downward spiral of physical activity in COPD." Pathophysiological mechanisms leading to this situation have been covered in detail in previous chapters of this book and will not be detailed here.

It is surprising that other determinants of physical activity that have been the focus of interest in the general population have hardly been considered in COPD patients. The Report of the Surgeon General about Physical Activity and Health [7] reviews several of the numerous theories and models on physical activity that have been used in behavioral and social sciences. Although diverse, there is agreement that the determinants of physical activity include the physiological (such as those abovementioned in the "downward spiral"), psychological (not limited to anxiety and depression, but also including expectancies or enjoyment with physical activity), and environmental (e.g., climate, culture, or family habits). Qualitative research in COPD patients has highlighted the importance of the patients' point of view, remarking that personal integrity as a motivating factor for regular activity needs to be considered when designing interventions [8]. Logically, the patient's point of view should also be considered in clinical research aimed at measuring the levels of activity or its effects, as well as in clinical practice during routine assessment of the COPD patient.

The potential role of external factors has been pointed out by a recent study that found different physical activity levels in COPD patients from Austria and Brazil, despite very similar sociodemographic, clinical, and functional variables [9]. In the general population, global and local environmental conditions, such as deprivation, urbanization, access to local amenities, or perceived local safety, interact with physical activity to determine health [10], and all should be considered when designing interventions.

Levels of Physical (In)Activity in COPD

Many studies have found that COPD patients have lower levels of physical activity than their age and gender-matched healthy subjects, irrespective of the tool used, and the geographic origin of the samples [1, 11–19]. However, this statement has not been consistent [20] and needs to be interpreted with caution in view of some limitations common to all mentioned studies, mainly confounding and selection bias. Probably, the most influential of these studies was the one published by Pitta *et al.* in 2005 [1] where 50 COPD and 25 healthy elderly subjects provided physical activities and movement intensity through an activity monitor. The COPD patients showed lower walking time, standing time, and movement intensity during walking, as well as higher sitting and lying times. In this study, the prevalence of osteoporosis, diabetes, depression, heart disease, and arterial hypertension was two- or threefold higher in patients with COPD. Unfortunately, the extent to which the differences could be attributed to COPD itself or to concomitant chronic diseases was not tested. Such a lack of adjustment for co-morbidities or other potential confounders is common to many available studies. As a result, the clinical implications of such research are affected, i.e., how doctors approach inactive COPD patients with co-morbidities.

Another common pitfall of the studies published thus far that compare physical activity in COPD with healthy subjects is that COPD patients have been recruited in hospital or pulmonary rehabilitation settings. Commonly, these COPD patients have lower physical activity levels than the entire COPD population, and furthermore, the control subjects are not truly representative of the general population. A hospital-based COPD study in Spain [21] found levels of physical activity comparable to the general population of the same age and gender [22]. Other large population-based samples, such as the participants in the European Prospective Investigation into Cancer and Nutrition (EPIC study) aged 50–64 years [23] or the US National Health Interview Survey subjects aged 65 years or older [24], also found levels of physical activity in COPD patients similar to the ones reported previously. The Copenhagen City Heart Study showed almost identical levels of physical activity between the general population and the mild and moderate population-based COPD sample, identifying differences only with the severe and very severe COPD stages (Fig. 10.2) [3, 4]. The latter is in agreement with two recent papers comparing COPD with chronic bronchitis or healthy controls that reported a decrease in physical activity comparing in those with moderate to severe disease [25, 26].

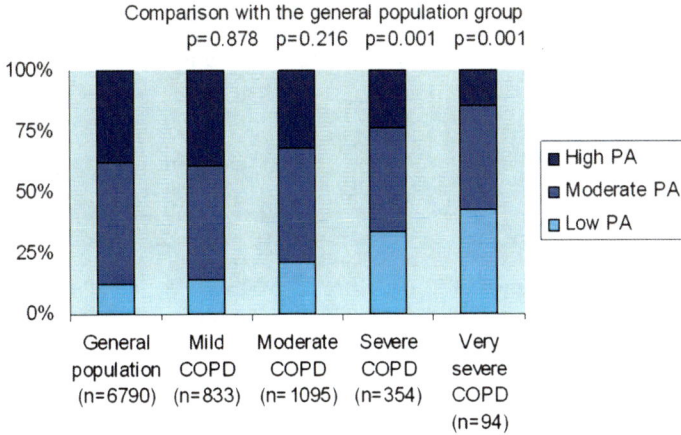

Fig. 10.2 Cumulative proportion of high, moderate and low physical activity in the general population and subjects with COPD, according to severity stage, in the Copenhagen City Heart Study [3, 4]

Effects of Physical (In)Activity in COPD

The first study that reported an effect of physical activity on COPD prognosis was the Study of the Risk Factors of COPD Exacerbation (EFRAM project), which included a mean of 1.1 year follow-up of 340 COPD patients recruited during an admission for an exacerbation in four tertiary hospitals in the Barcelona area, Spain [27]. The study was not designed specifically to assess the role of physical activity on COPD. Rather, it aimed to explain the risk factors of hospital admission for a COPD exacerbation. The study looked at a wide range of potential risk factors including socio-demographic variables, clinical and functional status, medical care and prescriptions, adherence to medication, lifestyle (including smoking and physical activity), health status, and social support [28]. One of the main findings was that the third of patients who reported a physical activity equivalent of walking 1 h daily or more had a 50% reduced risk of readmission over the year of follow-up, despite adjusting for previous admissions, PaO_2 and FEV_1, among other confounders. Similar reductions in the risk of admission for an exacerbation were found in the Copenhagen City Heart Study, where 2,386 subjects with COPD were identified from the general population (including mainly mild and moderate COPD) and followed up a mean of 12 years (Fig. 10.3) [3]. A limitation to both studies is the measure of physical activity through a self-reported questionnaire, which unavoidably involves some misclassification and therefore makes it more difficult to identify statistically significant differences where they exist [29]. A small study from Belgium obtained direct measure of physical activity by using accelerometers in COPD patients recruited at the emergency room and followed them for 1 year. Again, those with higher walking time had a lower risk of COPD admission in the

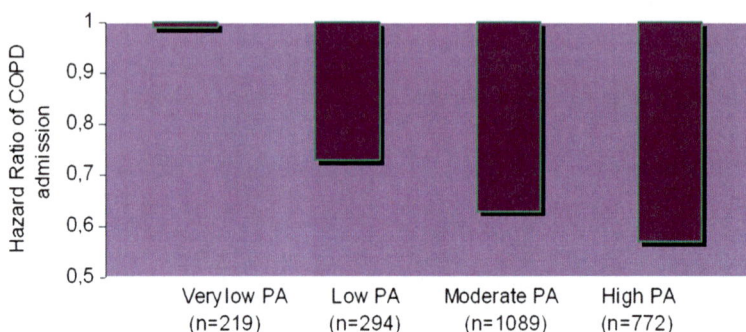

Fig. 10.3 Risk of admission for an exacerbation, according to physical activity levels, in 2,386 subjects with COPD from the Copenhagen City Heart Study [3]

year after [30]. One of the most important findings from these studies is that, despite different types of COPD patients, different methods to assess physical activity, and different settings and geographic areas, the amount of activity needed to obtain a significant reduction in the admission risk was relatively small (walking or cycling 2 h per week or more).

Another interesting finding has been that reduced activity levels in COPD may increase the risk of all-cause and respiratory mortality in these patients. This was observed in COPD subjects from the general population in Copenhagen [3], but has not been replicated thus far.

Other studies have tried to identify other effects of physical activity in COPD patients through cross-sectional study designs [31, 32]. Since this design makes it difficult to ascertain the direction of the associations, these studies will not be discussed here. In fact, the potential problem of reverse causation may be a concern even in longitudinal studies. Given that patients with COPD reduce their physical activity during and after an exacerbation [30] and given the long evolution of the disease, the actual levels of activity may have been influenced by previous exacerbations (or disease severity). Therefore, it may be difficult to distinguish whether activity is cause or effect of exacerbations. Recently, statistical methods specifically developed to deal with the methodological problems of reverse causation and time-dependent confounding [33] have been used to estimate the association between physical activity and COPD hospitalizations and death, and have provided very similar results to those obtained with standard analysis, supporting previous results and suggesting they were not due to time-dependent confounding [34].

Finally, it could be argued that experimental studies intervening on physical activity is the only way to assess what the effects are. In the absence of such experimental studies, a true effect could be potentially inferred from pulmonary rehabilitation programs, which include exercise training and physical activity advice. Indeed, a recent review of rehabilitation programs showed a positive impact on dyspnea, muscle function, and exercise capacity [35]. However, because most rehabilitation programs include multiple components, it is difficult to isolate the effects of physical activity.

Is Inactivity Reversible in COPD?

The previous sections have reported the current knowledge about determinants, levels, and effects of physical activity in COPD, as well as the limitations to existing research. However, such research would be useless in the absence of interventions that could maintain or increase the levels of physical activity in COPD patients. Unfortunately, research in this area is scarce.

One could argue that interventions on the determinants of physical activity could theoretically change the levels of activity. Both pharmacological and nonpharmacological treatments may improve some of the physiological (e.g., symptoms, or lung function) or psychological (e.g., quality of life, or anxiety) impairments. These treatments and their effects are widely covered in current guidelines for COPD [36, 37] and will not be detailed here. As examples, both bronchodilators and oxygen therapy may increase the level and the efficacy of exercise training by decreasing hyperinflation [38, 39]. Interestingly, evidence suggests that the effects of treatments on the actual level of physical activity will depend, in part, on the locus of symptom limitation, i.e., leg fatigue or dyspnea [40].

To date, there are few interventions in COPD whose primary outcome has been the level of physical activity. In one early study, 60 patients with COPD were randomized to a control group or an intervention of walking twice daily at speeds determined by treadmill exercise test results and cognitive and behavioral adherence interventions. In the 8 weeks of follow-up, total minutes walked ranged from 450 min per week for the control group to 1,800 min per week for the intervened group [41, 42]. More recently, the addition of active lifestyle counseling to a small pulmonary rehabilitation program, compared with pulmonary rehabilitation only, resulted in increased steps per day measured with a pedometer after 9 weeks [43]. Also, a secondary analysis of a dyspnea management intervention trial showed higher periods and duration of home walking in the subgroup whose intervention included exercise training, although differences were not statistically significant [44]. Finally, a systematic review that focused on outpatients found that the use of a pedometer is associated with significant increases in physical activity, although there are no data still available to ascertain the long-term effect [45]. In agreement with these findings, a recent noncontrolled experimental study with 35 stable COPD patients showed that a 12-week pedometer-based exercise counseling strategy was feasible and effectively enhanced daily physical activity [46].

Indirect but important evidence is also provided by pulmonary rehabilitation programs, which have been shown to increase levels of physical activity [35, 47]. However, the long-lasting effects of these programs are unknown. A recent pulmonary rehabilitation program in 29 COPD patients has shown that walking time in daily life did not improve significantly at 3 months, but only after 6 months. The authors concluded that long-lasting benefits may occur if we target behavior change in physical activity habits during daily life in COPD patients [48].

Summary

Physical activity is a potentially modifiable behavior that is reduced as a result of the pathophysiological impairments of COPD but whose maintenance can modify the evolution of COPD. Research about what are the determinants or effects of physical activity in COPD, or how it can be modified, is still scarce. Further research is needed with improved methodology using longitudinal studies with appropriate controls for confounding factors and selection bias.

References

1. Pitta F, Troosters T, Spruit MA, et al. Characteristics of physical activities in daily life in chronic obstructive pulmonary disease. Am J Respir Crit Care Med. 2005;171:972–7.
2. Barnes PJ, Celli BR. Systemic manifestations and comorbidities of COPD. Eur Respir J. 2009;33:1165–85.
3. Garcia-Aymerich J, Lange P, Benet M, et al. Regular physical activity reduces hospital admission and mortality in chronic obstructive pulmonary disease: a population-based cohort study. Thorax. 2006;61:772–8.
4. Garcia-Aymerich J, Lange P, Benet M, et al. Regular physical activity modifies smoking-related lung function decline and reduces risk of chronic obstructive pulmonary disease: a population-based cohort study. Am J Respir Crit Care Med. 2007;175:458–63.
5. Caspersen CJ, Powell KE, Christenson GM. Physical activity, exercise, and physical fitness: definitions and distinctions for health-related research. Public Health Rep. 1985;100:126–31.
6. ZuWallack R. How are you doing? What are you doing? Differing perspectives in the assessment of individuals with COPD. COPD. 2007;4:293–7.
7. U.S. Department of Health and Human Services. Physical activity and health: a report of the surgeon general. Atlanta, GA: U.S. Department of Health and Human Services, Centers for Disease Control and Prevention, National Center for Chronic Disease Prevention and Health Promotion; 1996.
8. Leidy NK, Haase JE. Functional status from the patient's perspective: the challenge of preserving personal integrity. Res Nurs Health. 1999;22:67–77.
9. Pitta F, Breyer MK, Hernandes NA, et al. Comparison of daily physical activity between COPD patients from Central Europe and South America. Respir Med. 2009;103:421–6.
10. Procter KL, Clarke GP, Ransley JK, et al. Micro-level analysis of childhood obesity, diet, physical activity, residential socioeconomic and social capital variables: where are the obesogenic environments in Leeds? Area. 2008;40:323–40.
11. Gosker HR, Lencer NH, Franssen FM, et al. Striking similarities in systemic factors contributing to decreased exercise capacity in patients with severe chronic heart failure or COPD. Chest. 2003;123:1416–24.
12. Walker PP, Burnett A, Flavahan PW, et al. Lower limb activity and its determinants in COPD. Thorax. 2008;63:683–9.
13. Sandland CJ, Singh SJ, Curcio A, et al. A profile of daily activity in chronic obstructive pulmonary disease. J Cardiopulm Rehabil. 2005;25:181–3.
14. Coronado M, Janssens JP, de Muralt B, et al. Walking activity measured by accelerometry during respiratory rehabilitation. J Cardiopulm Rehabil. 2003;23:357–64.
15. Mercken EM, Hageman GJ, Schols AM, et al. Rehabilitation decreases exercise-induced oxidative stress in chronic obstructive pulmonary disease. Am J Respir Crit Care Med. 2005;172:994–1001.
16. Schönhofer B, Ardes P, Geibel M, et al. Evaluation of a movement detector to measure daily activity in patients with chronic lung disease. Eur Respir J. 1997;10:2814–9.

17. Coronell C, Orozco-Levi M, Méndez R, et al. Relevance of assessing quadriceps endurance in patients with COPD. Eur Respir J. 2004;24:129–36.
18. Serres I, Gautier V, Varray A, et al. Impaired skeletal muscle endurance related to physical inactivity and altered lung function in COPD patients. Chest. 1998;113:900–5.
19. Lores V, García-Río F, Rojo B, et al. Recording the daily physical activity of COPD patients with an accelerometer: an analysis of agreement and repeatability. Arch Bronconeumol. 2006;42:627–32.
20. Janaudis-Ferreira T, Wadell K, Sundelin G, et al. Thigh muscle strength and endurance in patients with COPD compared with healthy controls. Respir Med. 2006;100:1451–7.
21. Garcia-Aymerich J, Felez MA, Escarrabill J, et al. Physical activity and its determinants in severe chronic obstructive pulmonary disease. Med Sci Sports Exerc. 2004;36:1667–73.
22. Tormo Díaz MJ, Navarro Sánchez C, Chirlaque López MD, et al. [Cardiovascular risk factors in the region of Murcia, Spain]. Rev Esp Salud Pública 1997;71:515–29.
23. Haftenberger M, Schuit AJ, Tormo MJ, et al. Physical activity of subjects aged 50–64 years involved in the European Prospective Investigation into Cancer and Nutrition (EPIC). Public Health Nutr. 2002;5:1163–76.
24. Yusuf HR, Croft JB, Giles WH, et al. Leisure-time physical activity among older adults: United States, 1990. Arch Intern Med. 1996;156:1321–6.
25. Watz H, Waschki B, Meyer T, et al. Physical activity in patients with COPD. Eur Respir J. 2009;33:262–72.
26. Troosters T, Sciurba F, Battaglia S, et al. Physical inactivity in patients with COPD, a controlled multi-center pilot-study. Respir Med. 2010;104(7):1005–11.
27. Garcia-Aymerich J, Farrero E, Felez MA, et al. Risk factors of readmission to hospital for a COPD exacerbation: a prospective study. Thorax. 2003;58:100–5.
28. Garcia-Aymerich J, Monso E, Marrades RM, et al. Risk factors for hospitalization for a chronic obstructive pulmonary disease exacerbation. EFRAM study. Am J Respir Crit Care Med. 2001;164:1002–7.
29. Ferrari P, Friedenreich C, Matthews CE. The role of measurement error in estimating levels of physical activity. Am J Epidemiol. 2007;166:832–40.
30. Pitta F, Troosters T, Probst VS, et al. Physical activity and hospitalization for exacerbation of COPD. Chest. 2006;129:536–44.
31. Watz H, Waschki B, Boehme C, et al. Extrapulmonary effects of chronic obstructive pulmonary disease on physical activity: a cross-sectional study. Am J Respir Crit Care Med. 2008;177: 743–51.
32. Garcia-Aymerich J, Serra I, Gómez FP, et al. Phenotype and course of COPD study group. Physical activity and clinical and functional status in COPD. Chest. 2009;136:62–70.
33. Robins JM, Hernan MA, Brumback B. Marginal structural models and causal inference in epidemiology. Epidemiology. 2000;11:550–60.
34. Garcia-Aymerich J, Lange P, Serra I, et al. Time-dependent confounding in the study of the effects of regular physical activity in chronic obstructive pulmonary disease: an application of the marginal structural model. Ann Epidemiol. 2008;18:775–83.
35. Nici L, Donner C, Wouters E, For the ATS/ERS Pulmonary Rehabilitation Writing Committee, et al. American Thoracic Society/European Respiratory Society statement on pulmonary rehabilitation. Am J Respir Crit Care Med. 2006;173:1390–413.
36. Celli BR, MacNee W, For the ATS/ERS Task Force. Standards for the diagnosis and treatment of patients with COPD: a summary of the ATS/ERS position paper. Eur Respir J. 2004;23: 932–46.
37. Global Initiative for Chronic Obstructive Lung Disease. Global strategy for the diagnosis, management, and prevention of chronic obstructive pulmonary disease (updated 2009). http://www.goldcopd.org. Accessed 30 Mar 2010.
38. Zuwallack RL. The roles of bronchodilators, supplemental oxygen, and ventilatory assistance in the pulmonary rehabilitation of patients with chronic obstructive pulmonary disease. Respir Care. 2008;53:1190–5.
39. Casaburi R, Kukafka D, Cooper CB, et al. Improvement in exercise tolerance with the combination of tiotropium and pulmonary rehabilitation in patients with COPD. Chest. 2005;127:809–17.

40. Deschenes D, Pepin V, Saey D, et al. Locus of symptom limitation and exercise response to bronchodilation in chronic obstructive pulmonary disease. J Cardiopulm Rehabil Prev. 2008; 28:208–14.
41. Atkins CJ, Kaplan RM, Timms RM, et al. Behavioral exercise programs in the management of chronic obstructive pulmonary disease. J Consult Clin Psychol. 1984;52:591–603.
42. Kaplan RM, Atkins CJ, Reinsch S. Specific efficacy expectations mediate exercise compliance in patients with COPD. Health Psychol. 1984;3:223–42.
43. de Blok BM, de Greef MH, ten Hacken NH, et al. The effects of a lifestyle physical activity counseling program with feedback of a pedometer during pulmonary rehabilitation in patients with COPD: a pilot study. Patient Educ Couns. 2006;61:48–55.
44. Donesky-Cuenco D, Janson S, Neuhaus J, et al. Adherence to a home-walking prescription in patients with chronic obstructive pulmonary disease. Heart Lung. 2007;36:348–63.
45. Bravata DM, Smith-Spangler C, Sundaram V, et al. Using pedometers to increase physical activity and improve health: a systematic review. JAMA. 2007;298:2296–304.
46. Hospes G, Bossenbroek L, Ten Hacken NH, et al. Enhancement of daily physical activity increases physical fitness of outclinic COPD patients: results of an exercise counseling program. Patient Educ Couns. 2009;75:274–8.
47. Ries AL, Bauldoff GS, Carlin BW, et al. Pulmonary rehabilitation: joint ACCP/AACVPR evidence-based clinical practice guidelines. Chest. 2007;131:4S–2.
48. Pitta F, Troosters T, Probst VS, et al. Are patients with COPD more active after pulmonary rehabilitation? Chest. 2008;134:273–80.

Chapter 11
Body Composition Abnormalities

Bram van den Borst and Annemie M.W.J. Schols

Abstract Chronic obstructive pulmonary disease (COPD) is a complex and debilitating disease. Although the degree of airflow limitation is currently the main clinical determinant used for disease staging, patients within the same stage have widely varying symptoms and mortality risks. In this Chapter, we discuss the observation that body composition plays an important role in the heterogeneity of COPD. Using clinical examples, we elaborate on cachexia, obesity and aging-related changes in body composition, and how these body composition phenotypes are related to disease burden and COPD progression. Potential mechanisms contributing to a changing body composition are discussed on the level of skeletal muscle, adipose tissue and bone tissue. Finally, an overview is presented on the potential of lifestyle and drug interventions on optimizing body composition in COPD.

Keywords COPD • Smoking • Body composition • Emphysema • Bronchitis • Phenotypes • Cachexia

Introduction

Chronic obstructive pulmonary disease (COPD) has been described as a chronic lifestyle-related disease characterized by an enhanced inflammatory response in the lungs to smoking or environmental pollution. As this textbook highlights, COPD is associated with a wide range of systemic consequences. This chapter focuses on

B. van den Borst (✉) • A.M.W.J. Schols
Department of Respiratory Medicine, NUTRIM School for Nutrition, Toxicology
and Metabolism, Maastricht University Medical Center+, Maastricht, The Netherlands
e-mail: b.vdborst@maastrichtuniversity.nl; a.schols@maastrichtuniversity.nl

L. Nici and R. ZuWallack (eds.), *Chronic Obstructive Pulmonary Disease: Co-Morbidities and Systemic Consequences*, Respiratory Medicine, DOI 10.1007/978-1-60761-673-3_11, © Springer Science+Business Media, LLC 2012

body composition abnormalities in COPD. Classically, COPD patients were divided into "pink puffers" and "blue bloaters," which was based on anthropometric characteristics. "Pink puffers" were mainly characterized by emphysema and were thin in appearance with a history of weight loss, while "blue bloaters" typically had chronic bronchitis and tended to be overweight [1]. While the classification of "pink puffers" and "blue bloaters" highlighted that COPD is characterized by different phenotypes; nowadays, new evidence calls for an extension of this simplified distinction.

In the past two decades, it has become clear that body composition is an important marker of extrapulmonary impairment in COPD. Illustrating its heterogeneity of disease presentation and natural course of the disease, COPD can be associated with severe weight loss, and also with obesity, both of which two body composition phenotypes have differential clinical consequences. Physiologically, the aging human body undergoes body composition changes that are characterized by loss of lean body mass, in particular of muscle mass, a process named sarcopenia. Alongside these physiological deteriorations with aging, multiple COPD-related factors including an adaptive lifestyle have the potential to aggravate these processes, ultimately causing muscle weakness, mobility limitation, and increased mortality. One key finding in the recent literature has been that skeletal muscle wasting is an important target to decrease COPD morbidity and mortality [2]. However, to further improve and individualize therapeutic strategies, a better understanding of underlying pathophysiological mechanisms of alterations in body composition in COPD is warranted.

Using clinical examples, we discuss body composition abnormalities in COPD in relation to disease burden in terms of physical performance and mortality. Next, we present an overview of determinants and mechanisms potentially underlying shifts in body composition in COPD. Finally, we outline the current and the future potential of lifestyle and therapeutic interventions to maintain or optimize body composition in COPD as part of integrated disease management.

Epidemiology

Weight Loss and Cachexia

Patient A: A 63 year-old patient was diagnosed with COPD 7 years ago. Two years later, she began to lose weight rapidly despite self-reported unchanged food intake. Her normal weight was 58 kg, and now she weighs only 40 kg, resulting in a current body mass index (BMI) of 15.2 kg/m^2. After having smoked 60 pack years, she remains unmotivated to quit. Thorough internal investigation did not yield any reasons for her extreme weight loss (e.g., malabsorption or cancer) other than the presence of COPD. During the last year, she had been admitted to the hospital twice for an infectious acute exacerbation of COPD. She takes calcium and vitamin D supplementation for osteoporosis. Her pulmonary medication consists of inhaled corticosteroids, β2-mimetics, and anticholinergics. Nonetheless, her clinical situation continues to deteriorate. She barely comes out of her house and she is too tired to perform any physical activities. Dyspnea is frequently increased and with an arterial oxygen tension of 6.9 kPa; she is at the brink of requiring long-term oxygen therapy. The forced expiratory volume in 1s (FEV_1) and diffusion capacity for carbon monoxide (DL_{CO}) measure 52% and 37% of predicted, respectively. Upon an incremental cycling test, the peak oxygen uptake (VO_2) is 57% of predicted and a drop in peripheral oxygen saturation of 9% is observed. Assessed by whole-body dual-energy X-ray absorptiometry (DXA), body composition measures reveal a fat-free mass index (FFMI) and fat mass index (FMI) of 12.1 and 3.1 kg/m^2, respectively, indicative of severe nutritional depletion.

Patient A has a clear history of severe weight loss and was diagnosed with COPD-related cachexia, also referred to as pulmonary cachexia [3]. Cachexia is defined as a complex debilitating metabolic syndrome associated with underlying disease, characterized by loss of muscle mass with or without loss of fat mass [4]. While the pathophysiology of cachexia is incompletely understood, it is clearly a poor prognostic factor that requires special clinical attention. Early studies in COPD have shown an inverse relationship between weight loss and a low body weight with survival, independent of the degree of airflow obstruction, smoking, gender, and arterial oxygen and carbon dioxide pressure. In patients with a BMI < 20 kg/m^2, both all-cause mortality and COPD mortality are higher than in patients with a normal weight, and mortality continues to decrease with increasing BMI [5], which is most pronounced in severe patients (FEV_1 < 50% predicted). These findings led to the hypothesis that weight gain would improve survival in COPD. Indeed, a large study confirmed the favorable effects of weight gain on survival in patients with severe COPD, providing a convincing starting point for clinicians to consider incorporation of weight management in clinical practice [6].

In terms of body composition, weight loss can either be attributable to a loss of fat mass (FM) or fat-free mass (FFM), or a combination. In parallel to whole-body weight loss, a decrease in bone mineral content (BMC) is common in COPD, especially in more severe COPD (FEV_1 < 50% predicted). Wasting of muscle mass ranging from 20 to 35% is prevalent in clinically stable COPD patients, and in moderate to severe COPD it has been related to impaired mobility and increased mortality [7], independent of airflow limitation. For example, in a landmark study comparing 99 COPD patients with age-matched healthy subjects, the COPD group had a lower lean mass and a lower BMC [8]. Moreover, the prevalence of involuntary weight loss in COPD patients with predominantly emphysema was 49%, while in patients with predominantly chronic bronchitis this was much lower, at 22% [9]. Also, BMI, FFMI, and FMI were lower in the emphysematous group compared to the chronic bronchitis group. This study highlighted that weight loss and muscle wasting in COPD may be more related to emphysema rather than chronic bronchitis, which was confirmed in later studies. Survival studies taking into account body compositional measures with weight loss revealed that loss of muscle mass is an independent predictor of mortality, irrespective of FM and BMI [10, 11]. Measures of lean mass are thus more informative with regard to survival than BMI alone, indicating a need for body composition measurements in the clinical assessment of COPD patients. With decreasing FFM and BMI, the odds of experiencing an acute exacerbation increase [12]. An exacerbation in COPD is typically characterized by enhanced levels of proinflammatory markers in the circulation, malnutrition, and physical inactivity and is often treated by high doses of prednisolone, all of which have been shown to have a negative impact on body mass. It was even demonstrated that COPD patients who recently experienced an exacerbation had the highest chance of having another exacerbation [12], which suggests that these patients with a low FFM and BMI may enter a downward spiral. Indeed, weight loss during hospitalization and low BMI on admission were related to a higher risk of readmission [13]. Therefore, to explore further therapeutic options, future attention should not only focus on clinically stable disease but also explore possibilities of improving the regenerative capacity after an exacerbation to restore muscle mass and fat mass.

Very little longitudinal data are available regarding the pattern and progression of wasting in COPD during clinically stable disease and whether a stepwise decline is seen with acute exacerbations [14]. Therefore, these studies are needed in order to be able to design individualized therapeutic strategies aimed at attenuating muscle wasting and weight loss and taking pulmonary disease progression into account.

Obesity

Patient B: A 58-year-old patient has had COPD for 4 years. She weighs 90 kg and her BMI is 33 kg/m^2. Her weight has been stable for decades. She has a job for 3 days a week and although she experiences mild dyspnea upon exertion, she is an active member of a walking club. Her COPD is controlled by her general practitioner and after having smoked 45 pack years, she has succeeded in quitting. She received antibiotics for suspected pneumonia once, but has never been admitted to the hospital for an acute exacerbation. While taking medication for hypertension, there is no history of diabetes or cardiovascular events. The FEV$_1$ and DL$_{CO}$ measure 48% and 81% of predicted, respectively. On incremental cycling test, the peak VO$_2$ is 89% of predicted and no peripheral desaturation is observed. A whole-body DXA scan revealed FFMI and FMI of 18.2 and 12.7 kg/m^2, respectively. While the body fat percentage lies in the 80th percentile, the FFMI is normal.

According to the classification of overweight and obesity based on BMI as defined by the World Health Organization, patient B is obese. While the cachectic patient A and obese patient B fall within the same GOLD classification based on FEV$_1$, patient B clearly experiences much less respiratory and physical discomfort. Literature on the coexistence of COPD and obesity is scarce, but available data suggest that these two lifestyle-related diseases are increasingly associated with each other in particular in earlier stages of COPD. For example, the prevalence of obesity was investigated in a large primary care population of patients with COPD in the Netherlands [15]. The overall prevalence of obesity in this population was 18%, with the highest prevalence in COPD patients with FEV$_1$ > 50% predicted (16–24%)

and the lowest in patients with $FEV_1 < 50\%$ predicted (6%). For comparison, the current prevalence of obesity in the general population in the Netherlands is 10% in adult men and 12% in adult women [16]. A much higher prevalence of obesity was reported in an adult cohort of patients with early-stage COPD in the USA [17]; 54% of the patients with COPD had a $BMI > 30 \text{ kg/m}^2$, which is considerably more than the overall 20–24% of obese individuals in the US (http://www.cdc.gov/BRFSS/). In fact, a significantly increased prevalence of (pre)obesity ($BMI > 28 \text{ kg/m}^2$) was reported in patients with chronic bronchitis (25%) compared with controls (16%) [18], while underweight was more prevalent in patients with emphysema. Thus, available data suggest that obesity is more prevalent in patients with COPD than in the general population, depending on the severity of chronic airflow limitation. However, studies with appropriate age- and sex-matched control groups are necessary to confirm these findings and to provide indications whether potential gender differences exist with regard to the prevalence of obesity in COPD.

In contrast with epidemiological data from the general population where obesity is associated with a largely decreased life expectancy [19], (pre)obesity in COPD is associated with improved outcome. This phenomenon is referred to as the "obesity paradox" and was identified in several other chronic disease states such as end-stage chronic kidney disease, chronic heart failure, and rheumatoid arthritis [20]. The relative risk for mortality was decreased in overweight and obese COPD patients with $FEV_1 < 50\%$ of predicted, while it is slightly increased in those with $FEV_1 > 50\%$ of predicted [5]. A possibly protective role for obesity in COPD was also observed in the early studies on the association between body weight and mortality [7, 21] and in severe COPD patients with long-term oxygen therapy [22]. In obese men with COPD, the annual decline in FEV_1 was significantly lower than in men of normal BMI range, while this effect was not observed in women [23]. This suggests a gender-specific protective role for obesity in the progression of chronic airflow limitation. Obese individuals not only have increased fat mass, but also slightly higher FFM, which may suggest that the improved survival of obese COPD patients may be explained by higher FFM reserves. However, it is not yet clear whether excessive fat mass or maintained muscle mass contributes to the survival advantage in chronic wasting diseases [20].

It has been suggested that abdominal obesity and fat deposition on the thorax exert lung-mechanistic consequences in simple obesity both at rest and during exercise, some of which were hypothesized to be beneficial in the COPD state. This may be relevant since abdominal obesity measured by waist circumference was almost twice as common in COPD patients as in age- and sex-matched controls [24]. Obese COPD patients consistently demonstrate less lung hyperinflation and have a large inspiratory capacity and inspiratory capacity/total lung capacity ratio than their lean counterparts matched for FEV_1. Interestingly, however, obese COPD patients were shown to have comparable exercise capacity with respect to with normal-weight COPD patients. In fact, the obese COPD patients had increased symptom-limited peak oxygen uptake, and dyspnea intensity ratings were lower. It was reasoned that the relatively reduced end-expiratory lung volume (EELV) at rest and throughout exercise were the most likely contributory factors to reduced dyspnea intensity in obese COPD individuals [25]. If obese COPD patients would experience less respiratory discomfort during exercise compared to normal-weight COPD patients, the respiratory mechanical effects of obesity may ultimately prevent COPD patients becoming severely physically inactive.

It is well recognized that the risk of cardiovascular mortality is increased in patients with chronic airflow limitation, independent of BMI [26]. Insulin resistance may contribute to the increased cardiovascular mortality in patients with COPD. It plays an important role in the pathogenesis of type 2 diabetes mellitus, and it clusters with a variety of risk factors for cardiovascular disease (CVD) such as abdominal obesity, dyslipidemia, and hypertension in the metabolic syndrome [27]. In a meta-analysis of longitudinal studies, the presence of the metabolic syndrome was strongly associated with cardiovascular morbidity and mortality [28]. Indeed, some studies suggest the presence of insulin resistance in COPD [29], especially in normal weight to obese patients [30] and those who are hypoxemic [31], but these findings need to be confirmed in larger samples.

So far, we have discussed obesity mostly in terms of increased whole-body fat mass, while, in fact, it has been shown that different adipose tissue compartments have distinct metabolic, inflammatory, and fatty acid buffering properties [32], and adipose tissue compartments may be enlarged disproportionally. The literature suggests that changes in body fat distribution, especially toward increased visceral fat mass, relate to increased risk of CVD [33]. As CVD is one of the major causes of death in COPD patients [34], more knowledge about potential fat mass redistributions in COPD is needed. While visceral fat is believed to play a major role in insulin resistance and inflammation, the role of the subcutaneous adipose tissue (either abdominal or thigh) may have a lower capacity of driving inflammation and may even play a protective role with respect to cardiovascular risk [33].

Many authors have demonstrated a low-grade systemic inflammation in COPD patients, which is believed to be related to multiple systemic consequences of the disease [35]. However, the origin of this systemic inflammatory load is unclear. The pulmonary overflow hypothesis states that increased permeability of pulmonary capillaries may enhance local pulmonary inflammatory markers to "spill over" into the circulation. However, there is no convincing evidence as yet published. Another potential site of production of inflammatory markers is the adipose tissue, as it has been described to be a potent producer of IL-6 and TNF-α [36], two cytokines frequently reported to be elevated in the circulation of COPD patients. In COPD patients who were screened for pulmonary rehabilitation, increased fat mass in the android/gynoid region (measured by whole-body DXA) was shown to be positively associated with circulating C-reactive protein (CRP) [37]. Although this study suggested a relation between centrally located fat mass and systemic inflammation, the lack of a control group precludes concluding whether these findings are disease-specific or represent a general metabolically driven inflammatory response in obesity. Furthermore, in contrast to DXA, more advanced imaging such as an abdominal computerized tomography scan can be utilized for the distinction between subcutaneous and visceral abdominal fat mass.

The pathophysiological mechanisms of the obesity paradox are yet to be unraveled. Also, the implications of obesity for the pharmacological and extrapulmonary management of patients with COPD are still unknown. Based on the evidence outlined above, it can be hypothesized that obesity exerts divergent effects in subgroups of COPD with different severities of disease. Obesity may protect against mortality in patients with advanced COPD in whom loss of FFM is a particularly important short-term risk factor for death. By contrast, in earlier stage COPD, the harmful long-term effects of obesity-related conditions such as low-grade systemic inflammation and insulin resistance may result in increased cardiovascular and all-cause mortality. Future research in this field should elucidate whether the heterogeneity of obesity-related effects in COPD can be explained by alterations in body fat distribution and potential gender differences.

Aging-Related Changes in Body Composition

Patient C: A 74-year-old patient was diagnosed with COPD many years ago. Although his body weight has remained stable for years at about 72 kg with a BMI of 22.3 kg/m², his weight has recently started to slowly decrease. Although the FEV_1 and DL_{CO} have been fairly stable around 53 and 68% of predicted, respectively, he notes that his functional status is progressively deteriorating. His daily 20-min walk is becoming increasingly difficult due to a feeling of whole-body weakness. He questions whether this is due to aging or if this is caused by the COPD. About once or twice a year, most often in the winter, his general practitioner prescribes oral prednisolone for 10 days because of respiratory distress. Measured in the spring, peak exercise capacity is 58% of predicted load, with a peak VO_2 of 63% of predicted, and a mild peripheral desaturation of 4% is noted. DXA revealed an FFMI and an FMI of 15.7 and 6.6 kg/m², respectively. The BMC is 2.3 kg, which is low.

Since COPD generally does not become clinically apparent until the age of approximately 50, physiological changes that occur with aging must be taken into account when discussing COPD-related abnormalities. Age-related sarcopenia is defined as the loss of muscle mass and muscle strength that is associated with aging [38]. More specifically, features include decreased muscle mass and cross-sectional area of muscle fibers, infiltration of muscle by fat and connective tissue, and decrease of particularly type II fiber size and number. The pathophysiology of sarcopenia in the elderly is complex, and a multitude of internal processes (e.g., reduction of anabolic hormones, increased apoptotic activity in myofibers, increases of proinflammatory cytokines, oxidative stress, and changes in mitochondrial function) and external processes (e.g., deficient energy, protein, and vitamin D intake) contribute to its development. Also, acute and chronic comorbidities that are increasingly prevalent with aging contribute to sarcopenia. Considering these age-related changes in body composition, it was suggested that observed changes in body composition in COPD patients reflect accelerated aging when occurring at younger ages. Cross-sectional studies in COPD have suggested that muscle wasting is not only present in underweight patients with advanced disease, but also in approximately 20–25% of normal-weight patients with less severe airflow obstruction. Thus, while a significant proportion of patients may remain relatively weight stable, a shift from less FFM to more FM may still be apparent. With aging, a progressive loss of subcutaneous adipose tissue and gain of visceral adipose tissue is observed, which is more pronounced in women [33]. However, whether this process is also accelerated in COPD needs to be investigated in future studies. Major advances have been made with respect to unraveling putative pathophysiological mechanisms of altered body composition and physical functioning in COPD from cross-sectional studies [39–42] and from longitudinal case studies without appropriate control groups [43–46]. However, since body composition changes, frailty, and dysregulation of inflammation are also common with aging [47, 48], inclusion of age-matched non-COPD control groups in longitudinal studies is crucial to unravel the effect of airflow obstruction on the pattern and progression of changes in lean mass, fat mass, BMC, and physical function. Such studies are currently lacking.

Pathophysiology

Muscle Wasting

Muscle wasting is a result of an imbalance between muscle protein synthesis and muscle protein breakdown. This can be due to a decreased protein synthesis and/or an increased protein breakdown. It is also possible that both processes are upregulated but to a different extent, resulting in either muscle atrophy or muscle hypertrophy. No conclusive studies have yet been presented regarding abnormal protein balance in muscle-wasted COPD patients with and without whole-body weight loss, probably partly because the studied patient groups were different with respect to COPD body composition phenotype. The regulation of muscle mass is complex and multimodal, but one of the most important denominators is physical activity. It stresses muscle fibers and switches on a hypertrophic signaling cascade resulting in larger myofibers and an increase in myonuclei count. A sedentary lifestyle is common in COPD and inversely related to FEV_1 [49].

Cigarette smoke exposure is considered the main risk factor in the pathogenesis of COPD. Research aimed at unraveling potential mechanisms suggests that smoking causes local pulmonary inflammation and also increased levels of circulating inflammatory mediators. For example, chronic cigarette exposure in mice resulted in low-grade systemic inflammation and decreased oxidative capacity of peripheral skeletal muscle, features that could resemble early signs of extrapulmonary manifestations observed in COPD patients [50]. Also in a human study, increased systemic levels of inflammatory markers were observed in current smokers [51]. Furthermore, non-COPD smokers were characterized by a significant reduction of oxidative fiber cross-sectional area, and it appeared that glycolytic activity was increased [52]. The basal rate of muscle protein synthesis is impaired in healthy

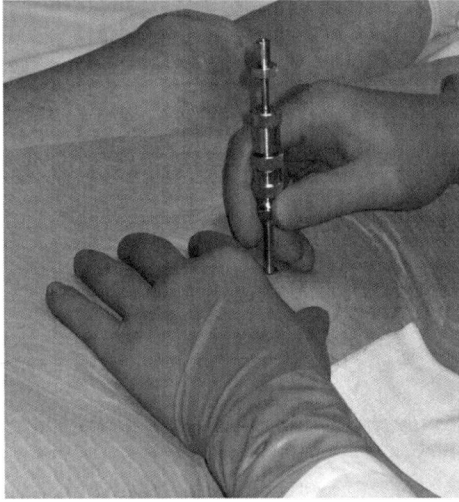

Fig. 11.1 The analysis of muscle biopsies from the quadriceps muscle has resulted in major advances in the understanding of muscle wasting in COPD

smokers compared with healthy nonsmokers, which coincides with increased expression of growth-inhibiting genes [53]. Smokers also have greater peripheral muscle fatigue than nonsmokers [54]. Systemic IL-6 levels are associated with reduced FEV_1, quadriceps strength, and exercise capacity in well-functioning elderly subjects with or without obstructive lung disease [42]. Altogether, these data suggest that smoking may enhance muscle wasting and accelerate the decline in physical functioning and that systemic inflammation could be a modulator. However, longitudinal data describing changes in body composition and physical functioning in the natural course of patients with COPD are lacking. Characterization and longitudinal follow-up of these populations would increase our knowledge with regard to the systemic effects of smoking and COPD such as accelerated sarcopenia and accelerated decline in physical functioning.

Major advances have been made in the understanding of muscle wasting in COPD through analyzing muscle biopsies (Fig. 11.1). Besides being obvious at the macroscopic level, muscle atrophy in COPD has recently been confirmed at the cellular level as well [55]. Atrophy of skeletal muscles in COPD appears to selectively affect glycolytic type IIA/IIX fibers [56]. Insulin-like growth factor-I (IGF-I) is an important mediator of anabolic pathways in skeletal muscle cells via Akt phosphorylation, and insulin/IGF-I signaling is also involved in suppression of protein degradation [57]. Proteolytic systems known to be suppressed by insulin/IGF-I signaling include the 26S-ubiquitin proteasome pathway (UPP) and lysosomal protein degradation (autophagy). Ongoing research in this field will determine whether modulation of these pathways will ultimately be beneficial to prevent or reverse muscle wasting.

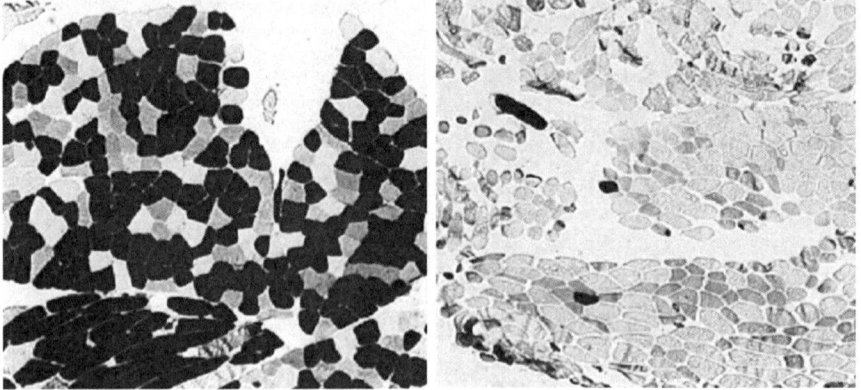

Fig. 11.2 Transversal sections of quadriceps muscle in which oxidative and glycolytic/anaerobic muscle fibres are stained *black* and *gray*, respectively, through adenine triphosphatase staining. The *left panel* is from a healthy person; the *right panel* is from a COPD patient and is characterized by a shift from oxidative-to-glycolytic muscle fiber type

The most prominent intrinsic muscular abnormality in COPD that is likely to be the cause of the above-mentioned impairment in cellular energy metabolism is the loss of muscle oxidative phenotype. A recent meta-analysis demonstrated a fiber-type I→II shift in lower limb skeletal muscle of patients with advanced COPD (Fig. 11.2), which was associated with the severity of airflow obstruction [40]. In parallel, reduced activities of enzymes involved in muscle oxidative metabolism and increased activities of glycolytic enzymes have been reported [58–60]. These alterations seem to be more pronounced in emphysematous patients [61–63] who, strikingly, are also more prone to weight loss [64]. Accordingly, loss of muscle oxidative phenotype is also reflected by decreased mitochondrial mass and/or mitochondrial function [65–67], which was found to be more pronounced in patients with low BMI [68]. These data suggest that the regulation of muscle oxidative phenotype and specifically mitochondrial biogenesis is altered in COPD, possibly predominantly in the cachectic subgroup [69]. The transcription factors peroxisome proliferator-activated receptor (PPAR) γ and β/δ and in particular their coactivator, PPAR-γ coactivator-1α (PGC-1α), are considered key regulators of muscle oxidative phenotype. Indeed, expression levels of these regulators are reduced in muscle biopsies of patients with COPD, including mitochondrial transcription factor A, a transcription factor that is encoded by the nuclear genome and switches on oxidative genes encoded by the mitochondrial genome [70]. The reduced expression of these regulators is more pronounced in cachectic patients, again suggesting that loss of muscle oxidative phenotype and muscle mass are somehow interrelated.

Alternatively, elevated exercise-induced oxidative stress, which has consistently been demonstrated for COPD [71–73], could be involved in muscle wasting as well, since reactive oxygen species (ROS) are obviously capable of inducing damage and subsequent muscle protein breakdown [74]. Hypoxemia may further increase ROS and also generate TNF-α and thereby induce pathways associated with muscle atrophy.

The suppressing effects of hypoxia on food intake may also play a role, and tissue hypoxia may lead to an imbalance between protein synthesis and protein breakdown. The protein myostatin is a potent inhibitor of skeletal muscle differentiation and growth, and hypoxia has recently been linked to its enhanced activity. This may also contribute to the loss of muscle mass under hypoxia. However, the observation that one patient with arterial hypoxemia becomes cachectic and the other does not indicates that it is not solely hypoxemia that underlies body composition shifts.

Energy Balance

Weight loss and fat wasting are generally the result of a negative energy balance. The normal adaptive response to (semi)starvation is to decrease resting energy metabolism. In contrast, increased resting energy requirements have been observed in COPD patients, as in most other chronic inflammatory wasting diseases [75]. While in many other diseases, a concomitant adaptive decrease in activity-induced energy expenditure results in an unchanged daily energy expenditure, ambulatory COPD patients are characterized by elevated activity-induced and daily energy expenditure [76, 77]. The oxygen cost of exercise has also been found to be higher in underweight COPD patients than in healthy subjects [78]. Without a corresponding increase in caloric intake, these patients inevitably lose weight [75]. It has been postulated that pulmonary pathology (airway obstruction and/or hyperinflation) increases the work of breathing and thus daily energy expenditure. It is difficult to reliably assess daily work of breathing, but indirect evidence for this hypothesis was provided by the clinical outcomes of two pulmonary intervention strategies aimed at improving breathing ability and lung function: lung volume reduction surgery and noninvasive positive pressure ventilation. Both resulted in spontaneous weight gain in underweight COPD patients [79, 80].

Impaired cellular and whole-body energy metabolism may also be due to intrinsic muscle abnormalities. Impaired cellular metabolism in limb muscles of patients with COPD is well-established. Studies using ^{31}P-NMR techniques revealed disturbed levels of energy-rich phosphates such as ATP and creatine phosphate in rest and their faster drop during acute exercise and recovery, indicative of impaired oxidative energy metabolism [81–83]. Consequently, the affected muscles rely more on anaerobic energy metabolism to produce ATP, which is much less efficient. Enhanced exercise-induced lactate and ammonia production have been reported for COPD [60, 84], lactate resulting from ATP production purely through glycolysis and ammonia from ATP production from ADP molecules. The latter renders AMP, which is further degraded to inosine monophosphate (IMP) and ammonia. In agreement with this mechanism, elevated intramuscular IMP levels have also been found at rest and after exercise in COPD [82, 85]. Moreover, acute stimulation of mitochondrial energy delivery by administration of dichloroacetate (an activator of the muscle pyruvate dehydrogenase complex) attenuates exercise-induced lactate and ammonia production in COPD [86].

Fat Cell Function

Adipose tissue is no longer considered a passive storage compartment of lipids, but now has been widely described as a source of inflammation. Chronic low-grade systemic inflammation is a hallmark of both obesity and COPD, and the link might reside within the adipose tissue. The expression and/or secretion of, for example, TNF-α, IL-6, and leptin are increased in the adipose tissue of obese, insulin-resistant individuals [87]. These factors are also systemically increased in COPD patients [88]. Enlarged adipocytes have been shown to have a more proinflammatory profile than normal-size adipocytes [89], and infiltrated macrophages appear to cross talk with the residing adipocytes enhancing the inflammatory load. These examples of adipose tissue dysfunction are observed primarily in simple obesity, insulin resistance, or diabetes mellitus, but little evidence exists for this in COPD. One study has demonstrated that the abdominal subcutaneous adipose tissue of severe COPD patients (mean FEV_1 24% predicted, mean BMI 19 kg/m^2) is characterized by increased gene expression of CD40, MKK4, and JNK as compared with less severe COPD patients (mean FEV_1 63% predicted, mean BMI 29 kg/m^2) [90]. These genes are implicated in the onset and maintenance of inflammatory reactions and are responsive to cellular stress. Interestingly, however, whereas adipocyte size in non-COPD individuals is positively associated with a proinflammatory state, this study showed that COPD patients with smaller-sized adipocytes had higher CD40, MKK4, and JNK expressions. This suggests that not only fat mass can be severely affected in COPD, but intrinsic adipose tissue abnormalities may exist as well. Therefore, attention should not be restricted only to adipose tissue in the obese COPD patient, but also expanded to patients who are vulnerable to develop sarcopenia.

Cytokines produced and secreted by adipocytes are called adipokines and have attracted growing interest with respect to the pathophysiology of COPD [91]. Various cross-sectional studies, mainly in nonobese COPD patients, demonstrate abnormalities in systemic adipokine levels such as leptin, adiponectin, visfatin, and ghrelin. Most adipokines are pleiotrophic proteins involved in a wide variety of body functions such as regulation of food intake, basal metabolism, and inflammation. Plasma leptin, known to strongly correlate with fat mass [92], has been shown to be decreased in cachectic COPD patients compared to normal-weight COPD patients [93]. Leptin is considered a mediator of nutritional status by inhibiting the trigger for food intake in the hypothalamus. However, leptin has also been shown to exert proinflammatory actions by stimulating the innate immune system [94] and may play a role in COPD both in the pulmonary compartment and systemically [95]. The functional relevance of alterations in circulating adipokines in COPD is not yet elucidated and requires further investigation.

In the recent years, experimental studies have reported that hypoxia may result in a proinflammatory state in adipose tissue. Hypertrophic adipocytes may outgrow the diffusion distance of oxygen, resulting in local hypoxic areas within the adipocytes. This effect is worsened when neovascularization is impaired such as in obesity [96]. While systemic oxygen levels are preserved in simple obesity, they are generally significantly lower in COPD patients, potentially causing adipose tissue hypoxia.

Whether adipose tissue in COPD contributes to the systemic inflammatory load and is mediated by hypoxia is uncertain and needs to be further studied.

Bone Demineralization

The WHO defines osteoporosis as a systemic skeletal disease characterized by a low bone mass and/or mircoarchitectural deterioration of bone tissue, leading to increased bone fragility and increased fracture risk [20]. Although the prevalence of osteoporosis (9–69%) and osteopenia (27–67%) in COPD varies widely between different studies, these figures are generally higher than in healthy individuals [41]. Risk factors for a decreasing bone mass and bone density in the general population are an increasing age, low body weight, chronic glucocorticoid therapy, hypovitaminosis D, and endocrine thyroid diseases. In addition, evidence suggests that proinflammatory cytokines can inhibit osteoblasts and stimulate osteoclasts, leading to a net destruction of the skeletal system [97]. Vitamin D, implicated in calcium uptake from the intestines and stimulating bone formation, is frequently decreased in COPD patients. This may at least partially explain lower bone mass in these patients [98, 99]. Low vitamin D plasma levels are associated with bone demineralization, are common in smokers with mild-to-moderate COPD (insufficiency 35%, and deficiency 31%) [100], and are related to lower FEV_1, independent of COPD status [101]. COPD severity is also strongly related to lower levels of physical activity [49] and may be associated with less sunlight exposure, which might also explain the relationship between low vitamin D, low bone mass, and FEV_1.

Genetics

It has been hypothesized that genetic factors may predispose certain individuals to lose body weight and/or fat-free mass, but this is a relatively unexplored area of research. One study found an altered distribution of interleukin (IL)-1β-511 single nucleotide polymorphism (SNP) genotypes in cachectic versus noncachectic COPD patients [102]. This suggests that susceptibility to inflammation may play a role. Another large study indicated a relationship between fat mass and obesity-associated (FTO) gene and a low BMI and FFMI [103]. Although the functional relevance of FTO gene polymorphisms has yet to be elucidated, this study suggests that this gene may be involved in the cachectic phenotype.

Lifestyle and Therapeutic Intervention

Tables 11.1 and 11.2 summarize the most important literature with regard to potential therapeutic strategies in COPD to optimize body composition. The majority of these therapeutic strategies demonstrate that success is only achieved when applied in combination with other modalities. This underlines the need for a multimodality

Table 11.1 Therapeutic strategies to optimize body composition in COPD: lifestyle interventions

Lifestyle interventions	Potential effect on body composition	Evidence in COPD?
Smoking cessation	Fat mass ↑	The effects of smoking cessation have been well-described in non-COPD individuals and consist of a particular increase in fat mass [104] but have not specifically been studied in COPD
Resistance training	Muscle mass ↑	Short-term progressive resistance training is mostly studied in combination with other training modalities in COPD and was found to improve muscle strength [105]
Constant work rate or interval training	Muscle endurance ↑ Fat mass ↓	Whole-body exercise improved muscle strength and fat-free mass in normal weight COPD patients [106]
Polyunsaturated fatty acids (PUFAs)	Exercise capacity ↑ by stimulation of PPAR transcription factor in muscle, leading to enhanced oxidative capacity Modulation of leukotrienes Inflammation ↓ via inhibiting leukocytes	PUFAs increased exercise capacity when added to a training program in severe COPD, but did not influence circulating cytokine levels [107]
Dietary fibers	Inflammation ↓ via suppression of transcriptional activity of NF-κB	A diet rich in fibers may reduce the risk of developing COPD [108], but no studies in COPD have specifically looked at dietary fiber intake and body composition
High protein diet	Muscle mass ↑ Satiety ↑ → fat mass ↓	Protein-rich supplements have been shown to be effective for the increase in muscle mass when combined with exercise training in underweight COPD patients [109]. Potential effects on satiety and energy balance have not been studied in COPD
Vitamin D	Bone mineral density ↑ Muscle strength ↑	Trials in COPD supplementing vitamin D have not yet been published
High-caloric diet	Body weight ↑, fat mass ↑	Caloric supplementation was able to increase body weight and fat mass in weight losing patients with severe COPD [110] and improved quality of life. Poor compliance and substitution instead of addition of the normal diet by nutritional supplements may hamper therapeutic efficacy
Weight losing diet	Fat mass ↓	Studies in COPD modulating nutrition so far primarily focused on those with under- or normal weight. No randomized controlled nutrition trials in obese COPD patients have yet been performed

PPAR Peroxisome proliferator-activated receptors, *COPD* Chronic obstructive pulmonary disease

Table 11.2 Therapeutic strategies to optimize body composition in COPD: drug interventions

Drug interventions	Potential effect on body composition	Evidence in COPD?
Anti-TNFα	Local and systemic inflammation ↓	In moderate-to-severe COPD, no effect on respiratory symptoms, FEV$_1$, 6-min walking distance, and exacerbations, while in cachectic patients 6-min walking distance did improve. More cases of cancer and pneumonia were observed under anti-TNFα treatment [111]
Anabolic steroids	Muscle mass ↑ via enhancement of erythropoietin and IGF signaling	Anabolic steroids in combination with a nutritional intervention may enhance fat-free mass in depleted COPD patients [112]. Anabolic steroids generally increased lean mass in COPD [113–115]
Testosterone	Muscle mass ↑ by reversing hypogonadism	Beneficial effects in combination with nutritional support and exercise, possibly via IGF signaling [116]
Phosphodiesterase-4 inhibitors	Increase intracellular cAMP activity → cellular inflammatory activity ↓	While designed to inhibit a local pulmonary inflammatory response, a side-effect of PDE4 inhibitors is weight loss (~2 kg), especially in those with BMI > 30 kg/m^2 [117, 118]
Statins	Systemic inflammation ↓ Oxidative stress in muscle ↓	Retrospective studies have indicated potential benefits in COPD patients [119], but controlled trials in COPD have not yet been completed
Growth hormone	Weight and muscle mass ↑ by stimulating anabolic signaling	Underweight COPD patients showed weight gain and increased muscle strength when growth hormone supplementation was combined with nutritional support [120], but another study showed no improvements in strength or exercise capacity [121]
Ghrelin	Increasing endogenous growth hormone levels	Ghrelin treatment improved body weight, muscle mass, and functional capacity in underweight COPD patients [122]

TNFα Tumor necrosis factor-alpha, *PDE4* Phosphodiesterase-4, *cAMP* Cyclic adenosine monophosphate, *BMI* Body mass index, *COPD* Chronic obstructive pulmonary disease

approach. While some of the drug trials have not primarily been designed to improve body composition, lessons can be learned from "side effects" of the treatment on, for example, muscle mass and fat mass.

Conclusions

COPD has been associated with severe weight loss, obesity, and accelerated sarcopenia. We have demonstrated that all of these body composition phenotypes are clinically associated with morbidity and mortality to varying degrees. Multiple

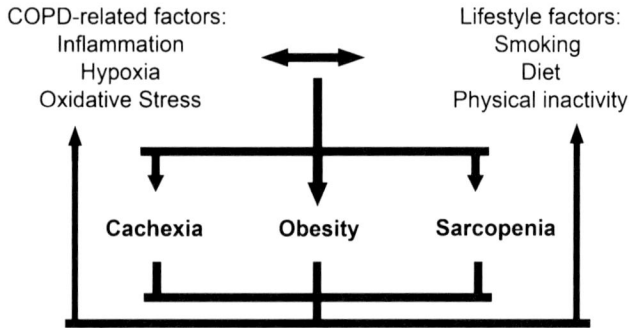

Fig. 11.3 Interrelationship between determinants and body composition phenotypes in COPD

factors have been implicated in body composition abnormalities in COPD and likely interrelate with each other in a synergistic manner (Fig. 11.3). While improving muscle mass favors survival in COPD, future research is necessary to unravel the pathophysiology of body composition alterations. Tailoring intervention strategies to the individual patient's phenotype and needs will result in the most optimal clinical outcome.

References

1. Franssen FM, O'Donnell DE, Goossens GH, Blaak EE, Schols AM. Obesity and the lung: 5. Obesity and COPD. Thorax. 2008;63(12):1110–7.
2. Schols AM. Nutritional rehabilitation: from pulmonary cachexia to sarcoPD. Eur Respir J. 2009;33(5):949–50.
3. Schols AM. Pulmonary cachexia. Int J Cardiol. 2002;85(1):101–10.
4. Evans WJ, Morley JE, Argiles J, Bales C, Baracos V, Guttridge D, et al. Cachexia: a new definition. Clin Nutr. 2008;27(6):793–9.
5. Landbo C, Prescott E, Lange P, Vestbo J, Almdal TP. Prognostic value of nutritional status in chronic obstructive pulmonary disease. Am J Respir Crit Care Med. 1999;160(6):1856–61.
6. Schols AM, Slangen J, Volovics L, Wouters EF. Weight loss is a reversible factor in the prognosis of chronic obstructive pulmonary disease. Am J Respir Crit Care Med. 1998;157 (6 Pt 1):1791–7.
7. Vestbo J, Prescott E, Almdal T, Dahl M, Nordestgaard BG, Andersen T, et al. Body mass, fat-free body mass, and prognosis in patients with chronic obstructive pulmonary disease from a random population sample: findings from the Copenhagen City Heart Study. Am J Respir Crit Care Med. 2006;173(1):79–83.
8. Engelen MP, Schols AM, Heidendal GA, Wouters EF. Dual-energy X-ray absorptiometry in the clinical evaluation of body composition and bone mineral density in patients with chronic obstructive pulmonary disease. Am J Clin Nutr. 1998;68(6):1298–303.
9. Engelen MP, Schols AM, Lamers RJ, Wouters EF. Different patterns of chronic tissue wasting among patients with chronic obstructive pulmonary disease. Clin Nutr. 1999;18(5):275–80.
10. Schols AM, Wouters EF. Nutritional considerations in the treatment of chronic obstructive pulmonary disease. Clin Nutr. 1995;14(2):64–73.

11. Marquis K, Debigare R, Lacasse Y, LeBlanc P, Jobin J, Carrier G, et al. Midthigh muscle cross-sectional area is a better predictor of mortality than body mass index in patients with chronic obstructive pulmonary disease. Am J Respir Crit Care Med. 2002;166(6):809–13.
12. Hurst JR, Vestbo J, Anzueto A, Locantore N, Mullerova H, Tal-Singer R, et al. Susceptibility to exacerbation in chronic obstructive pulmonary disease. N Engl J Med. 2010;363(12):1128–38.
13. Pouw EM, Ten Velde GP, Croonen BH, Kester AD, Schols AM, Wouters EF. Early non-elective readmission for chronic obstructive pulmonary disease is associated with weight loss. Clin Nutr. 2000;19(2):95–9.
14. van Wetering CR, van Nooten FE, Mol SJ, Hoogendoorn M, Rutten-Van Molken MP, Schols AM. Systemic impairment in relation to disease burden in patients with moderate COPD eligible for a lifestyle program. Findings from the INTERCOM trial. Int J Chron Obstruct Pulmon Dis. 2008;3(3):443–51.
15. Steuten LM, Creutzberg EC, Vrijhoef HJ, Wouters EF. COPD as a multicomponent disease: inventory of dyspnoea, underweight, obesity and fat free mass depletion in primary care. Prim Care Respir J. 2006;15(2):84–91.
16. Schokker DF, Visscher TL, Nooyens AC, van Baak MA, Seidell JC. Prevalence of over-weight and obesity in the Netherlands. Obes Rev. 2007;8(2):101–8.
17. Eisner MD, Blanc PD, Sidney S, Yelin EH, Lathon PV, Katz PP, et al. Body composition and functional limitation in COPD. Respir Res. 2007;8:7.
18. Guerra S, Sherrill DL, Bobadilla A, Martinez FD, Barbee RA. The relation of body mass index to asthma, chronic bronchitis, and emphysema. Chest. 2002;122(4):1256–63.
19. Peeters A, Barendregt JJ, Willekens F, Mackenbach JP, Al Mamun A, Bonneux L. Obesity in adulthood and its consequences for life expectancy: a life-table analysis. Ann Intern Med. 2003;138(1):24–32.
20. Kalantar-Zadeh K, Horwich TB, Oreopoulos A, Kovesdy CP, Younessi H, Anker SD, et al. Risk factor paradox in wasting diseases. Curr Opin Clin Nutr Metab Care. 2007;10(4): 433–42.
21. Wilson DO, Rogers RM, Wright EC, Anthonisen NR. Body weight in chronic obstructive pulmonary disease. The National Institutes of Health Intermittent Positive-Pressure Breathing Trial. Am Rev Respir Dis. 1989;139(6):1435–8.
22. Chailleux E, Laaban JP, Veale D. Prognostic value of nutritional depletion in patients with COPD treated by long-term oxygen therapy: data from the ANTADIR observatory. Chest. 2003;123(5):1460–6.
23. Watson L, Vonk JM, Lofdahl CG, Pride NB, Pauwels RA, Laitinen LA, et al. Predictors of lung function and its decline in mild to moderate COPD in association with gender: results from the Euroscop study. Respir Med. 2006;100(4):746–53.
24. Marquis K, Maltais F, Duguay V, Bezeau AM, LeBlanc P, Jobin J, et al. The metabolic syndrome in patients with chronic obstructive pulmonary disease. J Cardiopulm Rehabil. 2005;25(4):226–32. discussion 33–34.
25. Guenette JA, Jensen D, O'Donnell DE. Respiratory function and the obesity paradox. Curr Opin Clin Nutr Metab Care. 2010;13(6):618–24.
26. Hole DJ, Watt GC, Davey-Smith G, Hart CL, Gillis CR, Hawthorne VM. Impaired lung function and mortality risk in men and women: findings from the Renfrew and Paisley prospective population study. BMJ. 1996;313(7059):711–5. discussion 5–6.
27. Eckel RH, Grundy SM, Zimmet PZ. The metabolic syndrome. Lancet. 2005;365(9468): 1415–28.
28. Gami AS, Witt BJ, Howard DE, Erwin PJ, Gami LA, Somers VK, et al. Metabolic syndrome and risk of incident cardiovascular events and death: a systematic review and meta-analysis of longitudinal studies. J Am Coll Cardiol. 2007;49(4):403–14.
29. Bolton CE, Evans M, Ionescu AA, Edwards SM, Morris RH, Dunseath G, et al. Insulin resistance and inflammation – a further systemic complication of COPD. COPD. 2007;4(2): 121–6.
30. Koehler F, Doehner W, Hoernig S, Witt C, Anker SD, John M. Anorexia in chronic obstructive pulmonary disease – association to cachexia and hormonal derangement. Int J Cardiol. 2007;119(1):83–9.

31. Jakobsson P, Jorfeldt L. Oxygen supplementation increases glucose tolerance during euglycaemic hyperinsulinaemic glucose clamp procedure in patients with severe COPD and chronic hypoxaemia. Clin Physiol Funct Imaging. 2006;26(5):271–4.
32. Ibrahim MM. Subcutaneous and visceral adipose tissue: structural and functional differences. Obes Rev. 2009;11(1):11–8.
33. Zafon C. Fat and aging: a tale of two tissues. Curr Aging Sci. 2009;2(2):83–94.
34. Berry CE, Wise RA. Mortality in COPD: causes, risk factors, and prevention. COPD. 2010;7(5):375–82.
35. Wouters EF, Creutzberg EC, Schols AM. Systemic effects in COPD. Chest. 2002;121(5 Suppl):127S–30.
36. Ye J. Emerging role of adipose tissue hypoxia in obesity and insulin resistance. Int J Obes (Lond). 2009;33(1):54–66.
37. Rutten EP, Breyer MK, Spruit MA, Hofstra T, van Melick PP, Schols AM, et al. Abdominal fat mass contributes to the systemic inflammation in chronic obstructive pulmonary disease. Clin Nutr. 2010;29(6):756–60.
38. Muscaritoli M, Anker SD, Argiles J, Aversa Z, Bauer JM, Biolo G, et al. Consensus definition of sarcopenia, cachexia and pre-cachexia: Joint document elaborated by Special Interest Groups (SIG) "cachexia-anorexia in chronic wasting diseases" and "nutrition in geriatrics". Clin Nutr. 2010;29(2):154–9.
39. Eisner MD, Iribarren C, Yelin EH, Sidney S, Katz PP, Ackerson L, et al. Pulmonary function and the risk of functional limitation in chronic obstructive pulmonary disease. Am J Epidemiol. 2008;167(9):1090–101.
40. Gosker HR, Zeegers MP, Wouters EF, Schols AM. Muscle fibre type shifting in the vastus lateralis of patients with COPD is associated with disease severity: a systematic review and meta-analysis. Thorax. 2007;62(11):944–9.
41. Graat-Verboom L, Wouters EF, Smeenk FW, van den Borne BE, Lunde R, Spruit MA. Current status of research on osteoporosis in COPD: a systematic review. Eur Respir J. 2009;34(1):209–18.
42. Yende S, Waterer GW, Tolley EA, Newman AB, Bauer DC, Taaffe DR, et al. Inflammatory markers are associated with ventilatory limitation and muscle dysfunction in obstructive lung disease in well functioning elderly subjects. Thorax. 2006;61(1):10–6.
43. Scanlon PD, Connett JE, Wise RA, Tashkin DP, Madhok T, Skeans M, et al. Loss of bone density with inhaled triamcinolone in Lung Health Study II. Am J Respir Crit Care Med. 2004;170(12):1302–9.
44. Oga T, Nishimura K, Tsukino M, Sato S, Hajiro T, Mishima M. Exercise capacity deterioration in patients with COPD: longitudinal evaluation over 5 years. Chest. 2005;128(1):62–9.
45. Oga T, Nishimura K, Tsukino M, Sato S, Hajiro T, Mishima M. Longitudinal deteriorations in patient reported outcomes in patients with COPD. Respir Med. 2007;101(1):146–53.
46. Habraken JM, van der Wal WM, Ter Riet G, Weersink EJ, Toben F, Bindels PJ. Health-related quality of life and functional status in end-stage COPD: longitudinal study. Eur Respir J. 2011;37(2):280–8.
47. Koster A, Visser M, Simonsick EM, Yu B, Allison DB, Newman AB, et al. Association between fitness and changes in body composition and muscle strength. J Am Geriatr Soc. 2010;58(2):219–26.
48. Fulop T, Larbi A, Witkowski JM, McElhaney J, Loeb M, Mitnitski A, et al. Aging, frailty and age-related diseases. Biogerontology. 2010;11(5):547–63.
49. Garcia-Rio F, Lores V, Mediano O, Rojo B, Hernanz A, Lopez-Collazo E, et al. Daily physical activity in patients with chronic obstructive pulmonary disease is mainly associated with dynamic hyperinflation. Am J Respir Crit Care Med. 2009;180(6):506–12.
50. Gosker HR, Langen RC, Bracke KR, Joos GF, Brusselle GG, Steele C, et al. Extrapulmonary manifestations of COPD in a mouse model of chronic cigarette smoke exposure. Am J Respir Cell Mol Biol. 2008;40(6):710–6.

51. Levitzky YS, Guo CY, Rong J, Larson MG, Walter RE, Keaney Jr JF, et al. Relation of smoking status to a panel of inflammatory markers: the framingham offspring. Atherosclerosis. 2008;201(1):217–24.
52. Montes de Oca M, Loeb E, Torres SH, De Sanctis J, Hernandez N, Talamo C. Peripheral muscle alterations in non-COPD smokers. Chest. 2008;133(1):13–8.
53. Petersen AM, Magkos F, Atherton P, Selby A, Smith K, Rennie MJ, et al. Smoking impairs muscle protein synthesis and increases the expression of myostatin and MAFbx in muscle. Am J Physiol Endocrinol Metab. 2007;293(3):E843–8.
54. Wust RC, Morse CI, de Haan A, Rittweger J, Jones DA, Degens H. Skeletal muscle properties and fatigue resistance in relation to smoking history. Eur J Appl Physiol. 2008;104(1):103–10.
55. Plant PJ, Brooks D, Faughnan M, Bayley T, Bain J, Singer L, et al. Cellular markers of muscle atrophy in chronic obstructive pulmonary disease (COPD). Am J Respir Cell Mol Biol. 2010;42(4):461–71.
56. Gosker HR, Engelen MPKJ, van Mameren H, van Dijk PJ, van der Vusse GJ, Wouters EFM, et al. Muscle fiber type IIX atrophy is involved in the loss of fat-free mass in chronic obstructive pulmonary disease. Am J Clin Nutr. 2002;76:113–9.
57. Glass DJ. Skeletal muscle hypertrophy and atrophy signaling pathways. Int J Biochem Cell Biol. 2005;37(10):1974–84.
58. Green HJ, Bombardier E, Burnett M, Iqbal S, D'Arsigny CL, O'Donnell DE, et al. Organization of metabolic pathways in vastus lateralis of patients with chronic obstructive pulmonary disease. Am J Physiol Regul Integr Comp Physiol. 2008;295(3):R935–41.
59. Jakobsson P, Jorfeldt L, Henriksson J. Metabolic enzyme activity in the quadriceps femoris muscle in patients with severe chronic obstructive pulmonary disease. Am J Respir Crit Care Med. 1995;151(2 Pt 1):374–7.
60. Maltais F, Simard AA, Simard C, Jobin J, Desgagnes P, LeBlanc P. Oxidative capacity of the skeletal muscle and lactic acid kinetics during exercise in normal subjects and in patients with COPD. Am J Respir Crit Care Med. 1996;153(1):288–93.
61. Gosker HR, van Mameren H, van Dijk PJ, Engelen MPKJ, van der Vusse GJ, Wouters EFM, et al. Skeletal muscle fibre type shifting and metabolic profile in patients with COPD. Eur Respir J. 2002;19:617–26.
62. Maltais F, Sullivan MJ, LeBlanc P, Duscha BD, Schachat FH, Simard C, et al. Altered expression of myosin heavy chain in the vastus lateralis muscle in patients with COPD. Eur Respir J. 1999;13(4):850–4.
63. Satta A, Migliori GB, Spanevello A, Neri M, Bottinelli R, Canepari M, et al. Fibre types in skeletal muscles of chronic obstructive pulmonary disease patients related to respiratory function and exercise tolerance. Eur Respir J. 1997;10:2853–60.
64. Kurosaki H, Ishii T, Motohashi N, Motegi T, Yamada K, Kudoh S, et al. Extent of emphysema on HRCT affects loss of fat-free mass and fat mass in COPD. Intern Med. 2009;48(1):41–8.
65. Gosker HR, Hesselink MK, Duimel H, Ward KA, Schols AM. Reduced mitochondrial density in the vastus lateralis muscle of patients with COPD. Eur Respir J. 2007;30(1):73–9.
66. Picard M, Godin R, Sinnreich M, Baril J, Bourbeau J, Perrault H, et al. The mitochondrial phenotype of peripheral muscle in chronic obstructive pulmonary disease: disuse or dysfunction? Am J Respir Crit Care Med. 2008;178(10):1040–7.
67. Puente-Maestu L, Perez-Parra J, Godoy R, Moreno N, Tejedor A, Gonzalez-Aragoneses F, et al. Abnormal mitochondrial function in locomotor and respiratory muscles of COPD patients. Eur Respir J. 2009;33(5):1045–52.
68. Rabinovich RA, Bastos R, Ardite E, Llinas L, Orozco-Levi M, Gea J, et al. Mitochondrial dysfunction in COPD patients with low body mass index. Eur Respir J. 2007;29(4):643–50.
69. Franssen FM, Sauerwein HP, Rutten EP, Wouters EF, Schols AM. Whole-body resting and exercise-induced lipolysis in sarcopenic [corrected] patients with COPD. Eur Respir J. 2008;32(6):1466–71.

70. Remels AH, Schrauwen P, Broekhuizen R, Willems J, Kersten S, Gosker HR, et al. Peroxisome proliferator-activated receptor expression is reduced in skeletal muscle in COPD. Eur Respir J. 2007;30(2):245–52.
71. Barreiro E, Rabinovich R, Marin-Corral J, Barbera JA, Gea J, Roca J. Chronic endurance exercise induces quadriceps nitrosative stress in patients with severe COPD. Thorax. 2009; 64(1):13–9.
72. Couillard A, Maltais F, Saey D, Debigare R, Michaud A, Koechlin C, et al. Exercise-induced quadriceps oxidative stress and peripheral muscle dysfunction in patients with chronic obstructive pulmonary disease. Am J Respir Crit Care Med. 2003;167(12):1664–9.
73. Delample D, Durand F, Severac A, Belghith M, Mas E, Michel F, et al. Implication of xanthine oxidase in muscle oxidative stress in COPD patients. Free Radic Res. 2008;42(9):807–14.
74. Mercken EM, Gosker HR, Rutten EP, Wouters EF, Bast A, Hageman GJ, et al. Systemic and pulmonary oxidative stress after single leg exercise in COPD. Chest. 2009;136(5):1291–300.
75. Schols AM, Soeters PB, Mostert R, Saris WH, Wouters EF. Energy balance in chronic obstructive pulmonary disease. Am Rev Respir Dis. 1991;143(6):1248–52.
76. Baarends EM, Schols AM, Westerterp KR, Wouters EF. Total daily energy expenditure relative to resting energy expenditure in clinically stable patients with COPD. Thorax. 1997;52(9):780–5.
77. Slinde F, Ellegard L, Gronberg AM, Larsson S, Rossander-Hulthen L. Total energy expenditure in underweight patients with severe chronic obstructive pulmonary disease living at home. Clin Nutr. 2003;22(2):159–65.
78. Baarends EM, Schols AM, Akkermans MA, Wouters EF. Decreased mechanical efficiency in clinically stable patients with COPD. Thorax. 1997;52(11):981–6.
79. Vaughan P, Oey IF, Steiner MC, Morgan MD, Waller DA. A prospective analysis of the interrelationship between lung volume reduction surgery and body mass index. Eur J Cardiothorac Surg. 2007;32(6):839–42.
80. Budweiser S, Heinemann F, Meyer K, Wild PJ, Pfeifer M. Weight gain in cachectic COPD patients receiving noninvasive positive-pressure ventilation. Respir Care. 2006;51(2):126–32.
81. Green HJ, Burnett ME, D'Arsigny CL, O'Donnell DE, Ouyang J, Webb KA. Altered metabolic and transporter characteristics of vastus lateralis in chronic obstructive pulmonary disease. J Appl Physiol. 2008;105(3):879–86.
82. Pouw EM, Schols AMWJ, van der Vusse GJ, Wouters EFM. Elevated inosine monophosphate levels in resting muscle of patients with stable COPD. Am J Respir Crit Care Med. 1998;157(2):453–7.
83. Serres I, Hayot M, Prefaut C, Mercier J. Skeletal muscle abnormalities in patients with COPD: contribution to exercise intolerance. Med Sci Sports Exerc. 1998;30(7):1019–27.
84. Calvert LD, Singh SJ, Greenhaff PL, Morgan MD, Steiner MC. The plasma ammonia response to cycle exercise in chronic obstructive pulmonary disease. Eur Respir J. 2008;31(4): 751–8.
85. Steiner MC, Evans R, Deacon SJ, Singh SJ, Patel P, Fox J, et al. Adenine nucleotide loss in the skeletal muscles during exercise in chronic obstructive pulmonary disease. Thorax. 2005;60(11):932–6.
86. Calvert LD, Shelley R, Singh SJ, Greenhaff PL, Bankart J, Morgan MD, et al. Dichloroacetate enhances performance and reduces blood lactate during maximal cycle exercise in chronic obstructive pulmonary disease. Am J Respir Crit Care Med. 2008;177(10):1090–4.
87. Maachi M, Pieroni L, Bruckert E, Jardel C, Fellahi S, Hainque B, et al. Systemic low-grade inflammation is related to both circulating and adipose tissue TNFalpha, leptin and IL-6 levels in obese women. Int J Obes Relat Metab Disord. 2004;28(8):993–7.
88. Gan WQ, Man SF, Senthilselvan A, Sin DD. Association between chronic obstructive pulmonary disease and systemic inflammation: a systematic review and a meta-analysis. Thorax. 2004;59(7):574–80.
89. Skurk T, Alberti-Huber C, Herder C, Hauner H. Relationship between adipocyte size and adipokine expression and secretion. J Clin Endocrinol Metab. 2007;92(3):1023–33.

90. Tkacova R, Ukropec J, Skyba P, Ukropcova B, Pobeha P, Kurdiova T, et al. Increased adipose tissue expression of proinflammatory CD40, MKK4 and JNK in patients with very severe chronic obstructive pulmonary disease. Respiration. 2011;81(5):386–93.

91. Sood A. Obesity, adipokines, and lung disease. J Appl Physiol. 2010;108(3):744–53.

92. Schols AM, Creutzberg EC, Buurman WA, Campfield LA, Saris WH, Wouters EF. Plasma leptin is related to proinflammatory status and dietary intake in patients with chronic obstructive pulmonary disease. Am J Respir Crit Care Med. 1999;160(4):1220–6.

93. Yuan Y, Wang Z, Liu C. Preliminary investigation of effect of serum leptin on nutritional state of COPD patients. Zhonghua Jie He He Hu Xi Za Zhi. 2000;23(5):292–5.

94. La Cava A, Matarese G. The weight of leptin in immunity. Nat Rev Immunol. 2004;4(5): 371–9.

95. Vernooy JH, Drummen NE, van Suylen RJ, Cloots RH, Moller GM, Bracke KR, et al. Enhanced pulmonary leptin expression in patients with severe COPD and asymptomatic smokers. Thorax. 2009;64(1):26–32.

96. Cao Y. Adipose tissue angiogenesis as a therapeutic target for obesity and metabolic diseases. Net Rev Drug Discov. 2010;9(2):107–15.

97. McLean RR. Proinflammatory cytokines and osteoporosis. Curr Osteoporos Rep. 2009;7(4): 134–9.

98. Chishimba L, Thickett DR, Stockley RA, Wood AM. The vitamin D axis in the lung: a key role for vitamin D-binding protein. Thorax. 2010;65(5):456–62.

99. Quint JK, Wedzicha JA. Is vitamin D deficiency important in the natural history of COPD? Thorax. 2010;65(3):192–4.

100. Kunisaki KM, Niewoehner DE, Singh RJ, Connett JE. Vitamin D Status and longitudinal lung function decline in the Lung Health Study. Eur Respir J. 2010;37(2):238–43.

101. Black PN, Scragg R. Relationship between serum 25-hydroxyvitamin d and pulmonary function in the third national health and nutrition examination survey. Chest. 2005;128(6):3792–8.

102. Broekhuizen R, Grimble RF, Howell WM, Shale DJ, Creutzberg EC, Wouters EF, et al. Pulmonary cachexia, systemic inflammatory profile, and the interleukin 1beta – 511 single nucleotide polymorphism. Am J Clin Nutr. 2005;82(5):1059–64.

103. Wan ES, Cho MH, Boutaoui N, Klanderman BJ, Sylvia JS, Ziniti JP, Won S, Lange C, Pillai SG, Anderson WH, Kong X, Lomas DA, Bakke PS, Gulsvik A, Regan EA, Murphy JR, Make BJ, Crapo JD, Wouters EF, Celli BR, Silverman EK, Demeo DL. Genome-Wide Association Analysis of Body Mass in Chronic Obstructive Pulmonary Disease. Am J Respir Cell Mol Biol 2011;45(2):304–10.

104. Filozof C, Fernandez Pinilla MC, Fernandez-Cruz A. Smoking cessation and weight gain. Obes Rev. 2004;5(2):95–103.

105. O'Shea SD, Taylor NF, Paratz JD. Progressive resistance exercise improves muscle strength and may improve elements of performance of daily activities for people with COPD: a systematic review. Chest. 2009;136(5):1269–83.

106. Franssen FM, Broekhuizen R, Janssen PP, Wouters EF, Schols AM. Effects of whole-body exercise training on body composition and functional capacity in normal-weight patients with COPD. Chest. 2004;125(6):2021–8.

107. Broekhuizen R, Wouters EF, Creutzberg EC, Weling-Scheepers CA, Schols AM. Polyunsaturated fatty acids improve exercise capacity in chronic obstructive pulmonary disease. Thorax. 2005;60(5):376–82.

108. Varraso R, Willett WC, Camargo Jr CA. Prospective study of dietary fiber and risk of chronic obstructive pulmonary disease among US women and men. Am J Epidemiol. 2010;171(7): 776–84.

109. Slinde F, Gronberg AM, Engstrom CR, Rossander-Hulthen L, Larsson S. Individual dietary intervention in patients with COPD during multidisciplinary rehabilitation. Respir Med. 2002;96(5):330–6.

110. Weekes CE, Emery PW, Elia M. Dietary counselling and food fortification in stable COPD: a randomised trial. Thorax. 2009;64(4):326–31.

111. Rennard SI, Fogarty C, Kelsen S, Long W, Ramsdell J, Allison J, et al. The safety and efficacy of infliximab in moderate to severe chronic obstructive pulmonary disease. Am J Respir Crit Care Med. 2007;175(9):926–34.

112. Schols AM, Soeters PB, Mostert R, Pluymers RJ, Wouters EF. Physiologic effects of nutritional support and anabolic steroids in patients with chronic obstructive pulmonary disease. A placebo-controlled randomized trial. Am J Respir Crit Care Med. 1995;152(4 Pt 1): 1268–74.

113. Ferreira IM, Verreschi IT, Nery LE, Goldstein RS, Zamel N, Brooks D, et al. The influence of 6 months of oral anabolic steroids on body mass and respiratory muscles in undernourished COPD patients. Chest. 1998;114(1):19–28.

114. Yeh SS, DeGuzman B, Kramer T. Reversal of COPD-associated weight loss using the anabolic agent oxandrolone. Chest. 2002;122(2):421–8.

115. Creutzberg EC, Wouters EF, Mostert R, Pluymers RJ, Schols AM. A role for anabolic steroids in the rehabilitation of patients with COPD? A double-blind, placebo-controlled, randomized trial. Chest. 2003;124(5):1733–42.

116. Lewis MI, Fournier M, Storer TW, Bhasin S, Porszasz J, Ren SG, et al. Skeletal muscle adaptations to testosterone and resistance training in men with COPD. J Appl Physiol. 2007;103(4): 1299–310.

117. Fabbri LM, Calverley PM, Izquierdo-Alonso JL, Bundschuh DS, Brose M, Martinez FJ, et al. Roflumilast in moderate-to-severe chronic obstructive pulmonary disease treated with longacting bronchodilators: two randomised clinical trials. Lancet. 2009;374(9691):695–703.

118. Calverley PM, Rabe KF, Goehring UM, Kristiansen S, Fabbri LM, Martinez FJ. Roflumilast in symptomatic chronic obstructive pulmonary disease: two randomised clinical trials. Lancet. 2009;374(9691):685–94.

119. Janda S, Park K, FitzGerald JM, Etminan M, Swiston J. Statins in COPD: a systematic review. Chest. 2009;136(3):734–43.

120. Pape GS, Friedman M, Underwood LE, Clemmons DR. The effect of growth hormone on weight gain and pulmonary function in patients with chronic obstructive lung disease. Chest. 1991;99(6):1495–500.

121. Burdet L, de Muralt B, Schutz Y, Pichard C, Fitting JW. Administration of growth hormone to underweight patients with chronic obstructive pulmonary disease. A prospective, randomized, controlled study. Am J Respir Crit Care Med. 1997;156(6):1800–6.

122. Nagaya N, Itoh T, Murakami S, Oya H, Uematsu M, Miyatake K, et al. Treatment of cachexia with ghrelin in patients with COPD. Chest. 2005;128(3):1187–93.

Chapter 12
COPD, Comorbidity, and Disease-Specific Clinical Practice Guidelines

Kristina Frogale, Kerry M. Schnell, and Cynthia M. Boyd

Abstract Many recent studies suggest that individuals with chronic obstructive pulmonary disease (COPD) are predisposed to comorbidity. Data on the prevalence of individual comorbidities among patients with COPD are highly variable. This may partly be due to differences in the methods of data acquisition, which range from self-reported survey data to administrative database analysis. There is also variability in comorbidity selection and the patient demographics among studies. When trying to determine the best diagnostic or treatment modality for a given patient, physicians often look to disease-specific clinical guidelines for recommendations to guide clinical decisions. These guidelines evaluate the body of evidence behind clinical questions and formulate recommendations, with the intent to influence clinical decision making. The strength of a recommendation is partially based on the quality of evidence from which it is derived. Even the strongest recommendations, however, are meant to be interpreted within the context of individual patient preferences and goals of care. A physician must use his or her clinical judgment when applying these guidelines to medical practice. One important question that must always be asked is whether or not these recommendations apply to the patient in question who may be elderly or have multiple comorbidities.

K. Frogale (✉)
Johns Hopkins Bayview Medical Center, Baltimore, MD, USA
e-mail: kfrogale1@jhmi.edu

K.M. Schnell
School of Medicine, Johns Hopkins University, Baltimore, MD, USA
c-mail: kschnell1@jhmi.edu

C.M. Boyd
Department of Geriatric Medicine and Gerontology, Johns Hopkins Bayview Medical Center, Baltimore, MD, USA
e-mail: cyboyd@jhmi.edu

L. Nici and R. ZuWallack (eds.), *Chronic Obstructive Pulmonary Disease: Co-Morbidities and Systemic Consequences*, Respiratory Medicine, DOI 10.1007/978-1-60761-673-3_12,
© Springer Science+Business Media, LLC 2012

Keywords COPD • Comorbidity • Guidelines • Practice parameters • Evidence-based • Recommendations • Congestive heart failure • Diabetes • Osteoporosis

COPD and Comorbidity

Many recent studies suggest that individuals with COPD are predisposed to comorbidity. In 2006, the COPD foundation commissioned a national telephone survey of 1,003 individuals with a self-reported diagnosis of COPD and found that as many as 47% of patients with COPD endorse six or more comorbidities [1]. The patients were all age 40 or greater with a broad distribution of COPD disease severity, from mild to severe, as delineated by the Medical Research Council (MRC) dyspnea severity index. Multiple case-control studies further support this data regarding the prevalence of comorbidity [2, 3]. One study in the Netherlands acquired data from 28 general practices and evaluated 290 COPD patients (mean age of 66). More than half of the COPD patients exhibited only mild airway obstruction, with an FEV1 of greater than 70% predicted against 421 age-matched controls with no diagnosis of COPD. Despite the mild nature of much of the COPD in this patient group, patients with COPD were twice as likely to have three or more comorbidities when compared to age-matched controls [3]. This further suggests that there is an association between COPD and comorbidity, even in patients with mild COPD disease severity.

Data on the prevalence of individual comorbidities among patients with COPD is highly variable. This may partly be due to differences in the methods of data acquisition that range from self-reported survey data to administrative database analysis. There is also variability in comorbidity selection and the patient demographics among studies. A review of each comorbidity evaluated and its prevalence is outlined in Table 12.1, along with details regarding the study population.

Despite these differences, there appear to be some consistent trends. The relative prevalence of individual comorbidities tends to be higher among COPD patients, when compared to controls, particularly in regards to cardiovascular disease. The greatest difference is seen with congestive heart failure. A study of the Kaiser Permanente Medical Care Program administrative database that looked at COPD and its association with cardiovascular disease found that the prevalence of congestive heart failure was 7.2% in patients with COPD; sevenfold higher than matched controls. This association is further validated by a case control analysis of a smaller Health Maintenance Organization (HMO) database [La Comunidad Hispana (LHC) in New Mexico], which found that 13.5% of the 200 patients with COPD also had congestive heart failure, in contrast to only 2.5% of matched controls [2]. Interestingly, the 2006 COPD National Foundation survey only found the prevalence of congestive heart failure to be 5%. The most common comorbidities documented in the COPD National Foundation survey, irrespective of age or gender, were hypertension, hyperlipidemia, sinus problems, depression, diabetes, and coronary artery disease (angina and prior myocardial infarction). This was followed by osteoporosis, stroke, and congestive heart failure [1]. A study of the UK General

Table 12.1 A review of each comorbidity evaluated and its prevalence as well as details regarding the study population

Comorbidity	Barr et al. [1]	Sidney et al. [4]		van Manen et al. [3]		Mapel et al. [2]	
	Case n=1,003	Case n=45,960	Control n=45,966	Case n=290	Control n=421	Case n=200	Control n=200
Hypertension	55	18.2	11.2	22.7	21.4	45	36.5
Hyperlipidemia	52	8.7	7.1	–	–	–	–
Heart disease	–	–	–	13.1	11.0	22	14.5
Angina	22	1.0	0.2	–	–	–	–
Heart attack	19	1.8	0.4	–	–	–	–
CHF	5	7.2	0.9	–	–	13.5	2.5
Thrombosis	–	0.3	0.1	2.4	3.2	–	–
Arrhythmia	–	8.2	1.9	–	–	12.5	9.5
Diabetes	25	1.6	1.1	4.5	7.1	11	9.5
Depression	37			8.7	4.4	17	13
Gastritis/ulcers	–			7.2	1.5	32	17
Cancer	5			6.2	2.5	18	9.5
Sinus problems	59			12.4	2.5	–	–
Osteoporosis	14			–		–	–
Stroke	14	1.2	0.5	3.1	3.7	4.0	3.5
Locomotive d/o	–			36.1	28.6	–	–
Liver disease	–			0.3	0.5	1.5	1.0
Renal disease	–	0.6	0.2	0.3	0.2	1.5	1.0

CHF congestive heart failure

Practice Database revealed that COPD patients had a significantly increased risk of cardiac disease, with a relative risk of 4.01 when compared to matched controls [5]. However, there is also some data to suggest that musculoskeletal disorders such as osteoporosis, not cardiovascular disease, make up the most prevalent comorbidities in patients with COPD [3].

Further subgroup analysis within the COPD patient population looked to see if gender or age played a role in the prevalence of comorbidity. The 2006 COPD national survey found that for the most part, the prevalence of comorbidities was similar between men and women with COPD. Diseases found to be more common in women included depression (44 vs. 27%) and osteoporosis (39 vs. 12%), while heart attack appeared to be more common in men (27 vs. 14%) [1]. Although a smaller study, a case-control analysis in the Netherlands, which looked at 28 general practices, also found that women with COPD were more likely to have musculoskeletal disorders (as outlined under Table 12.1), as well as insomnia, and migraine, while men were more likely to have heart disease [3]. As a result, it may be necessary to take gender into consideration when treating patients with COPD, as there may be some variability in comorbidity.

COPD tends to be a disease of older adults and most studies looking at COPD and comorbidity have evaluated patients over the age of 40, with substantially higher mean ages. The Netherlands study included a further subgroup analysis and divided the COPD patient population into age brackets: 40–55, 55–70, and >70. The presence of one or more comorbidities increased with age, with a prevalence of 60.4% among patients aged 40–55, as compared to 82.4% among patients older than 70 years. The prevalence of hypertension and heart disease also increased with age [3]. This suggests that the burden of comorbidity is greater in elderly patients with COPD and should be taken into account when making treatment decisions.

There is also data to suggest a relationship between the presence of comorbidities and actual COPD disease severity. The 2006 COPD national survey specifically compared these two variables through use of the MRC dyspnea severity index (scale of 0–4). Sixty-one percent of the COPD patients studied reported moderate to severe COPD (MRC Dyspnea Index of greater than or equal to three). Interestingly, the mean MRC Dyspnea Index increased with the number of comorbid conditions, from 2.3 among those with 1–5 comorbid conditions, 2.8 with 6–10 comorbidities, 3.2 with 11–15 comorbidities, to 4.0 among those with 20–25 comorbidities [1]. These MRC dyspnea score differences indicate worsening functional status, with significant dyspnea even at rest in patients with an MRC dyspnea index score of 4.

As expected, the co-occurrence of COPD and comorbidity results in greater morbidity, mortality, as well as greater overall healthcare utilization [2, 4, 6]. The Kaiser Permanente study, which evaluated cardiovascular endpoints, found that heart failure was not only more common among patients with COPD but was also the leading cause of hospitalization for cardiovascular disease in this patient population. COPD patients had a relative risk of 3.75 of being hospitalized for heart failure compared to matched controls. This was followed by myocardial infarction (MI), with a relative risk of 1.89 for MI hospitalization [4]. Patients with COPD had a higher risk of incident hospitalization and mortality for each of the cardiovascular disease end points studied. Analysis of a smaller HMO database found that the discharge diagnosis of cardiovascular disease was twice as common among patients with COPD when compared to matched controls [2].

Understandably, COPD itself still remains the most common cause of hospitalization in this patient population, but it appears that comorbidity still plays a significant role in morbidity [2]. Studies indicate that comorbidities have an effect on length of COPD hospitalization. One such study found that the mean length of stay was 7.7 vs. 10.5 days if comorbidity was present [6]. This further translates into greater overall healthcare utilization. Patients with COPD also require more services, which are not all related to their pulmonary disease. As indicated by an HMO database, for example, patients with COPD were found to need greater specialty care, such as cardiology evaluation [2].

It is clear that there is a significant burden of comorbidity among this patient population. Therefore, it is imperative that physicians treat these patients within the context of their comorbidities. Each chronic condition contributes to the overall health of the patient and may influence decisions regarding treatment.

Clinical Practice Guidelines and Comorbidity

When trying to determine the best diagnostic or treatment modality for a given patient, physicians often look to disease-specific clinical guidelines for recommendations to guide clinical decisions [7]. These guidelines evaluate the body of evidence behind clinical questions and formulate recommendations, with the intent to influence clinical decision making. The strength of a recommendation is partially based on the quality of evidence from which it is derived. Even the strongest recommendations, however, are meant to be interpreted within the context of individual patient preferences and goals of care. A physician must use his or her clinical judgment when applying these guidelines to medical practice. One important question that must always be asked is whether or not these recommendations apply to the patient, who may be elderly or have multiple comorbidities.

This issue becomes particularly relevant in the era of pay-for-performance. Health insurers increasingly look to outcomes and quality of care when reimbursing physicians. While not their original intent, many clinical guidelines provide the basis for the "standard of care" from which quality measures are derived [8]. Multiple Medicare initiatives and demonstrations are moving away from the current fee-for-service insurance reimbursement model, as it promotes unnecessary spending, and incorporating pay-for-performance models. With pay-for-performance, the hope is that healthcare costs will be contained through the promotion of high quality, efficient care. Although the concept has face validity, it is difficult to establish quality measures that accurately represent the complexity of patient care for people with multimorbidity. As mentioned, clinical guidelines must always be interpreted within the context of the individual patient, and may not be applicable to the older, more complex patient. As a result, quality measures based on these disease-specific guidelines may deter physicians from treating patients with multiple comorbidities or those more prone to "poor outcomes." It may also lead to an inaccurate judgment of a physician's care for this population [9]. It is essential that clinical practice guidelines and quality of care measures that are based on them address the patient with comorbidity, as this represents a significant percentage of the patient population. This importance will increase given the increasing prevalence of chronic disease, multimorbidity, and the aging population [10].

In an effort to better understand the applicability of clinical practice guidelines to the patient with multiple comorbidities, a systematic review was undertaken. Clinical practice guidelines, as of March 2005, were reviewed for nine of the most common chronic diseases seen in primary care. The "most common" conditions were chosen based on prevalence data from the National Health Interview Survey and a nationally representative sample of Medicare beneficiaries [9–11]. A final list of chronic medical conditions included hypertension, COPD, osteoporosis, osteoarthritis, chronic heart failure, stable angina, atrial fibrillation, hypercholesterolemia, and diabetes mellitus. Clinical practice guidelines that focused on chronic aspects of the conditions were chosen for review; they were drawn from a variety of sources, including primary care, specialty, national, and international organizations [9].

Each clinical guideline underwent rigorous review by two reviewers. The reviews were based on standards for developing and rating the quality of clinical practice guidelines, with a particular emphasis on issues of relevance to older adults and people with multiple comorbidities [7, 12–17]. Each reviewer evaluated how well the guideline described whether the target population included older adults, people with multiple comorbidities, or older people with multiple comorbidities, whether or not it graded the quality of evidence for any of these populations, discussed therapeutic goals, discussed quality of life with incorporation of patient preferences, addressed duration of therapy necessary to achieve benefit in the context of overall life expectancy, and addressed competing risks and burden of treatment.

Interestingly, only four of the clinical practice guidelines (diabetes, osteoarthritis, atrial fibrillation, and angina) gave recommendations for older individuals with multiple comorbidities, and within that group, only the clinical practice guidelines addressing diabetes and atrial fibrillation discussed the quality of evidence for this patient population. Seven of the clinical practice guidelines made recommendations for treating the target disease in conjunction with a single other chronic disease, as outlined in Tables 12.2 and 12.3 [9]; however, the majority of older patients struggle with more than one comorbidity [18]. The clinical practice guidelines addressing chronic heart failure and hypercholesterolemia discussed treatment of multiple comorbidities in the setting of other cardiac diseases, but not of noncardiac diseases. In terms of treatment within the context of life expectancy, only the diabetes clinical practice guidelines addressed time needed to treat to achieve benefit.

None of the clinical practice guidelines discussed the burden of comprehensive treatment on patients or caregivers. Only three clinical practice guidelines (hypertension, angina, and hypercholesterolemia) acknowledged patients' financial burden. The clinical practice guideline for diabetes did mention the inconvenience and discomfort of self-monitoring blood glucose. The atrial fibrillation clinical practice

Table 12.2 Relevance of clinical practice guidelines for the treatment of older patients with diabetes mellitus, hypertension, osteoarthritis, osteoporosis, and COPD

Chronic disease addressed by guideline

	Diabetes	Hypertention	Osteoarthritis	Osteoporosis	COPD
Guideline addressed treatment for type of patient?	Older: yes Multiple comorbidities: yes Both: yes	Older: yes Multiple comorbidities: no Both: no	Older: yes Multiple comorbidities: yes Both: yes[a]	Older: no Multiple comorbidities: no Both: no	Older: no Multiple comorbidities: no Both: no
Quality of evidence discussed for type of patient	Older: yes Multiple comorbidities: yes Quality of evidence poor, requires extrapolation for nutrition recommendations	Older: yes Multiple comorbidities: no Quality of evidence good for treating hypertension in older patients	Older: no Multiple comorbidities: no	Older: no Multiple comorbidities: no	Older: no Multiple comorbidities: no
Specific recommendations for patients with one comorbid condition?	Yes Diseases: hypercholesterolemia, hypertension, congestive heart failure, chronic kidney disease, cardiovascular disease, peripheral vascular disease, benign prostatic hypertrophy	Yes Diseases: coronary artery disease, diabetes mellitus, metabolic syndrome, sleep apnea, chronic kidney disease, gout, left ventricular hypertrophy, erectile dysfunction, peripheral vascular disease, congestive heart failure, stroke, dementia,[b] renal transplantation, renal artery stenosis, urinary outflow obstruction	Yes Diseases/drugs: anticoagulants, glucocorticoids, peptic ulcer disease, chronic kidney disease, hypertension, congestive heart failure	No	No
Specific recommendations for patients with several comorbid conditions?	Yes	No	No	No	No
Time needed to treat to benefit from treatment in the context of life expectancy discussed?	Yes	No	No	No	No

With permission from Kinnunen et al. [6], copyright @ 2005 American Medical Association. All rights reserved [18]

[a]Limited to patients at highest risk of gastrointestinal tract bleeding with certain therapies

[b]Limited to the possible effects of antihypertensive treatment on preventing cognitive decline, not management of hypertensive patients with mild cognitive impairment or dementia

Table 12.3 Relevance of clinical practice guidelines for the treatment of older patients with atrial fibrillation, chronic heart failure, angina, and hypercholesterolemia

Chronic disease addressed by guidelines	Atrial fibrillation	Chronic heart failure	Angina	Hypercholesterolemia
Guideline addressed treatment for type of patient?	Older: yes Multiple comorbidities: yes Both: yes	Older: yes Multiple comorbidities: yes Both: no	Older: yes Multiple comorbidities: yes[a] Both: yes[a]	Older: yes Multiple comorbidities: yes[b] Both: no
Quality of evidence discussed for type of patient?	Older: yes Multiple comorbidities: yes	Older: yes Multiple comorbidities: no	Older: yes Multiple comorbidities: no	Older: yes[c] Multiple comorbidities: no
	Average age of patients in clinical trials younger than population average, trials excluded those at high risk for bleeding	Absence of older persons in large clinical trials	Few older patients were included in clinical trials for one possible intervention	
Specific recommendations for patients with one comorbid condition?	Yes	Yes	Yes	Yes
	Diseases: congestive heart failure, hypertension, diabetes mellitus, angina, left ventricular hypertrophy, Wolff–Parkinson–White syndrome, hypertrophic cardiomyopathy, hyperthyroidism, pregnancy, chronic obstructive pulmonary disease	Diseases: hypertension, diabetes mellitus, hypercholesterolemia, angina, atrial fibrillation, chronic obstructive pulmonary disease	Diseases: hypertension, diabetes mellitus, hypercholesterolemia, congestive heart failure, aortic valve stenosis, valvular heart disease, asthma, heart block, hypertrophic cardiomyopathy, atrial fibrillation, peripheral vascular disease, hyperthyroidism, chronic kidney disease, depression, migraines	Diseases: hypertension, diabetes mellitus, cardiovascular disease
Specific recommendations for patients with several comorbid conditions?	No	Yes: only for combination of cardiovascular diseases	Yes[a]	Yes: only for combination of diabetes mellitus and cardiovascular disease[b]
Time needed to treat to benefit from treatment in the context of life expectancy discussed?	No	No	No	No

With permission from Kinnunen et al. [6], copyright @ 2005 American Medical Association. All rights reserved [18]

[a] Limited to weighing severe comorbidity likely to limit life expectancy when considering treatment procedures that would lead to revascularization; asking patients in follow-up about presence of new comorbid illnesses; and the effect of severity of or treatment for comorbidities on angina. Older patients with severe angina and several comorbid illnesses may be satisfied with a reduction in symptoms that enables an improvement in physical disability

[b] Limited to multiple comorbid conditions that increase cardiovascular risk (no discussion of comorbidities other than combination of diabetes mellitus and cardiovascular disease)

[c] Secondary prevention trials included older persons. Guideline reports that PROSPER authors state that statin use can be extended to older persons. Conflicting data on cancer risk with statins; statins have no effect on cognition or progression of disability

guideline discussed quality of life regarding warfarin therapy, with its need for frequent monitoring and its potential drug interactions. Seven of the clinical practice guidelines discussed patients' preferences about medical care, but this was often without guidance. For example, there was little specific information on how best to incorporate patient preferences into the treatment plan through shared decision-making, such as what information should be communicated to patients regarding risks, benefits, and harms in order to elicit preferences. The clinical practice guideline for congestive heart failure discussed preferences, but only for end-of-life treatment.

To demonstrate the results of assuming applicability of disease-focused clinical practice guidelines to an older patient with multiple comorbidities, the group created a hypothetical elderly patient with multiple comorbidities and established a treatment regimen based on the most recent clinical practice guidelines for each disease state [9]. Whenever possible, the regimen was simplified and overall cost was addressed. The patient was a 79-year-old woman with osteoporosis, osteoarthritis, type 2 diabetes mellitus, hypertension, and COPD. According to the clinical guidelines, she would need to take 12 separate medications and the regimen would require a total of 19 doses per day, taken at five times during a typical day. There were 14 nonpharmacological activities recommended for this patient if all nutritional recommendations were pooled into one. Although it would be possible theoretically to compress monitoring into two to four primary care visits and one ophthalmologic visit per year, other work has demonstrated that most Medicare patients have several clinicians [19]. For example, studies indicate that patients with COPD not only utilize respiratory-related health resources, but also other specialty services, particularly related to concomitant cardiovascular disease [2]. An outline of this complex treatment regimen can be found in Tables 12.4 and 12.5 [9].

Along with the significant burden of polypharmacy and frequent monitoring, there were multiple potential interactions that could occur with concurrent adherence to all five clinical practice guidelines. These were divided into three different categories: interactions between a medication and a disease other than the target disease, between medication for different diseases, and between food and medications. These interactions are detailed in Table 12.6 [9]. In terms of financial burden, the patient's medications alone would cost her $406.45 per month or $4,877 annually, assuming no prescription drug coverage. Even with Medicare part D and the assumption that her income was above 150% of the federal poverty level (as it was for more than 60% of Medicare beneficiaries), she would pay $3,797 per year plus $373 for any future drug expenses for that year based on 2005 prices. This does not take into account the recommended nonpharmacological interventions that provide additional expense to the patient, informal caregivers, Medicare, and other insurers [9].

This review of multiple clinical guidelines along with the use of the hypothetical patient clearly demonstrates that clinical practice guideline recommendations are derived from disease-specific clinical evidence that does not account for the complexity of multiple comorbidities. At present, the physician must use his or her clinical judgment when applying these recommendations. The recommendations should always be interpreted within the context of the patient as a whole, which includes comorbid disease. In the next section, we will consider how guidelines may be made more relevant to this patient population.

Table 12.4 Treatment regimen based on clinical practice guidelines for a hypothetical 79-year-old woman with hypertension, diabetes mellitus, osteoporosis, osteoarthritis, and COPD

Time	Medications[a]	Other
7:00 a.m.	Ipratropium metered dose inhaler 70 mg/week of alendronate	Check feet Sit upright for 30 min on day when alendronate is taken Check blood sugar
8:00 a.m.	500 mg of calcium and 200 IU of vitamin D 12.5 mg of hydrochlorothiazide 40 mg of lisinopril 10 mg of glyburide 81 mg of aspirin 850 mg of metformin 250 mg of naproxen 20 mg of omeprazole	Eat breakfast 2.4 g/day of sodium 90 mmol/day of potassium Low intake of dietary saturated fat and cholesterol Adequate intake of magnesium and calcium Medical nutrition therapy for diabetes[b] DASH[b]
12:00 p.m.		Eat lunch 2.4 g/day of sodium 90 mmol/day of potassium Low intake of dietary saturated fat and cholesterol Adequate intake of magnesium and calcium Medical nutrition therapy for diabetes[b] DASH[b]
1:00 p.m.	Ipratropium metered dose inhaler 500 mg of calcium and 200 IU of vitamin D	
7:00 p.m.	Ipratropium metered dose inhaler 850 mg of metformin 500 mg of calcium and 200 IU of vitamin D 40 mg of lovastatin 250 mg of naproxen	Eat dinner 2.4 g/day of sodium 90 mmol/day of potassium Low intake of dietary saturated fat and cholesterol Adequate intake of magnesium and calcium Medical nutrition therapy for diabetes[b] DASH[b]
11:00 p.m.	Ipratropium metered dose inhaler	
As needed	Albuterol metered dose inhaler	

Clinical practice guidelines used (1) Joint National Committee on Prevention, Detection, Evaluation, and Treatment of High Blood Pressure VII.39. (2) ADA19–32; glycemic control is recommended; however, specific medicines are not described. (3) American College of Rheumatology33–36; recent evidence about the safety and appropriateness of cyclooxygenase inhibitors, particularly in individuals with comorbid cardiovascular disease, led us to omit them from the list of medication options, although they are discussed in the reviewed clinical practice guidelines. (4) National Osteoporosis Foundation40; this regimen assumes dietary intake of 200 IU of vitamin D. (5) National Heart, Lung, and Blood Institute and World Health Organization37, 38 Eat foods containing carbohydrate from whole grains, fruits, vegetables, and low-fat milk. Avoid protein intake of more than 20% of total daily energy; lower protein intake to about 10% of daily calories if overt nephropathy is present. Limit intake of saturated fat (10% of total daily energy) and dietary cholesterol (200–300 mg). Limit intake of *trans*unsaturated fatty acids. Eat two to three servings of fish per week. Intake of polyunsaturated fat should be about 10% of total daily energy With permission from Kinnunen et al. [6], copyright @ 2005 American Medical Association. All rights reserved [18]

ADA American Diabetes Association, *COPD* chronic obstructive pulmonary disease, *DASH* dietary approaches to stop hypertension

[a]Taken orally unless otherwise indicated. The medication complexity score of the regimen for this hypothetical woman is 14, with 19 doses of medications per day, assuming 2 as needed doses of albuterol metered dose inhaler plus 70 mg/week of alendronate

[b]DASH and ADA dietary guidelines may be synthesized, but the help of a registered dietitian is specifically recommended

Table 12.5 Recommendations based on clinical practice guidelines for a hypothetical 79-year-old woman with hypertension, diabetes mellitus, osteoarthritis, osteoporosis, and COPD

Patient tasks
Joint protection
Energy conservation
Exercise
Non-weight-bearing if severe foot disease present or weight-bearing for osteoporosis
Aerobic exercise for 30 min on most days
Muscle strengthening
Range of motion
Avoid environmental exposures that might exacerbate chronic obstructive pulmonary disease (COPD)
Wear appropriate footwear
Limit intake of alcohol
Maintain normal body weight (body mass index of between 18.5 and 24.9)

Clinician tasks
Administer vaccine
Pneumonia
Influenza annually
Check blood pressure at all clinician visits and sometimes at home[a]
Evaluate self-monitoring of blood glucose
Foot examination at all clinician visits if neuropathy present; otherwise check feet for
    protective sensation, structure, biomechanics, vascular status, and skin integrity annually
Laboratory tests
Microalbuminuria annually if not already present
Creatinine level and electrolytes at least 1–2 times per year
Cholesterol levels annually
Liver function biannually
Glycosylated hemoglobin level biannually to quarterly, depending on level of control
Referrals
Physical therapy
Ophthalmologic examination
Pulmonary rehabilitation
Dual-energy X-ray absorptiometry scan every other year
Patient education
High-risk foot conditions, foot care, and foot wear
Osteoarthritis
COPD medication and delivery system training
Diabetes mellitus

Clinical practice guidelines used (1) Joint National Committee on Prevention, Detection, Evaluation, and Treatment of High Blood Pressure VII.39. (2) ADA19–32; glycemic control is recommended; however, specific medicines are not described. (3) American College of Rheumatology33–36; recent evidence about the safety and appropriateness of cyclooxygenase inhibitors, particularly in individuals with comorbid cardiovascular disease, led us to omit them from the list of medication options, although they are discussed in the reviewed clinical practice guidelines. (4) National Osteoporosis Foundation40; this regimen assumes dietary intake of 200 IU of vitamin D. (5) National Heart, Lung, and Blood Institute and World Health Organization37, 38
    [a]Ambulatory blood pressure monitoring is helpful if "white coat hypertension" is suspected and no target organ damage, apparent drug resistance, hypotensive symptoms with antihypertensive medication, or episodic hypertension

Table 12.6 Potential treatment interactions for a hypothetical 79-year-old woman with five chronic diseases

Type of interaction				
Type of disease	Medications with potential interactions	Medication and other disease	Medications for different diseases	Medication and food
Hypertension	Hydrochlorothiazide, lisinopril	Diabetes: diuretics increase serum glucose and lipids[a]	Diabetes medications: hydrochlorothiazide may decrease effectiveness of glyburide	N/A
Diabetes	Glyburide, metformin, aspirin, and atorvastatin	N/A	Osteoarthritis medications: NSAIDs plus aspirin increase risk of bleeding; Diabetes medications: glyburide plus aspirin may increase the risk of hypoglycemia; aspirin may decrease effectiveness of lisinopril	Aspirin plus alcohol: increased risk of gastrointestinal tract bleeding; Atorvastatin plus grapefruit juice: muscle pain, weakness; Glyburide plus alcohol: low blood sugar, flushing, rapid breathing, tachycardia; Metformin plus alcohol: extreme weakness and heavy breathing; Metformin plus any type of food: medication absorption decreased
Osteoarthritis	NSAIDs	Hypertension: NSAIDs: raise blood pressure[b]; NSAIDs plus hypertension increase risk of renal failure	Diabetes medications: NSAIDs in combination with aspirin increase risk of bleeding; Hypertension medications: NSAIDs decrease efficacy of diuretics	N/A
Osteoporosis	Calcium, alendronate	N/A	Diabetes medications: calcium may decrease efficacy of aspirin; aspirin plus alendronate can cause upset stomach; Osteoporosis medications: calcium may lower serum alendronate level	Alendronate plus calcium: take on empty stomach (2 h from last meal); Alendronate: avoid orange juice; Calcium plus oxalic acid (spinach and rhubarb) or phytic (bran and whole cereals): eating these foods may decrease amount of calcium absorbed (2 h from last meal)
Chronic obstructive pulmonary disease	Short-acting-agonists	N/A	N/A	N/A

N/A no interaction is known, *NSAIDs* nonsteroidal anti-inflammatory drugs

[a]Thiazide-type diuretics may worsen hyperglycemia, but effect thought to be small and not associated with increased incidence of cardiovascular events.

[b]This interaction is noted to be particularly relevant for individuals with diabetes; no recommendation for treatment is given.

Clinical Practice Guidelines for COPD:
How Well Do They Address Comorbidity?

Many studies suggest a close association between COPD and multiple comorbidities, particularly those related to cardiovascular disease. These comorbidities may have a direct relationship with disease severity, as multiple studies demonstrate higher morbidity, mortality, and overall healthcare utilization in COPD patients with comorbidity [1, 2]. Therefore, the evaluation and treatment of patients with COPD must consciously occur within the context of their comorbidities. When making clinical decisions, physicians often look to disease-specific clinical practice guidelines for recommendations. However, Boyd and colleagues clearly demonstrated that the clinical practice guidelines for many common chronic medical conditions fail to address comorbidity in a meaningful way [9]. Strict adherence to multiple guidelines may result in significant patient burden, with polypharmacy and frequent monitoring, along with the risk of adverse interactions.

Since the systematic review by Boyd and colleagues in 2005, multiple COPD guidelines have been updated. As a result, the most recent COPD guidelines, as of October 2010, were critically reviewed based on a modification of the assessment adopted previously by Boyd and colleagues [9]. The following groups were involved in the COPD guidelines selected – the American Thoracic Society/European Respiratory Society (ATS/ERS) [20], the American College of Physicians (ACP) [21], the National Institute for Health and Clinical Excellence (NICE) [22], and the Global Initiative for Chronic Obstructive Lung Disease (GOLD) [23].

In an attempt to better understand how well these updated COPD guidelines address comorbidity, a series of questions were formulated. Each guideline was evaluated based on whether or not it addressed patients with one additional comorbidity vs. multimorbidity (two or more), whether it contained recommendations for ascertaining the presence of comorbidities, whether it addressed potential side effects or interactions, or expressed caution in regards to certain therapies in those with comorbidity, whether it contained treatment recommendations for patients with one or multiple comorbidities, and whether it discussed the level of evidence for these recommendations.

The ATS/ERS, GOLD, and NICE guidelines acknowledged that patients with COPD may suffer from comorbidity; however, only the GOLD 2009 guidelines reference data regarding the prevalence of multimorbidity. It quotes a study from the Netherlands that found that up to 25% of COPD patients older than 65 have 2 or more comorbidities and 17% have 3. It goes on to state that these patients are at an increased risk of myocardial infarction, angina, osteoporosis, respiratory infections, bone fracture, depression, diabetes, sleep disorders, anemia, and glaucoma. Both the NICE and ATS/ERS guideline address COPD and comorbidity within the context of cigarette smoking, stating that tobacco provides a shared risk factor for multiple other diseases, including atherosclerotic vascular disease, cancer, peptic ulcer, and osteoporosis. The ACP guidelines do not mention comorbidity or its relevance in treating patients with COPD.

The NICE, ATS/ERS, and GOLD guidelines not only mention the presence of comorbidity among this patient population but also recommend that these comorbidities be ascertained as part of the standard evaluation. According to the ATS/ERS guideline, as part of the past medical history, any comorbidities, such as those associated with the heart or peripheral vasculature, or neurologic comorbidities that share the same risk factor of tobacco exposure, should be obtained, along with depression and anxiety. However, no specific recommendations are given as to how to use this information, except that it may indicate the "need for appropriate treatment of these conditions." The NICE guidelines alert physicians to ask about depression and anxiety, but once again, no specific recommendations are given about the treatment of COPD patients with these comorbidities.

All three guidelines acknowledge the impact that comorbidity has on disease severity, morbidity, and mortality, either directly or indirectly. The GOLD guideline explicitly state that significant comorbidities must be taken into account in assessment of severity, need for hospitalization, and determining appropriate treatment. It goes on to state that morbidity from COPD may be affected by other comorbid conditions, such as musculoskeletal disease or diabetes mellitus, and that comorbidities can complicate the management of COPD. Although not directly stated, both the ATS/ERS and NICE guidelines imply this relationship between COPD and comorbidity. For example, the ATS/ERS guidelines acknowledge that COPD patients with comorbidities such as CHF, coronary artery disease, diabetes, chronic renal, or liver failure are at greater risk for relapse after an exacerbation and that these factors should be taken into consideration when determining the need for hospitalization. Along the same lines, the NICE guidelines state that patients with significant comorbidities such as cardiac disease or diabetes are more likely to require hospitalization for exacerbation treatment. In terms of mortality, the GOLD guidelines state that older age and diabetes are important risk factors for mortality in COPD patients hospitalized for an exacerbation.

This tendency toward increased risk of morbidity and mortality in the presence of comorbidities is further implied by the NICE, ATS/ERS, and GOLD guidelines when discussing multiple treatment modalities for stable COPD. The ATS/ERS guidelines indicate that caution should be used when prescribing nicotine replacement to COPD patients with underlying cardiac disease. This same caution is presented in regard to lung volume reduction surgery and bullectomy as cardiac disease is associated with an increased risk of poor outcomes. The NICE guidelines state that caution should be taken when undertaking lung transplantation in COPD patients with comorbidity, although cardiac disease is not mentioned explicitly. The GOLD guidelines mention that COPD patients are older and more likely to have comorbidities, so the risk of developing side effects from bronchodilator therapy is greater. Interestingly, all three guidelines mention comorbidity in the context of theophylline metabolism, as drug metabolism is affected by anticonvulsant drugs, CHF, and liver cirrhosis. According to the GOLD guidelines, caution should also be taken with air travel in COPD patients with comorbidity that impairs oxygen delivery, such as cardiac disease or anemia. It is not described what is meant by "caution" in many of these examples, particularly in terms of relaying information that should be communicated to patients about the actual risks of these possible adverse consequences.

It does appear, however, that there are certain comorbidities that are direct contraindications to therapy, as outlined by ATS/ERS, NICE, and GOLD guidelines. Both ATS/ERS and NICE guidelines state that pulmonary rehab is contraindicated in COPD patients with immobility, unstable angina, or those who have recently had an MI. GOLD guidelines suggest briefer periods of high-intensity exercise or the use of upper extremity exercise in patients with comorbidity. In regards to nicotine replacement, GOLD guidelines state that unstable coronary artery disease, untreated peptic ulcer disease, and recent MI or stroke, are contraindications to therapy. The ATS/ERS guidelines state that bupropion therapy is contraindicated in patients with seizure disorder or bulimia, and that this medication may worsen hypertension.

A few comorbidities are identified as indicators for certain testing. According to the ATS/ERS guidelines, during preflight assessment for air travel safety, candidates for the hypoxia inhalation test include those with comorbidities such as coronary artery disease, CHF, arrhythmia, other cardiac diseases, cerebrovascular disease, anemia, seizure disorder and other neurologic disease, and pulmonary vascular disease including pulmonary embolus. Both ATS/ERS and GOLD state that sleep studies may be indicated in patients with COPD and sleep apnea.

The quality of evidence behind these limited recommendations for COPD patient with comorbidity is only outlined in the NICE guidelines. The statements regarding theophylline metabolism, pulmonary rehab contraindications, risk of poor outcome with lung transplant and comorbidity, depression and COPD, and the relationship between comorbidity and COPD exacerbation severity, are all based on Grade D evidence.

This systematic review of recent COPD guidelines clearly reveals the lack of guidance provided for addressing COPD in the context of multiple comorbidities. Although the ATS/ERS, NICE, and GOLD guidelines address the need for caution when treating COPD patients with comorbidity, and acknowledge that these comorbidities may increase morbidity and mortality, often, there are no specific recommendations as to how to manage this increased risk of morbidity. A few specific comorbidities are outlined as direct contraindications to therapy, and certain comorbidities may provide impetus for further testing; however, there are significant knowledge gaps as to how the presence of two or more comorbidities can effect COPD management. As a result, it is unclear how these clinical guidelines can be used by physicians within a clinical setting, or how they can serve as a source of quality standards for treatment of this complex patient population. The GOLD guidelines state that "all comorbid conditions amplify the disability associated with COPD and can potentially complicate its management. Until more integrated guidance about disease management for specific comorbid problems becomes available, the focus should be on identification and management of these individual problems in line with local treatment guidance." [23] The statement, while highlighting the problem, only perpetuates the difficult situation clinicians find themselves in when considering patients with multiple coexisting conditions. It highlights the need for more applicable guidelines and integration across diseases to determine the highest priority recommendations for individuals with COPD and other specific comorbidities.

Future Direction

Evaluation of the current clinical guidelines for COPD clearly demonstrates a deficiency in addressing the needs of complex patients with multiple comorbidities. As patients with multimorbidity represent a large percentage of the patient population, and comorbidity is associated with increased morbidity and mortality, measures must be taken to improve guideline development. In order to do this, each component of guideline development must be critically evaluated. There are many factors that contribute to this problem, such as the paucity of clinical studies that address this patient population, and the greater need for collaboration in developing clinical guidelines.

Many professional organizations, such as the ATS, recognize the need for reevaluation of guideline development [24, 25]. In 2008, the ATS organized a workshop on "Integrating and Coordinating Efforts in Guideline Development," using COPD as an example. The meeting strongly emphasized the importance of collaboration. For example, clinical research summaries and appraisals from various organizations are often not available in a standardized format that is accessible to others. However, through networking of professional organizations, existing clinical evidence as well as current knowledge gaps in addressing patients with comorbidity could be presented in a standardized database, accessible to all participating organizations [24]. This would enable guideline developers to have access to a unified review of the latest clinical evidence.

Along with having a standardized database of the latest clinical research, it is important for guideline developers to identify the relevant clinical questions. Guidelines must provide practical information that can be applied within a physician's clinical practice. Questions should address the complexity of patients with multiple comorbidities, taking into account the risks and benefits of each treatment option and the patient's goals of care. One way to address this is through the composition of guideline panels. Panels should be multidisciplinary and incorporate the patient's perspective whenever possible. Once the relevant questions have been established, professional organizations should then collaborate in developing high-quality evidence summaries for each question [24].

Collaboration would also allow for use of a standardized approach to evidence review (the way in which evidence is graded and recommendations are developed). When grading evidence, developers should consider whether or not clinical trials address patients with comorbidity or if they apply only to a select patient population [24, 26]. Identification of evidence gaps regarding patients with comorbidity could then be used in planning future clinical trials.

As mentioned previously, review of current COPD guidelines demonstrates a significant knowledge gap in the management of patients with multiple comorbidities. Randomized control trials are frequently designed to exclude these more complex patients, as scientists try to elucidate whether or not an intervention works. A new approach to clinical evaluation, known as comparative effectiveness research (CER), takes this question a step further and asks whether or not an intervention will improve patient outcomes when translated into clinical practice, where it is applied to a heterogeneous patient population. This model uses observational and clinical trial methods to compare different care strategies provided by typical health care clinicians. The harms and benefits of a treatment are evaluated across different clinical settings, with different patient populations. Observational CER studies require access to a linked registry or administrative database that includes billing information, etc., from multiple clinical sites. This information provides data from real world settings, on a large-scale. As with any observational study, there will be confounding factors that are not accounted for, as well as risk of selection bias [27]. However, this observational study design still has the ability to evaluate guideline recommendations within the context of real treatment settings and can provide important insight into their applicability. As with any observational study, there will be confounding factors that are not accounted for as well as risk of selection bias, but the methodology may provide useful information to help evaluate guideline recommendations within the context of real treatment settings, and can provide important insight into their applicability. CER methodologies and translational research methodologies may be used to evaluate and to improve the care and outcomes of patients with COPD [27].

References

1. Barr RG, Celli BR, Mannino DM, et al. Comorbidities, patient knowledge, and disease management in a national sample of patients with COPD. Am J Med. 2009;122(4):348–55.
2. Mapel DW, Hurley JS, Frost FJ, Petersen HV, Picchi MA, Coultas DB. Health care utilization in chronic obstructive pulmonary disease. A case-control study in a health maintenance organization. Arch Intern Med. 2000;160(17):2653–8.
3. van Manen JG, Bindels PJ, IJzermans CJ, van der Zee JS, Bottema BJ, Schade E. Prevalence of comorbidity in patients with a chronic airway obstruction and controls over the age of 40. J Clin Epidemiol. 2001;54(3):287–93.
4. Sidney S, Sorel M, Quesenberry Jr CP, DeLuise C, Lanes S, Eisner MD. COPD and incident cardiovascular disease hospitalizations and mortality: Kaiser Permanente Medical Care Program. Chest. 2005;128(4):2068–75.
5. Soriano JB, Visick GT, Muellerova H, Payvandi N, Hansell AL. Patterns of comorbidities in newly diagnosed COPD and asthma in primary care. Chest. 2005;128(4):2099–107.
6. Kinnunen T, Saynajakangas O, Tuuponen T, Keistinen T. Impact of comorbidities on the duration of COPD patients' hospital episodes. Respir Med. 2003;97(2):143–6.
7. Hayward RS, Wilson MC, Tunis SR, Bass EB, Guyatt G. Users' guides to the medical literature. VIII. How to use clinical practice guidelines. A. Are the recommendations valid? The Evidence-Based Medicine Working Group. JAMA. 1995;274(7):570–4.
8. Garber AM. Evidence-based guidelines as a foundation for performance incentives. Health Aff (Millwood). 2005;24(1):174–9.
9. Boyd CM, Darer J, Boult C, Fried LP, Boult L, Wu AW. Clinical practice guidelines and quality of care for older patients with multiple comorbid diseases: implications for pay for performance. JAMA. 2005;294(6):716–24.
10. Anderson G, Horvath J. Chronic conditions: making the case for ongoing care. Princeton, NJ: Partnership for Solutions; 2002.

11. Current estimates from the National Health Interview Survey, 1994. Vital Health Stat 1995;10(193): 1–116.
12. Shiffman RN, Shekelle P, Overhage JM, Slutsky J, Grimshaw J, Deshpande AM. Standardized reporting of clinical practice guidelines: a proposal from the Conference on Guideline Standardization. Ann Intern Med. 2003;139(6):493–8.
13. Greer AL, Goodwin JS, Freeman JL, Wu ZH. Bringing the patient back in. Guidelines, practice variations, and the social context of medical practice. Int J Technol Assess Health Care. 2002;18(4):747–61.
14. Cluzeau FA, Littlejohns P, Grimshaw JM, Feder G, Moran SE. Development and application of a generic methodology to assess the quality of clinical guidelines. Int J Qual Health Care. 1999;11(1):21–8.
15. The AGREE Collaboration. Appraisal of Guidelines for Research and Evaluation (AGREE) Instrument. Vol 2005, 2001. http://www.agreecollaboration.org/pdf/agreeinstrumentfinal.pdf
16. Shaneyfelt TM, Mayo-Smith MF, Rothwangl J. Are guidelines following guidelines? The methodological quality of clinical practice guidelines in the peer-reviewed medical literature. JAMA. 1999;281(20):1900–5.
17. Graham ID, Calder LA, Hebert PC, Carter AO, Tetroe JM. A comparison of clinical practice guideline appraisal instruments. Int J Technol Assess Health Care. 2000;16(4):1024–38.
18. Weiss CO, Boyd CM, Yu Q, Wolff JL, Leff B. Patterns of prevalent major chronic disease among older adults in the United States. JAMA. 2007;298(10):1160–2.
19. Pham HH, Schrag D, O'Malley AS, Wu B, Bach PB. Care patterns in Medicare and their implications for pay for performance. N Engl J Med. 2007;356(11):1130–9.
20. American Thoracic Society/European Respiratory Society. ATS/ERS Standards for the Diagnosis and Management of Patients with COPD, 2004. http://www.thoracic.org/clinical/copd-guidelines/resources/copddoc.pdf.
21. Qaseem A, Snow V, Shekelle P, et al. Diagnosis and management of stable chronic obstructive pulmonary disease: a clinical practice guideline from the American College of Physicians. Ann Intern Med. 2007;147(9):633–8.
22. National Institute for Health and Clinical Excellence. Chronic obstructive pulmonary disease. Management of chronic obstructive pulmonary diseases in adults in primary and secondary care (partial update). NICE clinical guideline 101. Developed by the National Collaborating Centre for Acute and Chronic Conditions. http://guidance.nice.org.uk/CG101.
23. Rabe KF, Hurd S, Anzueto A, et al. Global strategy for the diagnosis, management, and prevention of chronic obstructive pulmonary disease: GOLD executive summary. Am J Respir Crit Care Med. 2007;176(6):532–55.
24. Schunemann HJ, Woodhead M, Anzueto A, et al. A vision statement on guideline development for respiratory disease: the example of COPD. Lancet. 2009;373(9665):774–9.
25. Guyatt GH, Oxman AD, Vist GE, et al. GRADE: an emerging consensus on rating quality of evidence and strength of recommendations. BMJ. 2008;336(7650):924–6.
26. Fabbri L, Boyd CM, Boschetto P, et al. How to deal with multiple comorbidities in guideline development: an official ATS/ERS Workshop Report. Manuscript submitted for publication, 2010.
27. Krishnan JA, Mularski RA. Acting on comparative effectiveness research in COPD. JAMA. 2010;303(23):2409–10.

Chapter 13
Pharmacologic Treatment Strategies

Rachael A. Evans, Robert G. Varadi, Kambiz Mirzaei, and Roger S. Goldstein

Abstract As COPD is characterized by only partially reversible airway obstruction, respiratory pharmacological agents focus primarily on addressing the airflow limitation, both by bronchodilatation and by reducing airway inflammation. However, the symptoms, morbidity and mortality associated with COPD are also associated with secondary impairments, such as skeletal muscle dysfunction, decreased bone density and alterations of mood. Patient management must also consider common co-morbidities such as cardiovascular disease and diabetes. Therefore pharmacological management must address both the consequences of the pulmonary disease, the secondary impairments and the co-morbidities.

This chapter provides discussion of 1) the currently recommended pulmonary pharmacological treatment, 2) the interaction between COPD and cardiovascular disease, and the implications for pharmacological management, 3) an overview of the management of osteoporosis in COPD, 4) the interaction between COPD and diabetes, and the implications for pharmacological management, 5) the management of mood disorders, 6) future treatment directions.

Keywords COPD • Pharmacology • Co-morbidity • Cardiovascular disease • Osteoporosis • Anxiety and depression • Diabetes

R.A. Evans(✉) • R.G. Varadi • R.S. Goldstein
Department of Respiratory Medicine, West Park Healthcare Centre, Toronto, ON, Canada
e-mail: rach27evans@hotmail.com; robert.varadi@westpark.org; rgoldstein@westpark.org

K. Mirzaei
Department of Pharmacy, West Park Healthcare Centre, Toronto, ON, Canada
e-mail: kambiz.mirzaei@westpark.org

L. Nici and R. ZuWallack (eds.), *Chronic Obstructive Pulmonary Disease: Co-Morbidities and Systemic Consequences*, Respiratory Medicine, DOI 10.1007/978-1-60761-673-3_13, © Springer Science+Business Media, LLC 2012

Introduction

Contemporary Pharmacological Management for COPD

Chronic obstructive pulmonary disease (COPD) is characterized by progressive airway obstruction, which is only partially reversible, resulting in progressive breathlessness [1]. The pathophysiology is complex and typically consists of a combination of bronchitis (hyperplasia and hypertrophy of the mucus glands, smooth muscle hypertrophy, mucosal edema, mucus plugging, and peribronchial fibrosis) as well as emphysema (alveolar wall destruction and bullous formation). These changes result in reduced airflow, hyperinflation, and gas trapping, initially on exertion but eventually also at rest, as the disease progresses. Respiratory pharmacological agents are designed primarily to improve airflow. They act either as bronchodilators, as with β_2-adrenoceptor agonists (β_2-agonists), anticholinergics acting on the muscarinic receptors (mainly M3 in the airways) and methylxanthines that mainly work through nonspecific inhibition of phosphodiasterase (PDE), or reduce airway inflammation as with inhaled or oral steroids.

The symptoms, morbidity, and mortality associated with COPD are not caused solely by the underlying pulmonary pathology but include important secondary impairments of skeletal muscle function [2], nutrition [3], bone density [4], mood [5], gonadal hormones [6], and hemoglobin [7]. Both systemic inflammation and deconditioning have been postulated as mechanisms behind some of these alterations [8]. Given that COPD tends to occur in older adults comorbidities such as atherosclerosis, diabetes, and benign prostatic hypertrophy are frequently present. Understanding the evidence and application of respiratory pharmacological management must include careful consideration of the potential interactions that these medications may have on comorbid conditions, or on medications designed to optimize comorbid conditions.

The commonly used pharmacological agents for COPD have altered considerably in the last decade to accommodate a reduced dosage frequency and combination therapy. There has also been considerable progress in our understanding of the longer term outcomes from these agents.

A typical stepwise approach to the management of COPD is shown in Fig. 13.1 [9]. Initial treatment is limited to short acting bronchodilators for occasional symptom relief. When short acting bronchodilators are required more frequently, treatment with long-acting β_2-agonists (LABA) or long-acting anticholinergics (LAAC) are preferable to provide lasting benefit at less frequent dosing intervals [10–12] and for their symptomatic and health benefits. Both LABA and LAAC reduce dyspnea [10, 13, 14], improve exercise capacity [13, 15], improve health status [12, 16, 17], and reduce exacerbation rate [18, 19]. International guidelines recommend LABAs for GOLD stage II–IV ($FEV_1 < 80\%$ predicted) [20] although their use in earlier stages has been considered.

The actions of LABA and LAAC and consequent improvements in health outcomes are not just from their bronchodilating effects. As β-adrenoceptors are

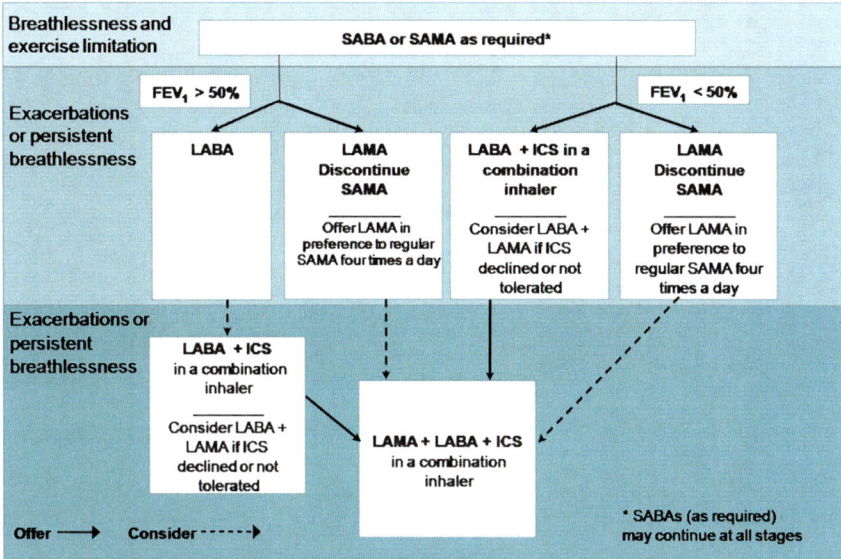

Fig. 13.1 Treatment strategy according to the severity of airflow reduction in COPD (with permission from NICE COPD guidelines [9]). *SABA* short acting beta agonist, *SAMA* short acting muscarinic antagonist, *LABA* long acting beta agonist, *LAMA* long acting muscarinic antagonist, *ICS* inhaled corticosteroid, *COPD* chronic obstructive pulmonary disease

expressed on neutrophils and macrophages, β_2-agonists can inhibit the release on inflammatory cytokines from these cells [21, 22] and can suppress airway inflammation when combined with inhaled corticosteroids (ICS) [23]. Muscarinic receptors are present on inflammatory cells so there is a potential for an anti-inflammatory effect of anticholinergics [24, 25], although tiotropium has not been shown to suppress airway or systemic inflammation [26].

Another interesting effect of β_2-agonists, relevant to the systemic manifestations of COPD, is their effect on skeletal muscle growth in animals [27]. Although suggested as a potential therapeutic agent for cachexia [28], their effect on skeletal muscle in COPD has yet to be investigated.

ICS are no longer recommended as single agents for patients with COPD [29] as monotherapy does not affect lung function decline [30] or mortality [31]. ICS are prescribed in combination with LABAs [32, 33] to reduce exacerbation frequency, improve health status, and reduce symptoms [31, 34]. Combined ICS and LABAs are thought to have a synergistic action and reduce airway inflammation [35] but not systemic inflammation [36]. Monotherapy with ICS may also increase the risk of pneumonia [31, 37].

Inhaled therapy has not shown a significant reduction in lung function decline [17, 29, 31]. Neither a large RCT of combined ICS/LABA(TORCH) [31] nor a large randomized controlled trial (RCT) of LAAC over 4 years (UPLIFT) [17] demonstrated any change in the rate of decline of FEV_1, although the therapies were associated with sustained initial improvements in airflow (Fig. 13.2).

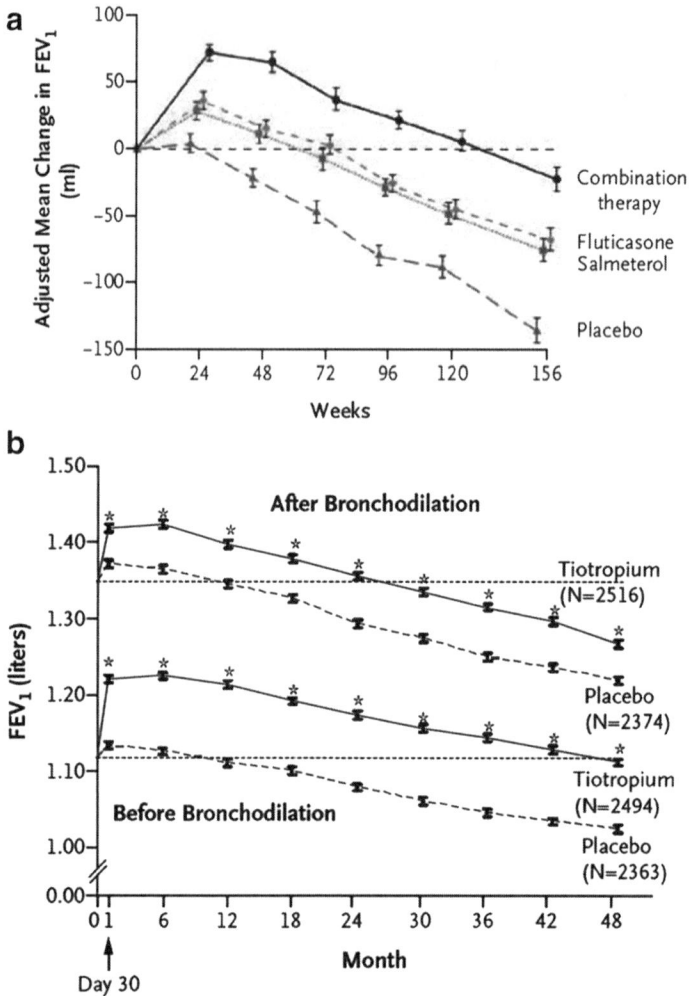

Fig. 13.2 Rate of lung function decline was unaltered for the four different treatment groups. Data taken from the TORCH (**a**) [17] and UPLIFT (**b**) [31] studies

Post hoc analysis revealed that lung function decline was reduced in a subgroup of patients with moderate to severe disease receiving ICS/LABA [38]. Combination LABA/ICS does not significantly impact on mortality [31]. They are mainly recommended for patients with a postbronchodilator $FEV_1 < 50\%$ predicted who have more than two exacerbations a year requiring either antibiotics or steroids [9]. In a predetermined secondary analysis of the UPLIFT trial, tiotropium was associated with a reduction in mortality for patients with moderate to severe disease (GOLD stages II–III) [39] and with a reduction in lung function decline in patients with GOLD stage II [40].

Most guidelines [9, 41], only add theophyllines for patients with severe disease due to their large side effect profile especially in older patients with significant comorbidities. However, there is evidence of an anti-inflammatory action [42] and they may enhance the effect of corticosteroids [43] especially during an acute exacerbation [44].

A combination of both LABA/ICS and LAAC is commonly prescribed for patients with severe COPD. Aaron et al. compared tiotropium with placebo or when added to LABA or a combination LABA/ICS (optimal study) [45]. Triple therapy was the best combination for lung function, health status, and hospitalization rates despite it not significantly reducing exacerbation rates. Similar results were shown with a different LABA/ICS combination with tiotropium, but a reduction in exacerbation rate was also demonstrated [46]. Currently, a combination of LABA/ICS with a LAAC is the optimal inhaled therapy for severe COPD.

Pharmacological Considerations with the Comorbidities and Secondary Impairments of COPD

Cardiovascular Disease

Prevalence and Implications of Cardiovascular Disease in COPD

COPD frequently coexists with cardiovascular disease, commonly coronary artery disease (CAD) [47] and chronic heart failure [48–50]. Some overlap is to be expected as these conditions increase in prevalence with age and have smoking as a common risk factor. The percentage of patients with both diseases ranges from 10 to 30% and the risk ratio of developing CHF in COPD compared to age-matched controls is 4.5 [51].

The presence of systemic inflammation, reported in patients with coronary heart disease [52, 53], chronic heart failure [54, 55], and COPD [56, 57] may be an important pathological mechanism contributing to cardiovascular complications; a common cause of death in COPD [31, 58]. Cardiovascular events increase in frequency as airflow obstruction progresses [59, 60]. The coexistence of heart and lung diseases is important as the combination is associated with a worse prognosis [61–63], a worse outcome after hospital admissions [64], more symptoms [65], and lower exercise capacity [66]. Cardiovascular disease in COPD (and COPD in heart disease) should therefore be actively managed.

Although there has been considerable progress in the pharmacological management of CHF and COPD individually, until recently little attention has been paid to management of the combined diseases [67]. This is relevant as the core pharmacological agents for CHF and COPD such as β-blockers for CHF and β-agonists for COPD may have opposing actions and also involve complex interactions with β-adrenoceptors.

β-Adrenoreceptors ($β_1$, $β_2$, and $β_3$) are subtyped according to their affinity for epinephrine and norepinephrine; $β_1$ receptors have equal affinity, whereas $β_2$ have a greater affinity for epinephrine and $β_3$ have a much lower affinity for both. Their activation causes G protein-mediated activation of adenylyl cyclase that increases cyclic AMP. Despite $β_1$ receptors being predominantly in the myocardium, they account for 10 and 30% of the β receptors in the submucosal glands and alveolar walls, respectively [68]. Similarly 23% of β-adrenoceptors in the healthy heart are $β_2$ [69]. Activation of the β-adrenoceptors results in calcium flux across the cell membrane, in the myocardium, with both inotropic and chronotropic effects. In the airways, β-adrenoceptor activation promotes smooth muscle relaxation. $β_3$ Receptors are located on adipose tissue and skeletal muscle where they are involved in lipolysis and thermogenesis, respectively.

Understanding the adrenoceptors has relevance for the pharmacological application of their agonists and antagonists. With repetitive stimulation, desensitization of the cells occurs via receptor sequestration, downregulation, and impaired coupling between the receptors and the G proteins [70]. For example, the effect of LABAs in asthma can change over time from their initial actions of bronchodilation and reducing airway hyperresponsiveness (AHR) to increasing AHR, airway inflammation, and possibly increase mortality [70–75], whether this occurs in COPD is unknown. Genetic variants of the adrenoceptors (haplotypes and genotypes) appear to also determine the effects of certain drugs [76–78].

Effect of the Pharmacological Treatment of COPD on the Cardiovascular System

Initial evidence suggested that $β_2$-agonists may have a deleterious effect on the cardiovascular system in patients with COPD [79], but more recent evidence supports there being no increased risk of all cause mortality (Fig. 13.3) or cardiovascular mortality (3% in the salmeterol group compared to 5% in the placebo group in the TORCH study) [31].

$β_2$-Agonists are not highly selective and therefore $β_1$-receptors in the myocardium may also be activated and although $β_2$-agonists for COPD are typically inhaled, systemic effects of tremor and tachycardia are not uncommon. In a large ($n = 220,000$) retrospective review of patients with COPD or asthma, those receiving $β_2$-agonists had an increased risk of hospital admissions from supraventricular tachycardia as well as from myocardial infarction (MI) [80].

Inhaled anticholinergics are not lipid soluble and are therefore less likely to cause the tachycardia associated with $β_2$-agonists. However, a higher rate of cardiovascular events, including hospitalization has been reported in smokers receiving ipratropium bromide [80, 81]. Retrospective reviews of ipratropium in COPD suggested an increased risk of all cause mortality [82] and cardiovascular events [83]. In 2008, a meta-analysis by Singh et al. of 17 RCTs of tiotropium vs. placebo for at least 30 days reported that tiotropium was associated with increased cardiovascular deaths, MI, and stroke [84] and a study (INSPIRE) that compared a combination

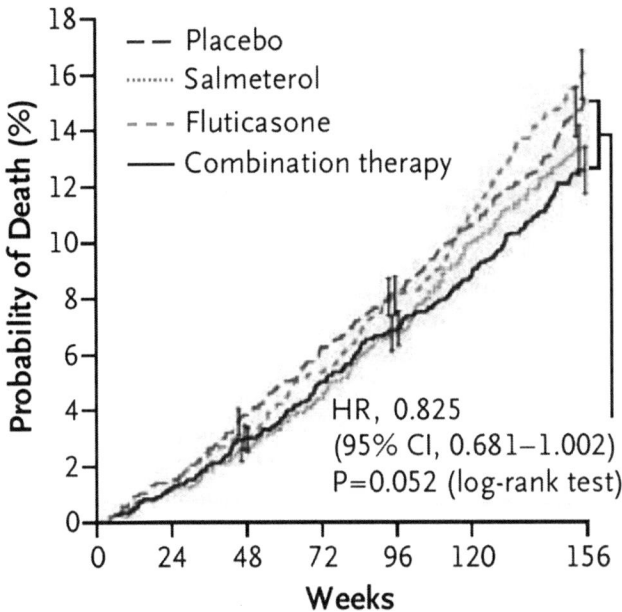

Fig. 13.3 Risk of death associated with the four different inhaled treatments (data taken from the TORCH study results) [31]

LABA/ICS with tiotropium reported a lower all-cause mortality and cardiovascular mortality for the combination LABA/ICS [85].

However, a subsequent meta-analysis including 19 studies and a systematic review that included data from a large prospective RCT of tiotropium vs. placebo (the UPLIFT trial) [86, 87] did not confirm any increase in risk with LAAC, in fact they reported a lower all risk for cardiovascular events. Whether tiotropium is associated with an increased risk of stroke has not been investigated prospectively, but was not identified in a retrospective study [88].

The safety of tiotropium has also been assessed from data generated from the UPLIFT study [17]. Tiotropium was reported to decrease all cause mortality, cardiovascular mortality, and cardiovascular events [89]. As these were a priori secondary outcomes, the results need to be confirmed.

The potential effects of ICS on cardiovascular mortality are reported in observational studies and a meta-analysis with conflicting results. One large observational study showed a significant reduction in mortality with ICS and interestingly the majority of this was achieved by a reduction in cardiovascular deaths with little change in respiratory-related deaths [90]. A meta-analysis of seven trials of ICS showed a reduction in all cause mortality, but only a trend toward a reduction in cardiovascular mortality [91]. It has been suggested that very low doses of ICS have been associated with a reduced risk of acute myocardial infarction in COPD [92] but a large prospective RCT did not support this observation for mortality (Fig. 13.3) or cardiovascular mortality (Fig. 13.4) [31].

Fig. 13.4 Cardiovascular
deaths for the four different
treatment groups using data
from the TORCH study
results [31]. *LABA* long
acting beta agonist, *ICS*
inhaled corticosteroid

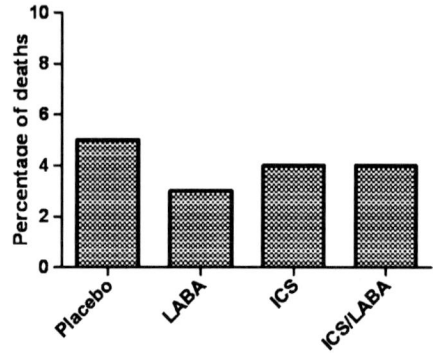

Effect of the Pharmacological Treatment for COPD on Cardiovascular Disease

Although there has been much concern over the use of beta blockade in COPD little attention had been paid to the safety of inhaled bronchodilators in patients with coexisting cardiovascular disease. β_2-Agonists, through nonselective stimulation, may down regulate β_1-receptors [93], a phenomenon associated with worsening heart failure [94]. Beta blockade with suppression of the sympathetic nervous system is a key treatment for chronic heart failure [95, 96] as it causes a reduction in mortality long term. Therefore, β_2-agonists with the associated reflex tachycardia may be potentially harmful to patients with CHF. A retrospective report using data from RCT of Candesartan vs. placebo [Candesartan in Heart failure – Assessment of Reduction in Mortality and morbidity (CHARM)] stratified a large cohort of CHF patients into four groups according to their bronchodilator or β-blocker use (see Fig. 13.5) [97]. Patients with CHF who received a bronchodilator, but no β-blocker had the worst survival.

The lower survival might have reflected the confounding effect of severe COPD, but it is noteworthy that the combination of a β-blocker and a bronchodilator led to a lower mortality rate than that seen with a bronchodilator alone.

Support for a deleterious effect of β_2-agonists in cardiovascular disease also comes from a retrospective case-controlled review of patients post-myocardial infarction, in which a β-agonist prescription within 3 months was associated with an increased risk among those with a history of cardiovascular disease [79]. Au et al. also reported a dose response increased risk of heart failure hospitalization as well as all-cause mortality in those with left ventricular systolic dysfunction who were using β-agonists (Fig. 13.6) [98].

Whereas β_2-agonists help relieve dyspnea in COPD, clinicians need to be aware that they may not be completely safe when administered to patients with coexisting cardiovascular disease. The safety of LABA, combination LABA/ICS, and LAACs in patients with COPD with coexisting cardiovascular disease needs to be prospectively assessed.

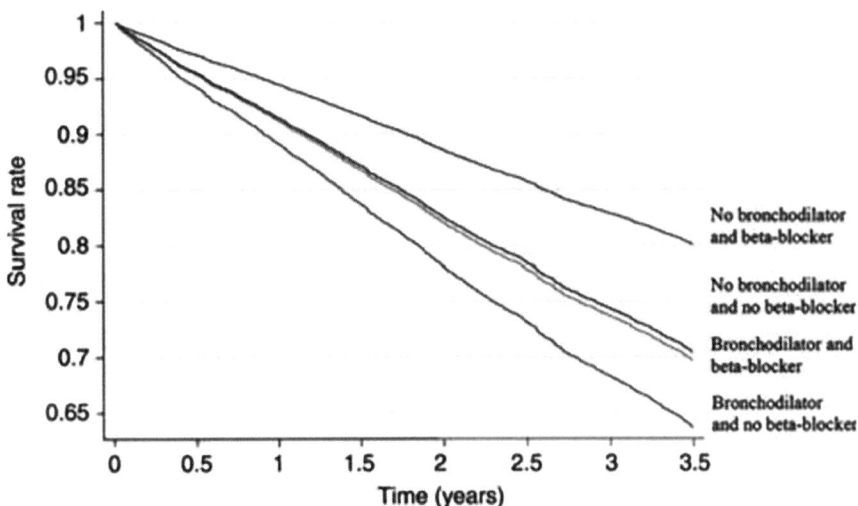

Fig. 13.5 Survival rate for patients with CHF according to bronchodilator and β-blocker use (with permission from Hawkins et al. [48])

Fig. 13.6 Risk of death associated with inhaled β-agonist use in patients with LVSD (modified from Au et al. [79]). Number of canisters of a beta-agonist used per month. *LVSD* left ventricular systolic dysfunction

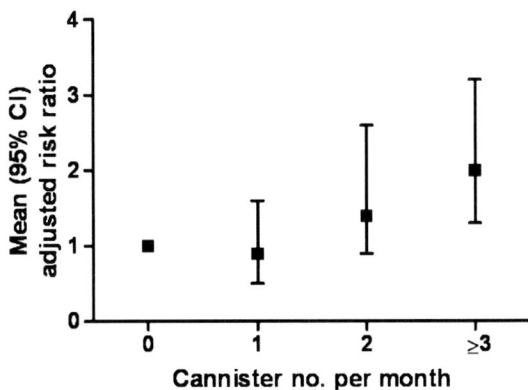

Treating Cardiovascular Disease in Patients with Coexistent COPD

Although β-blockers were historically thought to be harmful for patients with CHF, the advent of cardioselective β_1-blockers (bisoprolol and metoprolol) and the non-selective β-blockers with alpha(α) receptor antagonism (carvedilol) has revolution-ized the treatment of CHF such that they are now key components in the treatment for coronary heart disease and chronic heart failure and have been associated with a reduction in mortality for both [99–103].

β-Blockers were contraindicated in patients with airways disease because of their potential to cause bronchoconstriction [104], especially the nonselective agents such as propranolol and oxprenolol [105]. However, newer cardioselective agents have removed these initial concerns [106]. A meta-analysis of 19 single-dose studies showed that there was an initial reduction in FEV_1 with cardioselective β-blockers, but no increase in respiratory symptoms [107]. Over 4 weeks, there was no significant difference in FEV_1 symptoms or inhaler use with cardioselective β-blockers compared with placebo, but an increased response to $β_2$-agonists. A meta-analysis for reversible disease reported similar findings [108], and both concluded that cardioselective β-blockers do not produce adverse effects in the short term and should not be withheld in patients with comorbidities in which they are known to be beneficial.

Despite these recommendations, fewer than 20% of patients with both heart failure and COPD are receiving β-blockers [48]. In a retrospective review of an RCT of Candesartan vs. placebo (CHARM), the patients receiving bronchodilators were less likely to be receiving β-blockers even under study conditions [97]. Similarly, in patients with COPD and acute coronary syndromes, those receiving β-blockers (the minority) had a better prognosis [109] than those without.

The next question is which β-blocker to use in patients with CHF and COPD. The selectivity of β-blockers is variable [110] and the differences in effect on FEV_1 between the three β-blockers recommended for heart failure (carvedilol, metoprolol, and bisoprolol) has been tested in patients with both COPD and CHF compared to CHF only [111]. The FEV_1 significantly increased when carvedilol was replaced with either cardioselective agent, but interestingly this phenomenon was also seen in patients with CHF and no COPD. There is insufficient literature as to the preferred β-blocker for optimal pulmonary and cardiac function in patients with both CHF and COPD.

Long-term prospective data on the effects of cardioselective β-blockers on pulmonary function and clinical outcomes are lacking. However, retrospective data from a large cohort of patients with COPD who were prescribed β-blockers showed a reduction in hospitalizations, but a small increase in emergency departments with cardioselective agents not seen with nonselective β-blockers. Data from patients with asthma showed a higher rate of emergency visits and hospitalizations for those taking β-blockers indicating the potential difference for reversible disease. A retrospective report from inpatients with exacerbations of COPD taking β-blockers actually had a lower mortality than those not taking them, despite these patients being older and having more cardiovascular disease.

Other retrospective data have suggested that β-blockers may decrease the risk of mortality and exacerbation rate in COPD [112]. Although the mechanisms by which β-blockers reduce mortality in CHF are multifactorial, the reduction in the overactivation of the sympathetic nervous system has a major role. The activation of the sympathetic nervous system, renin–angiotensin system and subsequent increased secretion on brain natriuretic peptide (BNP), atrial natriuretic peptide (ANP), antidiuretic hormone (ADH), and others is termed neurohumeral activation is behind the pathogenesis of CHF and is a major target for the pharmacological agents used. Anker et al describe the evidence to suggest neurohumeral overactivation also exists in patients with COPD [113], which similarly is associated with a worse prognosis [114] providing a potential mechanism for the role of β-blockers in COPD. There is now debate for the use of β-blockers for patients with asthma supporting a more direct role in reversible disease. β-Receptor density increases with the long-term use of β-blockers and it is arguable (supported by animal data) that with time β-blockers may reduce airway hyperresponsiveness [115].

In summary, if patients with COPD have coexisting cardiovascular disease necessitating treatment with β-blockers these should be prescribed [110, 116]. When initiating β-blockers in COPD there may be an initial worsening of symptoms, but if these do not persist and are not clinically important, the medication should be continued. Cardioselective agents should probably be used, started at a low dose and titrated upward. The caveats are that long-term safety data for β-blockers in COPD are still lacking and the strongest evidence is for patients who do not have substantially reversible disease.

There is emerging evidence supporting a possible role for other traditionally "cardiac" drugs for COPD [117]. It is becoming clear that the improved cardiovascular outcome from the "statin" agents relates both to their lipid-lowering effects and their anti-inflammatory effects [118]. Observational studies have suggested that patients with COPD who are prescribed "statins" have a reduced exacerbation rate [117, 119], but this needs to be investigated prospectively.

ACE inhibitors are now a key component for the pharmacological treatment of CHF with a clear reduction in mortality [120]. An interesting observation from a large study was that ACE inhibition was associated with less weight loss in patients with heart failure [121] and it has been a suggested that the effects may have occurred by preventing skeletal muscle wasting [122]. Angiotensin is involved in proteolysis [123] so there may be a role for angiotensin receptor blockers for cachexia, a major problem for some patients with COPD. Mancini et al. also reported retrospectively a reduced exacerbation rate in patients with COPD receiving ACE inhibitors [117]. At present, these findings are at an observational stage, but it is likely that the mechanisms will be tested prospectively [124].

Therefore, pharmacologic treatment of COPD should not solely be from a pulmonary focus, but should include agents necessary to manage comorbid cardiovascular disease. The potential for interactions between medications for pulmonary and cardiovascular disease should be considered.

Osteoporosis

Osteoporosis is a leading cause of bony fractures, hospitalization, morbidity, and mortality worldwide [125]. It is generally defined as a disease characterized by low bone mass and microarchitectural deterioration of bone tissue, which predisposes to so-called fragility fractures [126]. These are fractures resulting from trauma that would not under normal circumstances cause serious injury, such as a fall from one's own height. Women, and particularly postmenopausal women, are disproportionately affected. More than 280,000 hip fractures occur each year in the United States; the lifetime risk of hip fracture has been estimated at 18% in women and 6% in men [127]. A great many of these patients do not live out the following year: the

1-year mortality after hip fracture is about 30% [128]. Vertebral fractures often do not come to immediate clinical attention, but can be associated with chronic back pain and functional impairment, as well as loss of pulmonary function [129, 130].

Though definitive diagnosis of osteoporosis requires examination of bone histology, the gold standard for clinical diagnosis is the finding of low BMD by dual-energy X-ray absorptiometry (DXA). The World Health Organization (WHO) gives an operational definition of osteoporosis based on the patient's BMD as compared to a reference sex-matched young adult population [125]. A patient whose BMD is more than 2.5 standard deviations below the young-adult mean (referred to as T-score<-2.5) is defined as having osteoporosis, while one whose BMD falls between 1 and 2.5 standard deviations below the mean ($-2.5<$T-score<-1) is said to have osteopenia or abnormally low BMD. Hip BMD most strongly predicts the risk of hip fracture and is the preferred site for BMD assessment [131].

Prevalence studies have reported osteoporosis in 24–69% of patients with COPD, depending on the population studied, setting, and diagnostic tool employed [132]. When compared to age-matched control subjects, the prevalence of osteoporosis was about three times as great in those with COPD [132]. Osteoporosis risk factors commonly encountered in patients with COPD include advanced age, female sex, postmenopausal status, more severe lung function impairment, malnutrition, low BMI and fat-free mass, smoking, excessive alcohol consumption, inactivity, and use of corticosteroids [133].

Who Should Be Treated?

Treatment should be tailored to the patient's risk of fracture. Though no COPD-specific instruments are available, several groups have developed tools to estimate fracture risk in the general population. The WHO has developed FRAX™, a fracture risk assessment tool to estimate the 10-year probability of hip and major osteoporotic fracture based on simple and commonly collected clinical variables, which can be supplemented by hip BMD [134]. The tool has been validated in a number of large cohorts and has been modified for use in many countries. An official online FRAX calculator has been made available at http://www.shef.ac.uk/FRAX/. The American National Osteoporosis Foundation (NOF) suggests treatment based on a history of hip or vertebral fracture, or the presence of osteoporosis based on BMD (T-score<-2.5) [135]. For those without fracture history and with intermediate BMD values, use of the FRAX calculator is recommended.

Management of Osteoporosis in COPD

The management of osteoporosis in COPD consists of improving bone density and reducing fracture rates through risk factors modification and through pharmacotherapy.

Smoking Cessation

Smoking cessation is at the heart of COPD treatment, and all patients should be counseled to stop smoking. The deleterious effects of cigarette smoking on bone health persist in former smokers [136]. There is observational evidence to support improvements in bone density through smoking cessation. In a cross-sectional study, former smokers were found to have BMD intermediate between active and never smokers [137]. In a large prospective cohort of older Americans followed over 16 years, the magnitude of BMD loss correlated well with smoking cessation: remote quitters had lesser decline in hip BMD than more recent quitters, while active smokers had lost the most [138]. While these studies relied on self-reported smoking cessation, Oncken and colleagues examined data from a clinical trial of smoking cessation, in which exhaled CO measurements were used to confirm abstinence from tobacco [139]. Those who sustained abstinence for 1 year demonstrated significant improvement in hip BMD, compared to continued smokers who had little change in BMD. Smoking cessation can significantly reduce rates of hip fracture, but this effect may only become apparent after 10 years of follow-up [140].

Exercise

Pulmonary rehabilitation incorporating exercise training significantly improves symptoms, exercise tolerance, mood, and quality of life in patients with COPD [141]. Although not yet well studied, rehabilitation may yield similar benefits to bone health as well. Exercise programs that combine multiple modalities of exercise, such as strength, endurance, balance, and flexibility, can reduce the rate of falls in the general elderly population [142]. Exercises that focus on improving balance, such as Tai Chi, seem especially effective. Even simple leisure activity appears to be protective of falls and fractures. In the Nurses Health Study, women who reported walking more than 4 h a week, even without any other exercise or training, had nearly half as many hip fractures over 12 years than did women who walked less than 1 h per week [143]. Though data in chronic lung disease are sparse, resistance training of the back muscles has been shown to improve vertebral BMD after lung transplantation [144, 145]. Exercise and physical activity should be counseled for all patients with COPD and osteoporosis, though the optimal type or modality of exercise remains to be determined.

Corticosteroids

The association between systemic corticosteroids and osteoporosis is well recognized. Corticosteroid-induced bone loss is mediated through a number of different mechanisms, producing a negative calcium balance, decreasing bone formation, and increasing resorption [146, 147]. Loss of BMD is most pronounced in the first year of therapy, while the risk of osteoporotic fractures increases out of proportion to the BMD decline [148–151]. Major osteoporosis guidelines generally consider corticosteroids to be a major risk when used for at least 3 months at a daily dose of at least 5–7.5 mg of prednisone (or equivalent) [134, 152, 153]. Patients who are expected to need at least 3 months of treatment should be started on osteoporosis pharmacotherapy, as discussed below.

A general principle in treatment is to limit exposure to systemic corticosteroids as much as possible. Extrapolating data from the rheumatology literature, it may be safer to treat patients with higher corticosteroid doses in short bursts, as is recommended for acute COPD exacerbations, than to limit the dose but extend the duration. One group showed that BMD was unchanged after 1 year of intermittent pulse methylprednisolone therapy for rheumatoid arthritis, while significant BMD loss was noted with daily oral prednisone [154]. After discontinuing systemic corticosteroids in chronic users, BMD may actually improve and fracture risk may return to baseline with time [155].

The impact of ICS on bones is far more controversial. Several observational and experimental studies in both COPD and asthma have reported increased rates of osteoporosis and fractures in ICS users [156–160]. However, a similar number of groups have found no such association [161–164]. Drawing any definitive conclusions is difficult, owing to differences in study design, ICS selection and duration of use, and potential for confounding by disease severity. Overall, it appears that ICS have less impact on bone health than oral corticosteroids, but solid recommendations on modifying ICS therapy to prevent or treat osteoporosis cannot be made.

Calcium and Vitamin D

All patients with COPD should ensure adequate intake of calcium and vitamin D. There is a strong association between adequacy of dietary calcium intake and a positive calcium balance, which is necessary to avoid bone loss [165]. Vitamin D enhances gut absorption of calcium and prevents PTH-induced bone turnover and loss. Several studies have demonstrated that higher serum vitamin D levels are associated with greater BMD in women and men; conversely, low levels have been associated with higher rates of fracture [166–168]. In temperate climates, seasonal variations in serum vitamin D levels parallel those in incidence of hip fractures, with a winter extreme seen in both [169].

Through 2009, Cochrane Library reviewers identified 45 clinical trials investigating calcium/vitamin D supplementation in the prevention of osteoporotic fractures [170]. The combination effectively reduced hip fracture rates when compared to placebo. However, this benefit was strongest in unselected populations – those in whom a history of osteoporotic fracture was not required. In studies that mandated prior fracture as an inclusion criterion, no significant difference was detected. It can be inferred from these data that calcium and vitamin D alone are not sufficient therapy for those patients at higher fracture risk.

For patients receiving systemic corticosteroid therapy, the American College of Rheumatology recommends a daily intake of at least 1,000 mg of calcium and at least

800 U of vitamin D through diet and/or supplements [153]. Calcium and vitamin D alone may be able to blunt the loss of BMD in patients receiving low-dose corticosteroids, equivalent to less than 6 mg of prednisone daily [171]. However, they are insufficient for patients receiving higher doses. In a large clinical trial, patients were administered calcium with or without calcitriol, a more potent vitamin D analogue, within 4 weeks of starting systemic corticosteroid therapy [172]. The mean starting dose was equivalent to prednisone 25 mg daily, and the mean daily dose over the first year was 13.5 mg. Patients in either group lost 1–4% in vertebral and femoral neck BMD over 1 year. Similarly, patients receiving a minimum daily corticosteroid dose of 7.5 mg of prednisone were treated with calcium and low-dose vitamin D, with or without weekly alendronate [149]. Those in the control arm of calcium and vitamin D supplements alone demonstrated slight declines in BMD by about 1%, while those also receiving alendronate saw increases in BMD by 2–3%.

There is a two- to threefold increase in risk of hypercalcemia with vitamin D supplementation, highest in those receiving calcitriol. Increased incidence of gastrointestinal intolerance and of renal stones has also been reported [170]. Calcium interferes with the absorption and bioavailability of many medications, including bisphosphonates, oral corticosteroids, and quinolone antibiotics. These interactions can be minimized simply by administering the medication at least 2 h before or 6 h after the dose of an oral calcium supplement.

Bisphosphonates

The bisphosphates, synthetic analogs of pyrophosphate, are potent modifiers of bone metabolism. They are avidly taken up at sites of active bone turnover; there, they interfere with osteoclastic bone resorption, either by impairing osteoclast function or by inducing apoptosis, thus preserving bone density [173]. Their therapeutic benefit is countered by their tendency to interfere with the formation of hydroxyapatite crystals, the central mineral component of bone, thereby inhibiting mineralization and leading to osteomalacia. Etidronate, for instance, inhibits both resorption and mineralization to a similar extent, limiting its use for the management of osteoporosis. The newer generations of bisphophonates, such as alendronate and risedronate, are far more potent inhibitors of resorption than of mineralization and have become the preferred agents.

Bisphosphonates currently form the mainstay of treatment of osteoporosis. Their beneficial effects on bone density and fracture rates have been well established in large well-designed clinical trials. Improvements in femoral neck and vertebral BMD by at least 3–5% relative to placebo are seen over 2–3 years of treatment in patients with established osteoporosis [174, 175]. The clinical benefits have been best demonstrated in secondary prevention studies involving over 26,000 postmenopausal women (Fig. 13.7). Treatment with the equivalent of alendronate 10 mg or risedronate 5 mg daily reduces vertebral fracture rates by about 40% and nonvertebral fracture rates (especially hip) by at least 20% [176, 177]. These benefits have proven sustainable over time. In women who discontinue treatment after

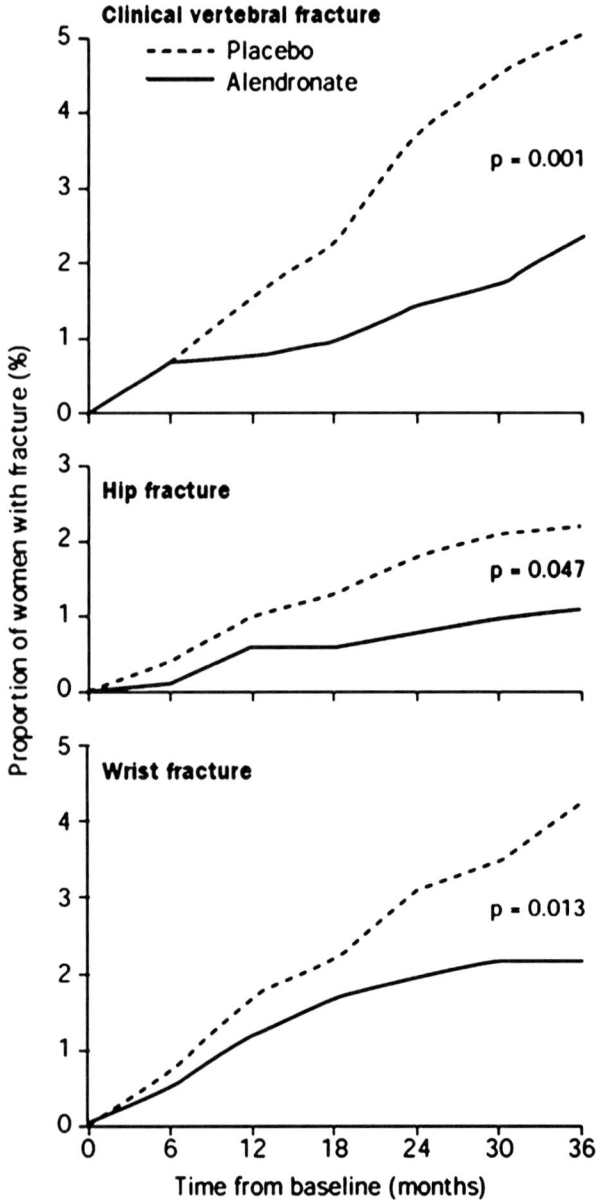

Fig. 13.7 In postmenopausal women with a vertebral fracture at baseline, treatment with alendronate significantly reduced the incidence of various osteoporotic fractures (with permission from Black et al. [174])

5 years, BMD and markers of bone turnover remain better than baseline values after a further 5 years' follow-up [178]. Bisphosphonates have been less well studied in men, but the benefits in secondary prevention of fractures appear to be similar to those in women [179].

There is substantial evidence that bisphosphonates can blunt the loss of bone density seen with systemic corticosteroid therapy. Though the bulk of data are derived from studies of patients with rheumatologic diagnoses, a substantial minority were being treated for asthma. In a meta-analysis of 13 clinical trials, bisphosphonates led to improvements in hip and lumbar spine BMD by 2 and 4%, respectively [180]. The most impressive benefits are seen when bisphosphonates were initiated early in the course of corticosteroid treatment when the steroid-induced loss of BMD is most rapid. Therefore, it is recommended that patients being started on a long course (at least 3 months) of corticosteroids should be prescribed a potent bisphosphonate as early as possible.

It should be noted that, in the majority of studies, bisphosphonates were coadministered with calcium and vitamin D supplements. As such, all patients being treated with a bisphosphonate should receive calcium/vitamin D supplementation as well.

Bisphosphonates have poor oral bioavailability and should not be taken with food. Since calcium supplements may decrease the absorption of bisphosphonate derivatives, their administration should be separated by at least 2 h. Once absorbed, bisphosphonates may persist in bone for many years [181]. Major toxicities include hypocalcemia and gastrointestinal complications including severe esophagitis. Patients should be instructed to remain upright for at least 30 min after ingestion of a dose. Though some concerns have been raised about a possible link between bisphosphonate use and esophageal cancer, a large cohort study found no evidence for such an association [182]. There appears to be a small but significant increased risk of atrial fibrillation [183]. Osteonecrosis or avascular necrosis of the jaw is a very rare but severe complication of bisphosphonate therapy that tends to occur predominantly in patients treated for malignancy [184].

Hormonal Agents

Menopause and its attendant estrogen deficiency are accompanied by rapid bone loss due to increased bone resorption. Estrogen replacement therapy (ERT), particularly when administered early in menopause, increases BMD and reduces hip, vertebral, and other osteoporotic fracture rates [185, 186]. However, the Women's Health Initiative and other studies have shown ERT to increase the risk of CAD, stroke, venous thromboembolism (VTE), and breast cancer [185]. Furthermore, there appears to be accelerated loss of BMD after ERT is stopped [187]. Estrogen replacement is generally reserved for those women who have significant menopausal symptoms and are intolerant of other osteoporosis treatments. The combination of ERT and bisphosphonates has additive effects on improving BMD, though no significant impact on fractures has been detected [188, 189].

Raloxifene is a tissue-selective estrogen receptor modulator (SERM). Owing to proestrogenic effects in bone, it leads to improvements in BMD, bone turnover, and risk of fractures [190–192]. Unlike estrogen, raloxifene reduces rates of breast cancer and does not increase cardiovascular event rates, although it too is associated with higher rates of fatal strokes and VTE [190]. It has proven less potent in bone protection than alendronate and is therefore considered second-line therapy for women who are intolerant of bisphosphonates [193].

Testosterone deficiency has been identified in men with COPD, especially in those treated with corticosteroids [194]. Among other effects, reductions in testosterone levels have been associated with low BMD [195]. Correcting testosterone deficiency in younger patients with hypogonadism improves BMD [196]. Although the bone-protective effects of androgens in elderly men are less clear, they appear to have greatest benefit in those with more profound hypogonadism, as evidenced by lower testosterone levels [197–199]. Therapeutic use of androgens is limited by numerous side effects, the most important of which in elderly men is prostatic hyperplasia [200].

Calcitonin

Calcitonin is a calcium-regulatory hormone secreted by the thyroid C-cells. Its main effects are to reduce calcium absorption in the gut, increase renal calcium excretion, and impair osteoclastic bone resorption [201]. Calcitonin has modest effects on BMD and fracture risk in both postmenopausal and corticosteroid-associated osteoporosis, although to a much lesser extent than bisphosphonates [202, 203]. A unique feature of calcitonin is its analgesic effect in vertebral fractures, which makes it an attractive choice of antiresorptive in patients with pain related to osteoporotic fractures [204].

Salmon calcitonin, which is far more potent in humans than its human analogue, can be delivered by intranasal spray or subcutaneous injection. While bioavailability is lower by nasal route, it has the advantage of fewer gastrointestinal and dermatologic side effects and therefore better tolerance [205]. Its respiratory side effects, including nasal irritation and rhinitis/sinusitis, are generally mild.

Diabetes Mellitus

Diabetes is a common comorbidity in COPD with a reported prevalence of 14% [206, 207] and is associated with a higher risk of hospitalization and mortality [208–210]. Diabetes is independently associated with reduced airflow and an inflammatory mechanism has been postulated [211, 212]. Smoking is associated with increased glucose levels and insulin resistance, further supporting the necessity of smoking cessation for these patients.

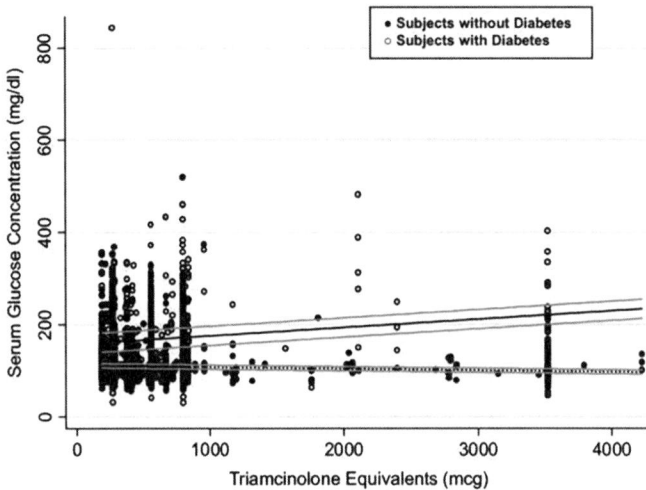

Fig. 13.8 Serum glucose concentration and inhaled corticosteroid use [213] with permission. Gray lines represent the 95% confidence interval of the mean. The inhaled corticosteroid dosage has been converted into triamcinolone equivalents. The solid regression line is for patients with diabetes and the dotted line represents those without diabetes

The core treatments for COPD, β-agonists, and corticosteroids, both alter glucose metabolism; β-agonists increase glycogenolysis and steroids cause an increase in serum glucose levels. The latter occurs by effects on (1) the liver by stimulating the formation of glucose and depositing glucose as glycogen and (2) the periphery by reducing the utilization of glucose, increasing protein and lipid breakdown, thus promoting gluconeogenesis. Corticosteroids worsen control in patients with known diabetes and precipitate hyperglycemia in patients who are predisposed.

ICS are systemically absorbed and can worsen glycemic control in type II diabetes. One large study ($n = 1,698$) showed a dose response of an increase serum glucose level of 2.65 mg/dl for every 100 μg increase in ICS (Fig. 13.8) [213]. There was no change in patients not known to be diabetic. In a small study ($n = 10$), HbA1C was unchanged after 6 weeks of treatment with inhaled fluticasone 440 mcg bid [214]. It would seem sensible to advise patients with type II diabetes, starting ICS treatment, that their diabetic medication may need adjustment.

Long-term, low-dose oral steroids (<10–15 mg) for stable COPD are no longer advocated [215]. Although high-dose steroids (>30 mg) are associated with an improvement in FEV_1, their long-term side effects preclude this option for most patients. After 3 weeks of treatment with high-dose steroids, an increase in blood glucose levels of 1.72 mg/dl has been reported. Glucose intolerance improves after cessation of oral steroids [216].

Short courses of steroids (5–14 days) are the mainstay of treatment for exacerbations of COPD (AECOPD) [1, 217]. A recent systemic review of steroids for the treatment of AECOPD [218] reported an increased risk of hyperglycemia

(OR: 4.95; 95% CI 2.47–9.91). There is surprisingly little guidance regarding glucose monitoring during the initiation of high-dose prednisone. Two retrospective AECOPD studies have reported a worse outcome associated with hyperglycemia [219], and a prospective study reported hyperglycemia to be associated with a worse outcome for AECOPD [220]. This is similar to findings for myocardial infarction, stroke, pneumonia, and critically ill patients.

Inhaled insulin has been under investigation as an alternative approach to the traditional subcutaneous administration of insulin for diabetics [221]. Although diabetes is common in COPD, there are challenges for this route of administration. In asthma there is lower absorption of inhaled insulin compared to healthy controls, which can be increased by the prior administration of inhaled terbutaline [222]. The variability of airway function in patients with airway diseases is of concern for the diabetic control using inhaled insulin [223].

Consideration is also needed for the effect of the inhaled medication on the airways. A three year study of inhaled insulin vs. subcutaneous insulin showed a small reduction in FEV_1 and DLCO in patients without preexisting lung disease, which improved after the six months washout at the end of the trial [224]. In patients with asthma using inhaled insulin, no changes in spirometry at 1 year were reported despite an initial reduction in FEV_1 and DLCO [225].

The long-term effect of inhaled therapy on lung function is under review [141–143] for COPD and ARDS [226]. This work highlights the expanding role of the inhaled route for nonpulmonary pharmacological agents.

Benign Prostatic Hyperplasia

Benign prostatic hyperplasia (BPH) is very common and increases with age. It is present in >40% of men over the age of 50 [227] and >30% of this group suffer from lower urinary tract symptoms. Urinary retention is not infrequent in BPH and more than 10% of these episodes may be drug related. Anticholinergics can worsen symptoms of BPH and precipitate acute urinary retention (AUR), increasing the post-void urine residual (PVR). Therefore, current guidelines for BPH exclude them. As BPH and COPD occur in similar age groups, inhaled anticholinergics especially LAACs are a concern.

There is little prospective literature on the effect of inhaled anticholinergics in patients with BPH; as such, patients have often been excluded from LAAC in COPD trials. A small study showed no difference in urinary flow rate or postvoid residual volume and no episodes of AUR over a 3-month period [228]. The adverse events recorded from the UPLIFT trial ($n = 5,992$) showed no significant increase in worsening symptoms from BPH with tiotropium 1.18 (0.9–1.54), but patients with significant symptomatic prostatic hyperplasia or bladder neck obstruction were excluded (those controlled on medication were included).

Patients with BPH also have bladder instability requiring anticholinergic therapy. A systematic review and meta-analysis of oral anticholinergics in BPH (five RCTs) revealed no significant change in urinary flow rate, an increase in postvoid residual volume, but no increase in AUR. The authors concluded that oral anticholinergics are safe in patients with BPH and bladder instability. Although it would seem sensible to advise patients with BPH that their symptoms may worsen with tiotropium, the evidence supports initiation of tiotropium in COPD for patients whose symptoms of BPH are controlled. As tiotropium (LAAC) is excreted via the kidney, it should be used with caution in patients with a creatinine clearance ≤50 mL/min.

Management of Anxiety and Depression in COPD

Anxiety

Anxiety is the apprehensive anticipation of stressful situations associated with unease and symptoms of tension. It manifests itself as restlessness, decreased concentration, rapid speech, palpitations, and dyspnea. Although many patients with severe COPD report some symptoms of anxiety, a much smaller number have a general anxiety disorder, defined by excessive anxiety for more than 6 months resulting in impaired social function. Panic attack episodes of acute anxiety with fears and dyspnea occur in many patients with COPD with a few suffering from a panic disorder characterized by repeated panic attacks.

The disparity of prevalence information for anxiety (as with depression) relates to the type of patient studied, the definition and type of anxiety, and the study design. Anxiety is more prevalent among women, those with depression, and those with poor self-efficacy. It is unrelated to age, education, or the number of comorbidities but may be triggered by dyspnea, anger, or frustration. Anxiety reduces health-related quality of life and increases hospitalization and emergency department visits. In the multicenter Nordic study [229], following an acute exacerbation, anxiety (HADS) [230] was noted in 15% men and 20% women, depression in 10% men and 6% women and both in 15% of men and 24% of women. COPD is associated with an increased risk of anxiety (odds ratio 1.85, 95% CI, 1.1–3.2) and among stable patients with COPD, the prevalence of anxiety was 15 vs. 6% in a referent non-COPD population [231].

Depression

Depression is a mood disorder characterized by a decrease in mood, interest, and concentration accompanied by feelings of sadness, irritability, and hopelessness. The most common manifestations of depression are social withdrawal and a decreased ability to enjoy work or leisure. Physical symptoms include poor quality of sleep, reduction in appetite, and an increase in fatigue. The diagnosis is made more difficult as there is an overlap between symptoms of COPD (dyspnea, fatigue, poor sleep, and reduced appetite) and symptoms of a secondary psychological impairment.

Table 13.1 Prevalence and odds of depression in patients with COPD compared with referents

	n	Depressive Symptoms	OR (95% CI)
COPD Subjects[†]			
FEV_1 ≥80% predicted	283	26.5%	3.1 (1.7–5.6)
FEV_1 ≥50–80% predicted	549	25.9%	2.9 (1.7–5.1)
FEV_1 ≥30–50% predicted	258	28.7%	4.6 (2.5–8.4)
FEV_1 <30% predicted	112	34.8%	8.0 (4.1–15.7)
Referents	302	5.6%	1.0 (referent)

[†]Comparing the whole COPD group to referents in multivariate analysis adjusted for the same covariates yields an odds ratio for depressive symptoms of 3.6 (95% CI, 2.1–6.1)

Sadness and loss are frequently present in severe COPD, especially post-hospitalization [232]. This is different from an adjustment disorder – excessive distress for the stimulus – or from a major depressive disorder, which may have no relationship to COPD. Depression is more likely if there is a family history of depression, a lack of social support, and a reduced economic status. It impairs health-related quality of life and increases length of stay following an exacerbation. Depressed patients are also more likely to refuse resuscitation than those without depression.

In 1,202 COPD patients and 302 matched referents, Omachi and colleagues [233] noted that COPD patients are at an increased risk for depression (odds ration 3.6, 95% CI, 2, 1–6.1, $p < 0.001$). Depressive symptoms are associated with a reduction in health-related quality of life (odds ratio 3.6, 95% CI, 2.7–4.8, $p < 0.01$). Of note (Table 13.1), depressive symptoms are more prevalent as airflow is reduced.

The importance of managing depression has been emphasized by Ng and colleagues who noted it in 44% of 376 subjects [234]. Depression increases length of stay and mortality (Hazard Ratio 1.93, 95% CI, 1.04–3.58) (Fig. 13.9).

Pharmacologic Treatment of Anxiety and Depression in COPD

Despite the paucity of research related to the use of anxiolytics (Table 13.2) or antidepressants (Table 13.3) in COPD, clinicians must select, from a wide variety of medication classes and chemical families. Anxiolytics come from:

- Selective serotonin reuptake inhibitors (SSRIs)
- Serotonin–norepinephrine reuptake inhibitors (SNRIs)
- Benzodiazepines
- Tricyclic antidepressants (TCAs)
- Monoamine oxidase inhibitors (MAOIs)
- Reversible inhibitors of monoamine oxidase-A (RIMAs)
- Noradrenergic and specific serotonergic antidepressants (NaSSAs)
- Atypical antipsychotics
- Antiepileptics

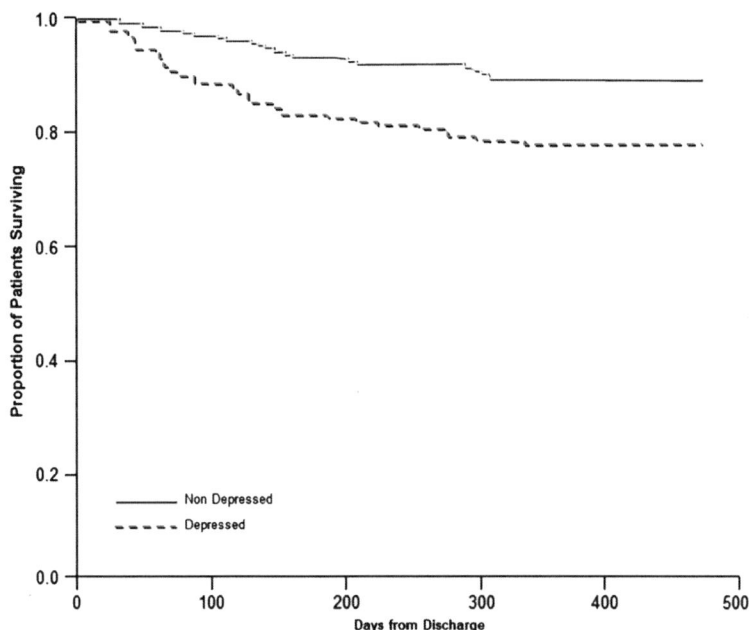

Fig. 13.9 Depressive symptoms and COPD: mortality after discharge by depression status at baseline. Note: the relationship between depression as measured by the Hospital Anxiety Depression Scale (HADS) and mortality in patients with COPD (with permission from Ng et al. [234])

- β-Adrenergic antagonists
- Azapirones

Antidepressants belong to SSRIs, SNRIs, TCAs, MAOIs, NaSSAs, 5HT2 antagonists/serotonin reuptake inhibitors, aminoketones (bupropion), and second generation antipsychotics.

Choosing the most appropriate medication for patients with COPD is influenced by the stage of COPD, the presence of comorbidities, the patient's treatment history, and compatibility with current medications. An assessment of the type of anxiety or depression is also needed, as well as drug tolerability and patient preferences.

Medications used to treat COPD sometimes cause anxiety or adverse effects that resemble anxiety. Such medications include short- and long-acting inhaled β_2-adrenergic agonists, which may cause tremor, nervousness, tachycardia, and palpitations, as well as theophylline and aminophylline, which may cause nausea, vomiting, abdominal cramps, headaches, nervousness, tremor, insomnia, and tachycardia. Corticosteroids may induce depression-like manifestations and mood changes. Therefore, optimization of the pharmacologic treatment of the patient with COPD is important prior to prescribing an antianxiety or antidepression medication.

SSRIs have been used effectively in the treatment of anxiety disorders in COPD patients [243–246], and are the first choice for treating a major depressive disorder in adults [247, 248]. They are tolerable and provide patients and clinicians with the ease of dosing. Considering their efficacy and the ease with which interactions with

Table 13.2 Pharmacologic treatment of anxiety in COPD

First author	Study design	Intervention	Measurement instruments	Results
Argyropoulou [235]	RCT (n = 16)	Buspirone (20 mg) vs. placebo for 2 weeks	Symptom Check List 90-R 6MWD and WRmax	↓Anxiety and depression ↑increased 6MWD and WRmax
Singh [236]	RCT (n = 11)	Buspirone (30–60 mg) vs. placebo for 6 weeks	State-Trait Anxiety Inventory 12MWD and WRmax	No differences in anxiety or exercise capacity
Silvertooth [237]	RCT (n = 19)	Citalopram (20–40 mg) vs. placebo for 12 weeks	Hamilton Anxiety Rating Scale	No between group differences
Borson [238]	RCT (n = 30)	Nortriptyline vs. placebo for 12 weeks	Patient-Rated Anxiety Scale	↓Anxiety

WRmax maximum work-rate, *12MWD* 12-min walking distance, *COPD* chronic obstructive pulmonary disease

Adapted from Hill et al. [5]

Table 13.3 Pharmacological treatment of depression

First author	Study design	Intervention	Measurement instruments	Results
Gordon [239]	RCT (n=6)	Desipramine vs. placebo for 8 weeks	Beck, Zung Self-Rating Scale	↓Depression in both groups
Light [240]	RCT (n=9)	Doxepine vs. placebo for 6 weeks	12MWD, Beck, Trait-State Anxiety Inventory	No impact in either group
Borson [238]	RCT (n=30)	Nortriptyline vs. placebo for 12 weeks	12MWD, PFSS Scale, Hamilton Depression, Patient-Rated Anxiety Scale	↓Anxiety in study group no change in depression
Strom [241]	RCT (n=30)	Protriptyline vs. placebo for 12 weeks	Dyspnea Scale, SIP, Anxiety and Depression: MoodCheck List; HADS	No impact in either group
Lacasse [232]	RCT (n=15)	Paroxetine vs. placebo for 12 weeks	CRQ, Geriatric Depression Scale	CRQ emotion and mastery in study group. No difference in depression scores
Eiser [242]	RCT (n=23)	Paroxetine vs. placebo for 6 weeks	SGRQ, 6MWD, HADS, Beck, Montgomery Depression Scale	No impact in either group

RCT randomized controlled trial, *CRQ* chronic respiratory questionnaire, *SGRQ* St. George's Respiratory Questionnaire, *6MWD* 6-min walking distance, *HADS* Hospital Anxiety and Depression Scale, *SIP* sickness impact profile
Adapted from Hill et al. [5]

other comorbidities such as diabetes, hypertension, CAD, and congestive heart failure (CHF) can be managed, SSRIs are popular for treating anxiety, panic disorders, and major depression in COPD patients.

SNRIs are also possible choices although Venlafaxine is associated with dose-dependent increases in blood pressure and must therefore be used with caution in patients with hypertension [244].

The main side effects of SSRIs are nausea, agitation, insomnia, decreased appetite, and an increased risk of GI bleeding. As SSRIs are substrate inhibitors of cytochrome P450 isoenzymes, their use may increase serum levels of many commonly used drugs such as theophylline, antiepileptics, calcium channel antagonists, macrolide antibiotics, and statins. This means that a complete interaction profile needs to be reviewed.

There is usually a delay in response to SSRIs, which may be accompanied by initial agitation, that may be managed with high potency low dose Benzodiazepines [247, 249], but caution should be exercised in COPD patients since Benzodiazepines may reduce respiratory drive and should only be used in the absence of respiratory depression and if other antianxiety medications are not sufficient to control the condition [246]. Although Benzodiazepines will also induce muscle relaxation, sedation, analgesia, and anxiolysis in patients receiving mechanical ventilation [250], they may impair weaning from the ventilator [251, 252].

TCAs have also been used in the treatment of depression in COPD patients. In a 12 week randomized controlled study of 30 patients, nortriptyline was clearly superior to placebo for the treatment of depression, improving dyspnea, physical comfort, and day-to-day function [238].

Although SSRIs are the preferred treatment for patients with diabetes mellitus and depression [253] or anxiety, in some instances SSRIs (and TCAs) may affect fasting blood glucose (FBG) levels [254–256]. Although in comorbid diabetes mellitus and depression, evidence supports the use of fluoxetine for good glucose control with sertraline as an attractive alternative, in the absence of information on diabetes mellitus and depression in COPD, caution is advised.

As with anxiety, depressed patients prescribed TCAs may also have the metabolic syndrome of obesity and dyslipidemia, such that close monitoring of glycemic control may be required. In one report of 1,217 depressed or anxious subjects and 629 controls, the prevalence of the metabolic syndrome increased with worse symptoms of depression [248]. As the use of TCAs also increases the risk of metabolic syndrome, independently of the severity of the depression, caution should be exercised when COPD patients with the metabolic syndrome are managed with TCA medications.

Argyropoulou et al. reported on a RCT of 16 COPD patients who received either Buspirone 20 mg or placebo for a 2-week period [235]. The authors reported a decrease in anxiety and an increase in 6MWD and maximum exercise capacity among the Buspirone-treated group. Singh et al. reported on an RCT of 11 individuals assigned to Buspirone 30–60 mg vs. placebo over a 6-week period [236]. Outcome measures included the State-Trait Anxiety Inventory, the 12-min walk test distance, and maximum exercise capacity. Unfortunately, no differences were identified in either anxiety or exercise capacity. Silvertooth and colleagues reported that an RCT of Citalopram 20–40 mg daily vs. placebo over a 12-week period did not influence anxiety in either control or treated subjects [237]. Borson et al. noted a reduction in anxiety among patients receiving 12 weeks of nortriptyline vs. controls [238]. This work was recently summarized in a review article [5].

The pharmacologic treatment of depression is limited by the small number of RCTs (Table 13.2). Gordon and colleagues randomized six subjects to receive Desipramine or placebo for 8 weeks and reported a decrease in depression in both groups [239]. Light et al. randomized nine subjects to receive Doxipene or placebo for 6 weeks and reported that depression did not change in either group [240]. Neither Borson et al. [238] nor Strom et al. [241] noted an impact of TCAs on depression in their RCTs, but Lacasse and colleagues [232] in a 12-week RCT of Pyroxene reported a between group difference in the emotional and mastery domains of the Chronic Respiratory Questionnaire. This was in contrast to a 6-week study by Eisner et al. who found no effect of Pyroxene on depression in treated or control subjects [242].

Although psychological comorbidities are frequently present in COPD, reports of pharmacologic management are limited. Cardiovascular comorbidities in COPD have encouraged clinicians to favor SSRIs over TCAs [257] as sertraline in treatment of patients with acute MI or unstable angina has been evaluated to be safe [258]. Imipramine is contraindicated immediately post-myocardial infarction or in the presence of acute CHF. Even when used for a short time to treat depression in patients with heart disease, postural hypotension and prolongation of the QTc interval, arrhythmias, and even heart block must be considered [259]. TCA medications often have the side effect of a dry mouth, which can aggravate the dry mouth associated with use of LAAC in COPD. As the use of short-acting and long-acting β-selective agonists may influence heart rate and rhythm, the dose of TCA used should be modest and increased over time, with periodic ECG monitoring.

Buspirone, a partial 5HT1A-receptor agonist has been used for the treatment of anxiety in patients with COPD with conflicting results [246]. MAOIs are usually avoided in COPD patients because of their adverse effects on comorbid conditions such as diabetes and heart diseases, such as weight gain, changes in cardiac conduction, postural hypotension [253] and the possibility of severe drug interactions. Mirtazapine, which is also an appetite stimulant, may be considered if depressed patients also suffer from anorexia or if dyspnea is severe enough to interfere with eating [244].

Nonselective β-blockers, such as propranolol, which is used in treating a Social Anxiety Disorder especially when there is a specific task-related anxiety, has been avoided in COPD patients with cardiovascular disease because of concerns relating to adverse pulmonary effects. Cardioselective β-blockers are not contraindicated, but their role as anxiolytics needs to be explored.

In addition to pharmacologic approaches, cognitive behavioral therapy (CBT) and exercise should be combined. In fact, exercise, education, and stress management will have an impact on depression even in the absence of pharmacologic management [260, 261], so clinical trials of combined pharmacologic and nonpharmacologic therapy are warranted.

Future and Novel Therapies for COPD

Despite large advances in the understanding of COPD beyond it being a single organ disease, there are still few existing pharmacological therapies that convincingly reduce mortality, in part due to the under-recognition of COPD comorbidities. Increasing knowledge of the molecular mechanisms of inflammation in the pathology of COPD will inform new therapies. There is some evidence that existing therapies may have anti-inflammatory, not just bronchodilator, properties [25, 262]. Interest in anti-inflammatory drugs for COPD is ongoing. One potential therapeutic target are the peroxisome proliferator-activated receptors (PPARs), which are a group of transcription factors that have a key role in energy homeostasis. They have been implicated in systemic inflammation and skeletal muscle dysfunction in COPD [263, 264]. PPAR agonists are available (Rosiglitazone), but further agents are being developed and they may have a role in suppressing airway smooth muscle inflammation [118, 265].

Other anti-inflammatory drugs such as anti-TNFα have been ineffective in COPD overall but there may be certain subgroups who benefit [266]. PDE4 inhibitors such as roflumilast are probably the most advanced of the other anti-inflammatory targets. Despite a small reduction in lung function over one year, there was no reduction in moderate to severe exacerbation rate and the side effect profile was high [267]. A further RCT confirmed these findings, but a subgroup analysis of patients with very severe disease showed a significant reduction in acute exacerbations of COPD (AECOPD) with Roflumilast [268]. The major limitation of this treatment appears to be the side effect profile and further work needs to examine if there is a subgroup of patients that might benefit [269].

Macrolide antibiotics have also received interest over recent years for their anti-inflammatory actions. They reduce proinflammatory cytokines from monocytes and epithelial cells by inhibiting nuclear factor-kappa B (NF-κB) [270]. An RCT of erythromycin vs. placebo for 12 months in COPD demonstrated a reduction in AECOPD in the treated group [271]. Other potential anti-inflammatory agents for COPD, such as glygosaminoglycans (heparin), antioxidants, mitogen-activated protein kinase, and NF-κB inhibitors, have been highlighted in two detailed reviews [272, 273].

COPD is a fascinating condition whose management is made more challenging by the increased awareness of its attendant multiple comorbidities. Pharmacological expertise is very helpful in considering both the impact that medications for comorbidities may have on COPD and the impact that COPD medications may have on one or more comorbid conditions.

References

1. Celli BR, MacNee W. Standards for the diagnosis and treatment of patients with COPD: a summary of the ATS/ERS position paper. Eur Respir J. 2004;23(6):932–46.
2. Maltais F, LeBlanc P, Jobin J, Casaburi R. Peripheral muscle dysfunction in chronic obstructive pulmonary disease. Clin Chest Med. 2000;21(4):665–77.

3. Schols AM. Nutritional and metabolic modulation in chronic obstructive pulmonary disease management. Eur Respir J Suppl. 2003;46:81s–6.

4. Ionescu AA, Schoon E. Osteoporosis in chronic obstructive pulmonary disease. Eur Respir J Suppl. 2003;46:64s–75.

5. Hill K, Geist R, Goldstein RS, Lacasse Y. Anxiety and depression in end-stage COPD. Eur Respir J. 2008;31(3):667–77.

6. Van Vliet M, Spruit MA, Verleden G, Kasran A, Van Herck E, Pitta F, et al. Hypogonadism, quadriceps weakness, and exercise intolerance in chronic obstructive pulmonary disease. Am J Respir Crit Care Med. 2005;172(9):1105–11.

7. Similowski T, Agusti A, MacNee W, Schonhofer B. The potential impact of anaemia of chronic disease in COPD. Eur Respir J. 2006;27(2):390–6.

8. Agusti A, Soriano JB. COPD as a systemic disease. COPD. 2008;5(2):133–8.

9. NICE COPD guidelines. http://guidance.nice.org.uk/CG101. 2010.

10. Mahler DA, Donohue JF, Barbee RA, Goldman MD, Gross NJ, Wisniewski ME, et al. Efficacy of salmeterol xinafoate in the treatment of COPD. Chest. 1999;115(4):957–65.

11. Dahl R, Greefhorst LA, Nowak D, Nonikov V, Byrne AM, Thomson MH, et al. Inhaled formoterol dry powder versus ipratropium bromide in chronic obstructive pulmonary disease. Am J Respir Crit Care Med. 2001;164(5):778–84.

12. Vincken W, Van Noord JA, Greefhorst AP, Bantje TA, Kesten S, Korducki L, et al. Improved health outcomes in patients with COPD during 1 yr's treatment with tiotropium. Eur Respir J. 2002;19(2):209–16.

13. O'Donnell DE, Fluge T, Gerken F, Hamilton A, Webb K, Aguilaniu B, et al. Effects of tiotropium on lung hyperinflation, dyspnoea and exercise tolerance in COPD. Eur Respir J. 2004;23(6):832–40.

14. Di Marco F, Milic-Emili J, Boveri B, Carlucci P, Santus P, Casanova F, et al. Effect of inhaled bronchodilators on inspiratory capacity and dyspnoea at rest in COPD. Eur Respir J. 2003;21(1):86–94.

15. Brouillard C, Pepin V, Milot J, Lacasse Y, Maltais F. Endurance shuttle walking test: responsiveness to salmeterol in COPD. Eur Respir J. 2008;31(3):579–84.

16. Mahler DA. The effect of inhaled beta2-agonists on clinical outcomes in chronic obstructive pulmonary disease. J Allergy Clin Immunol. 2002;110(6 Suppl):S298–303.

17. Tashkin DP, Celli B, Senn S, Burkhart D, Kesten S, Menjoge S, et al. A 4-year trial of tiotropium in chronic obstructive pulmonary disease. N Engl J Med. 2008;359(15):1543–54.

18. Stockley RA, Whitehead PJ, Williams MK. Improved outcomes in patients with chronic obstructive pulmonary disease treated with salmeterol compared with placebo/usual therapy: results of a meta-analysis. Respir Res. 2006;7:147.

19. Niewoehner DE, Rice K, Cote C, Paulson D, Cooper Jr JA, Korducki L, et al. Prevention of exacerbations of chronic obstructive pulmonary disease with tiotropium, a once-daily inhaled anticholinergic bronchodilator: a randomized trial. Ann Intern Med. 2005;143(5):317–26.

20. Rabe KF, Hurd S, Anzueto A, Barnes PJ, Buist SA, Calverley P, et al. Global strategy for the diagnosis, management, and prevention of chronic obstructive pulmonary disease: GOLD executive summary. Am J Respir Crit Care Med. 2007;176(6):532–55.

21. Yoshimura T, Kurita C, Nagao T, Usami E, Nakao T, Watanabe S, et al. Inhibition of tumor necrosis factor-alpha and interleukin-1-beta production by beta-adrenoceptor agonists from lipopolysaccharide-stimulated human peripheral blood mononuclear cells. Pharmacology. 1997;54(3):144–52.

22. Barnes PJ. Effect of beta-agonists on inflammatory cells. J Allergy Clin Immunol. 1999;104(2 Pt 2):S10–7.

23. Bourbeau J, Christodoulopoulos P, Maltais F, Yamauchi Y, Olivenstein R, Hamid Q. Effect of salmeterol/fluticasone propionate on airway inflammation in COPD: a randomised controlled trial. Thorax. 2007;62(11):938–43.

24. Grando SA, Kawashima K, Kirkpatrick CJ, Wessler I. Recent progress in understanding the non-neuronal cholinergic system in humans. Life Sci. 2007;80(24–25):2181–5.

25. Bateman ED, Rennard S, Barnes PJ, Dicpinigaitis PV, Gosens R, Gross NJ, et al. Alternative mechanisms for tiotropium. Pulm Pharmacol Ther. 2009;22(6):533–42.

26. Powrie DJ, Wilkinson TM, Donaldson GC, Jones P, Scrine K, Viel K, et al. Effect of tiotropium on sputum and serum inflammatory markers and exacerbations in COPD. Eur Respir J. 2007;30(3):472–8.

27. Rajab P, Fox J, Riaz S, Tomlinson D, Ball D, Greenhaff PL. Skeletal muscle myosin heavy chain isoforms and energy metabolism after clenbuterol treatment in the rat. Am J Physiol Regul Integr Comp Physiol. 2000;279(3):R1076–81.

28. Koopman R, Ryall JG, Church JE, Lynch GS. The role of beta-adrenoceptor signaling in skeletal muscle: therapeutic implications for muscle wasting disorders. Curr Opin Clin Nutr Metab Care. 2009;12(6):601–6.

29. Yang IA, Fong KM, Sim EH, Black PN, Lasserson TJ. Inhaled corticosteroids for stable chronic obstructive pulmonary disease. Cochrane Database Syst Rev 2007;(2):CD002991.

30. Soriano JB, Sin DD, Zhang X, Camp PG, Anderson JA, Anthonisen NR, et al. A pooled analysis of FEV_1 decline in COPD patients randomized to inhaled corticosteroids or placebo. Chest. 2007;131(3):682–9.

31. Calverley PM, Anderson JA, Celli B, Ferguson GT, Jenkins C, Jones PW, et al. Salmeterol and fluticasone propionate and survival in chronic obstructive pulmonary disease. N Engl J Med. 2007;356(8):775–89.

32. Nannini LJ, Cates CJ, Lasserson TJ, Poole P. Combined corticosteroid and long-acting beta-agonist in one inhaler versus inhaled steroids for chronic obstructive pulmonary disease. Cochrane Database Syst Rev 2007;(4):CD006826.

33. Nannini L, Cates CJ, Lasserson TJ, Poole P. Combined corticosteroid and long-acting beta-agonist in one inhaler versus placebo for chronic obstructive pulmonary disease. Cochrane Database Syst Rev 2007;(4):CD003794.

34. Calverley PM, Boonsawat W, Cseke Z, Zhong N, Peterson S, Olsson H. Maintenance therapy with budesonide and formoterol in chronic obstructive pulmonary disease. Eur Respir J. 2003;22(6):912–9.

35. Barnes PJ. Scientific rationale for inhaled combination therapy with long-acting beta2-agonists and corticosteroids. Eur Respir J. 2002;19(1):182–91.

36. Sin DD, Man SF, Marciniuk DD, Ford G, FitzGerald M, Wong E, et al. The effects of fluticasone with or without salmeterol on systemic biomarkers of inflammation in chronic obstructive pulmonary disease. Am J Respir Crit Care Med. 2008;177(11):1207–14.

37. Singh S, Loke YK. Risk of pneumonia associated with long-term use of inhaled corticosteroids in chronic obstructive pulmonary disease: a critical review and update. Curr Opin Pulm Med. 2010;16(2):118–22.

38. Celli BR, Thomas NE, Anderson JA, Ferguson GT, Jenkins CR, Jones PW, et al. Effect of pharmacotherapy on rate of decline of lung function in chronic obstructive pulmonary disease: results from the TORCH study. Am J Respir Crit Care Med. 2008;178(4):332–8.

39. Celli B, Decramer M, Kesten S, Liu D, Mehra S, Tashkin DP. Mortality in the 4-year trial of tiotropium (UPLIFT) in patients with chronic obstructive pulmonary disease. Am J Respir Crit Care Med. 2009;180(10):948–55.

40. Decramer M, Celli B, Kesten S, Lystig T, Mehra S, Tashkin DP. Effect of tiotropium on outcomes in patients with moderate chronic obstructive pulmonary disease (UPLIFT): a prespecified subgroup analysis of a randomised controlled trial. Lancet. 2009;374(9696):1171–8.

41. GOLD guidelines updated 2009. http://www.goldcopd.com/GuidelinesResources.asp?l1=2&l2=0. 2010.

42. Culpitt SV, de Matos C, Russell RE, Donnelly LE, Rogers DF, Barnes PJ. Effect of theophylline on induced sputum inflammatory indices and neutrophil chemotaxis in chronic obstructive pulmonary disease. Am J Respir Crit Care Med. 2002;165(10):1371–6.

43. Barnes PJ. Theophylline in chronic obstructive pulmonary disease: new horizons. Proc Am Thorac Soc. 2005;2(4):334–9.

44. Cosio BG, Iglesias A, Rios A, Noguera A, Sala E, Ito K, et al. Low-dose theophylline enhances the anti-inflammatory effects of steroids during exacerbations of COPD. Thorax. 2009;64(5):424–9.

45. Aaron SD, Vandemheen KL, Fergusson D, Maltais F, Bourbeau J, Goldstein R, et al. Tiotropium in combination with placebo, salmeterol, or fluticasone-salmeterol for treatment of chronic obstructive pulmonary disease: a randomized trial. Ann Intern Med. 2007;146(8):545–55.
46. Welte T, Miravitlles M, Hernandez P, Eriksson G, Peterson S, Polanowski T, et al. Efficacy and tolerability of budesonide/formoterol added to tiotropium in patients with chronic obstructive pulmonary disease. Am J Respir Crit Care Med. 2009;180(8):741–50.
47. Topsakal R, Kalay N, Ozdogru I, Cetinkaya Y, Oymak S, Kaya MG, et al. Effects of chronic obstructive pulmonary disease on coronary atherosclerosis. Heart Vessels. 2009;24(3):164–8.
48. Hawkins NM, Jhund PS, Simpson CR, Petrie MC, Macdonald MR, Dunn FG, et al. Primary care burden and treatment of patients with heart failure and chronic obstructive pulmonary disease in Scotland. Eur J Heart Fail. 2010;12(1):17–24.
49. Rutten FH, Moons KG, Cramer MJ, Grobbee DE, Zuithoff NP, Lammers JW, et al. Recognising heart failure in elderly patients with stable chronic obstructive pulmonary disease in primary care: cross sectional diagnostic study. BMJ. 2005;331(7529):1379.
50. Mascarenhas J, Lourenco P, Lopes R, Azevedo A, Bettencourt P. Chronic obstructive pulmonary disease in heart failure. Prevalence, therapeutic and prognostic implications. Am Heart J. 2008;155(3):521–5.
51. Curkendall SM, DeLuise C, Jones JK, Lanes S, Stang MR, Goehring Jr E, et al. Cardiovascular disease in patients with chronic obstructive pulmonary disease, Saskatchewan Canada cardiovascular disease in COPD patients. Ann Epidemiol. 2006;16(1):63–70.
52. Lavie CJ, Milani RV, Verma A, O'Keefe JH. C-reactive protein and cardiovascular diseases – is it ready for primetime? Am J Med Sci. 2009;338(6):486–92.
53. Willerson JT. Systemic and local inflammation in patients with unstable atherosclerotic plaques. Prog Cardiovasc Dis. 2002;44(6):469–78.
54. Wisniacki N, Taylor W, Lye M, Wilding JP. Insulin resistance and inflammatory activation in older patients with systolic and diastolic heart failure. Heart. 2005;91(1):32–7.
55. Torre-Amione G. Immune activation in chronic heart failure. Am J Cardiol. 2005;95(11A): 3C–8.
56. Garcia-Rio F, Miravitlles M, Soriano JB, Munoz L, Duran-Tauleria E, Sanchez G, et al. Systemic inflammation in chronic obstructive pulmonary disease: a population-based study. Respir Res. 2010;11(1):63.
57. Higashimoto Y, Iwata T, Okada M, Satoh H, Fukuda K, Tohda Y. Serum biomarkers as predictors of lung function decline in chronic obstructive pulmonary disease. Respir Med. 2009;103(8):1231–8.
58. Sin DD, Man SF. Why are patients with chronic obstructive pulmonary disease at increased risk of cardiovascular diseases? The potential role of systemic inflammation in chronic obstructive pulmonary disease. Circulation. 2003;107(11):1514–9.
59. Hole DJ, Watt GC, Davey-Smith G, Hart CL, Gillis CR, Hawthorne VM. Impaired lung function and mortality risk in men and women: findings from the Renfrew and Paisley prospective population study. BMJ. 1996;313(7059):711–5.
60. Sin DD, Man SF. Chronic obstructive pulmonary disease as a risk factor for cardiovascular morbidity and mortality. Proc Am Thorac Soc. 2005;2(1):8–11.
61. Boudestein LC, Rutten FH, Cramer MJ, Lammers JW, Hoes AW. The impact of concurrent heart failure on prognosis in patients with chronic obstructive pulmonary disease. Eur J Heart Fail. 2009;11(12):1182–8.
62. De Blois J, Simard S, Atar D, Agewall S. COPD predicts mortality in HF: the Norwegian Heart Failure Registry. J Card Fail. 2010;16(3):225–9.
63. Macchia A, Monte S, Romero M, D'Ettorre A, Tognoni G. The prognostic influence of chronic obstructive pulmonary disease in patients hospitalised for chronic heart failure. Eur J Heart Fail. 2007;9(9):942–8.
64. Dunlay SM, Redfield MM, Weston SA, Therneau TM, Hall LK, Shah ND, et al. Hospitalizations after heart failure diagnosis a community perspective. J Am Coll Cardiol. 2009;54(18): 1695–702.

65. Staszewsky L, Wong M, Masson S, Barlera S, Carretta E, Maggioni AP, et al. Clinical, neurohormonal, and inflammatory markers and overall prognostic role of chronic obstructive pulmonary disease in patients with heart failure: data from the Val-HeFT heart failure trial. J Card Fail. 2007;13(10):797–804.

66. Sirak TE, Jelic S, Le Jemtel TH. Therapeutic update: non-selective beta- and alpha-adrenergic blockade in patients with coexistent chronic obstructive pulmonary disease and chronic heart failure. J Am Coll Cardiol. 2004;44(3):497–502.

67. Le Jemtel TH, Padeletti M, Jelic S. Diagnostic and therapeutic challenges in patients with coexistent chronic obstructive pulmonary disease and chronic heart failure. J Am Coll Cardiol. 2007;49(2):171–80.

68. Carstairs JR, Nimmo AJ, Barnes PJ. Autoradiographic visualization of beta-adrenoceptor subtypes in human lung. Am Rev Respir Dis. 1985;132(3):541–7.

69. Bristow MR, Ginsburg R, Umans V, Fowler M, Minobe W, Rasmussen R, et al. Beta 1- and beta 2-adrenergic-receptor subpopulations in nonfailing and failing human ventricular myocardium: coupling of both receptor subtypes to muscle contraction and selective beta 1-receptor down-regulation in heart failure. Circ Res. 1986;59(3):297–309.

70. Brodde OE. Beta-1 and beta-2 adrenoceptor polymorphisms: functional importance, impact on cardiovascular diseases and drug responses. Pharmacol Ther. 2008;117(1):1–29.

71. Nguyen LP, Omoluabi O, Parra S, Frieske JM, Clement C, Ammar-Aouchiche Z, et al. Chronic exposure to beta-blockers attenuates inflammation and mucin content in a murine asthma model. Am J Respir Cell Mol Biol. 2008;38(3):256–62.

72. Currie GP, Lee DK, Lipworth BJ. Long-acting beta2-agonists in asthma: not so SMART? Drug Saf. 2006;29(8):647–56.

73. Wijesinghe M, Perrin K, Harwood M, Weatherall M, Beasley R. The risk of asthma mortality with inhaled long acting beta-agonists. Postgrad Med J. 2008;84(995):467–72.

74. Liao MM, Ginde AA, Clark S, Camargo Jr CA. Salmeterol use and risk of hospitalization among emergency department patients with acute asthma. Ann Allergy Asthma Immunol. 2010;104(6):478–84.

75. Weatherall M, Wijesinghe M, Perrin K, Harwood M, Beasley R. Meta-analysis of the risk of mortality with salmeterol and the effect of concomitant inhaled corticosteroid therapy. Thorax. 2010;65(1):39–43.

76. Taylor DR. Pharmacogenetics of beta2-agonist drugs in asthma. Clin Rev Allergy Immunol. 2006;31(2–3):247–58.

77. Sandilands A, Yeo G, Brown MJ, O'Shaughnessy KM. Functional responses of human beta1 adrenoceptors with defined haplotypes for the common 389R>G and 49S>G polymorphisms. Pharmacogenetics. 2004;14(6):343–9.

78. Kaye DM, Smirk B, Williams C, Jennings G, Esler M, Holst D. Beta-adrenoceptor genotype influences the response to carvedilol in patients with congestive heart failure. Pharmacogenetics. 2003;13(7):379–82.

79. Au DH, Curtis JR, Every NR, McDonell MB, Fihn SD. Association between inhaled beta-agonists and the risk of unstable angina and myocardial infarction. Chest. 2002;121(3):846–51.

80. Macie C, Wooldrage K, Manfreda J, Anthonisen N. Cardiovascular morbidity and the use of inhaled bronchodilators. Int J Chron Obstruct Pulmon Dis. 2008;3(1):163–9.

81. Anthonisen NR, Connett JE, Enright PL, Manfreda J. Hospitalizations and mortality in the Lung Health Study. Am J Respir Crit Care Med. 2002;166(3):333–9.

82. Lee TA, Pickard AS, Au DH, Bartle B, Weiss KB. Risk for death associated with medications for recently diagnosed chronic obstructive pulmonary disease. Ann Intern Med. 2008;149(6):380–90.

83. Ogale SS, Lee TA, Au DH, Boudreau DM, Sullivan SD. Cardiovascular events associated with ipratropium bromide in COPD. Chest. 2010;137(1):13–9.

84. Singh S, Loke YK, Furberg CD. Inhaled anticholinergics and risk of major adverse cardiovascular events in patients with chronic obstructive pulmonary disease: a systematic review and meta-analysis. JAMA. 2008;300(12):1439–50.

85. Wedzicha JA, Calverley PM, Seemungal TA, Hagan G, Ansari Z, Stockley RA. The prevention of chronic obstructive pulmonary disease exacerbations by salmeterol/fluticasone propionate or tiotropium bromide. Am J Respir Crit Care Med. 2008;177(1):19–26.

86. Rodrigo GJ, Castro-Rodriguez JA, Nannini LJ, Plaza MV, Schiavi EA. Tiotropium and risk for fatal and nonfatal cardiovascular events in patients with chronic obstructive pulmonary disease: systematic review with meta-analysis. Respir Med. 2009;103(10):1421–9.

87. Hilleman DE, Malesker MA, Morrow LE, Schuller D. A systematic review of the cardiovascular risk of inhaled anticholinergics in patients with COPD. Int J Chron Obstruct Pulmon Dis. 2009;4:253–63.

88. Grosso A, Douglas I, Hingorani AD, MacAllister R, Hubbard R, Smeeth L. Inhaled tiotropium bromide and risk of stroke. Br J Clin Pharmacol. 2009;68(5):731–6.

89. Celli B, Decramer M, Leimer I, Vogel U, Kesten S, Tashkin DP. Cardiovascular safety of tiotropium in patients with COPD. Chest. 2010;137(1):20–30.

90. Macie C, Wooldrage K, Manfreda J, Anthonisen NR. Inhaled corticosteroids and mortality in COPD. Chest. 2006;130(3):640–6.

91. Sin DD, Wu L, Anderson JA, Anthonisen NR, Buist AS, Burge PS, et al. Inhaled corticosteroids and mortality in chronic obstructive pulmonary disease. Thorax. 2005;60(12):992–7.

92. Huiart L, Ernst P, Ranouil X, Suissa S. Low-dose inhaled corticosteroids and the risk of acute myocardial infarction in COPD. Eur Respir J. 2005;25(4):634–9.

93. Qing F, Rahman SU, Hayes MJ, Rhodes CG, Ind PW, Jones T, et al. Effect of long-term beta2-agonist dosing on human cardiac beta-adrenoceptor expression in vivo: comparison with changes in lung and mononuclear leukocyte beta-receptors. J Nucl Cardiol. 1997;4(6):532–8.

94. Bristow MR, Ginsburg R, Minobe W, Cubicciotti RS, Sageman WS, Lurie K, et al. Decreased catecholamine sensitivity and beta-adrenergic-receptor density in failing human hearts. N Engl J Med. 1982;307(4):205–11.

95. Hunt SA, Abraham WT, Chin MH, Feldman AM, Francis GS, Ganiats TG, et al. 2009 focused update incorporated into the ACC/AHA 2005 Guidelines for the Diagnosis and Management of Heart Failure in Adults: a report of the American College of Cardiology Foundation/American Heart Association Task Force on Practice Guidelines: developed in collaboration with the International Society for Heart and Lung Transplantation. Circulation. 2009;119(14): e391–479.

96. Dickstein K, Cohen-Solal A, Filippatos G, McMurray JJ, Ponikowski P, Poole-Wilson PA, et al. ESC guidelines for the diagnosis and treatment of acute and chronic heart failure 2008: the Task Force for the diagnosis and treatment of acute and chronic heart failure 2008 of the European Society of Cardiology. Developed in collaboration with the Heart Failure Association of the ESC (HFA) and endorsed by the European Society of Intensive Care Medicine (ESICM). Eur Heart J. 2008;29(19):2388–442.

97. Hawkins NM, Wang D, Petrie MC, Pfeffer MA, Swedberg K, Granger CB, et al. Baseline characteristics and outcomes of patients with heart failure receiving bronchodilators in the CHARM programme. Eur J Heart Fail. 2010;12(6):557–65.

98. Au DH, Udris EM, Fan VS, Curtis JR, McDonell MB, Fihn SD. Risk of mortality and heart failure exacerbations associated with inhaled beta-adrenoceptor agonists among patients with known left ventricular systolic dysfunction. Chest. 2003;123(6):1964–9.

99. Cruickshank JM, McAinsh J. Atenolol and ischaemic heart disease: an overview. Curr Med Res Opin. 1991;12(8):485–96.

100. Leren P. Ischaemic heart disease: how well are the risk profiles modulated by current beta blockers? Cardiology. 1993;82 Suppl 3:8–12.

101. Hjalmarson A, Goldstein S, Fagerberg B, Wedel H, Waagstein F, Kjekshus J, et al. Effects of controlled-release metoprolol on total mortality, hospitalizations, and well-being in patients with heart failure: the Metoprolol CR/XL Randomized Intervention Trial in congestive heart failure (MERIT-HF). MERIT-HF Study Group. JAMA. 2000;283(10):1295–302.

102. Eichhorn EJ, Bristow MR. The carvedilol prospective randomized cumulative survival (COPERNICUS) trial. Curr Control Trials Cardiovasc Med. 2001;2(1):20–3.

103. The Cardiac Insufficiency Bisoprolol Study II(CIBIS-II): a randomised trial. Lancet 1999; 353(9146):9–13.
104. Tattersfield AE. Beta adrenoceptor antagonists and respiratory disease. J Cardiovasc Pharmacol. 1986;8 Suppl 4:S35–9.
105. Fogari R, Zoppi A, Tettamanti F, Poletti L, Rizzardi G, Fiocchi G. Comparative effects of celiprolol, propranolol, oxprenolol, and atenolol on respiratory function in hypertensive patients with chronic obstructive lung disease. Cardiovasc Drugs Ther. 1990;4(4):1145–9.
106. Dorow P, Bethge H, Tonnesmann U. Effects of single oral doses of bisoprolol and atenolol on airway function in nonasthmatic chronic obstructive lung disease and angina pectoris. Eur J Clin Pharmacol. 1986;31(2):143–7.
107. Salpeter S, Ormiston T, Salpeter E. Cardioselective beta-blockers for chronic obstructive pulmonary disease. Cochrane Database Syst Rev 2005;(4):CD003566.
108. Salpeter S, Ormiston T, Salpeter E. Cardioselective beta-blockers for reversible airway disease. Cochrane Database Syst Rev 2002;(4):CD002992.
109. Olenchock BA, Fonarow GG, Pan W, Hernandez A, Cannon CP. Current use of beta blockers in patients with reactive airway disease who are hospitalized with acute coronary syndromes. Am J Cardiol. 2009;103(3):295–300.
110. Matera MG, Martuscelli E, Cazzola M. Pharmacological modulation of beta-adrenoceptor function in patients with coexisting chronic obstructive pulmonary disease and chronic heart failure. Pulm Pharmacol Ther. 2010;23(1):1–8.
111. Jabbour A, Macdonald PS, Keogh AM, Kotlyar E, Mellemkjaer S, Coleman CF, et al. Differences between beta-blockers in patients with chronic heart failure and chronic obstructive pulmonary disease: a randomized crossover trial. J Am Coll Cardiol. 2010;55(17):1780–7.
112. Rutten FH, Zuithoff NP, Hak E, Grobbee DE, Hoes AW. Beta-blockers may reduce mortality and risk of exacerbations in patients with chronic obstructive pulmonary disease. Arch Intern Med. 2010;170(10):880–7.
113. Andreas S, Anker SD, Scanlon PD, Somers VK. Neurohumoral activation as a link to systemic manifestations of chronic lung disease. Chest. 2005;128(5):3618–24.
114. Leuchte HH, Baumgartner RA, Nounou ME, Vogeser M, Neurohr C, Trautnitz M, et al. Brain natriuretic peptide is a prognostic parameter in chronic lung disease. Am J Respir Crit Care Med. 2006;173(7):744–50.
115. Callaerts-Vegh Z, Evans KL, Dudekula N, Cuba D, Knoll BJ, Callaerts PF, et al. Effects of acute and chronic administration of beta-adrenoceptor ligands on airway function in a murine model of asthma. Proc Natl Acad Sci USA. 2004;101(14):4948–53.
116. Cazzola M, Matera MG. Beta-blockers are safe in patients with chronic obstructive pulmonary disease, but only with caution. Am J Respir Crit Care Med. 2008;178(7):661–2.
117. Mancini GB, Etminan M, Zhang B, Levesque LE, FitzGerald JM, Brophy JM. Reduction of morbidity and mortality by statins, angiotensin-converting enzyme inhibitors, and angiotensin receptor blockers in patients with chronic obstructive pulmonary disease. J Am Coll Cardiol. 2006;47(12):2554–60.
118. Barnes PJ, Celli BR. Systemic manifestations and comorbidities of COPD. Eur Respir J. 2009;33(5):1165–85.
119. Soyseth V, Brekke PH, Smith P, Omland T. Statin use is associated with reduced mortality in COPD. Eur Respir J. 2007;29(2):279–83.
120. Jessup M, Abraham WT, Casey DE, Feldman AM, Francis GS, Ganiats TG, et al. 2009 focused update: ACCF/AHA Guidelines for the Diagnosis and Management of Heart Failure in Adults: a report of the American College of Cardiology Foundation/American Heart Association Task Force on Practice Guidelines: developed in collaboration with the International Society for Heart and Lung Transplantation. Circulation. 2009;119(14):1977–2016.
121. Anker SD, Negassa A, Coats AJ, Afzal R, Poole-Wilson PA, Cohn JN, et al. Prognostic importance of weight loss in chronic heart failure and the effect of treatment with angiotensin-converting-enzyme inhibitors: an observational study. Lancet. 2003;361(9363):1077–83.
122. Springer J, Filippatos G, Akashi YJ, Anker SD. Prognosis and therapy approaches of cardiac cachexia. Curr Opin Cardiol. 2006;21(3):229–33.

123. Song YH, Li Y, Du J, Mitch WE, Rosenthal N, Delafontaine P. Muscle-specific expression of IGF-1 blocks angiotensin II-induced skeletal muscle wasting. J Clin Invest. 2005;115(2): 451–8.

124. Mancini GB. Clarion call for trials assessing "cardiopulmonary" agents to reduce morbidity and mortality in inflammatory lung diseases. Chest. 2007;131(4):950–1.

125. WHO Scientific Group on the Prevention and Management of Osteoporosis. Prevention and management of osteoporosis: report of a WHO scientific group. Geneva: World Health Organisation; 2000.

126. Consensus development conference: diagnosis, prophylaxis, and treatment of osteoporosis. Am J Med 1993; 94(6):646–50

127. Melton III LJ. Who has osteoporosis? A conflict between clinical and public health perspectives. J Bone Miner Res. 2000;15(12):2309–14.

128. LaVelle DG. Fractures and dislocations of the hip. In: Canale ST, Beaty JH, editors. Campbell's Operative Orthopaedics. Philadelphia, PA: Mosby Elsevier; 2008. p. 3237–308.

129. Nevitt MC, Ettinger B, Black DM, Stone K, Jamal SA, Ensrud K, et al. The association of radiographically detected vertebral fractures with back pain and function: a prospective study. Ann Intern Med. 1998;128(10):793–800.

130. Schlaich C, Minne HW, Bruckner T, Wagner G, Gebest HJ, Grunze M, et al. Reduced pulmonary function in patients with spinal osteoporotic fractures. Osteoporos Int. 1998;8(3):261–7.

131. Cummings SR, Bates D, Black DM. Clinical use of bone densitometry: scientific review. JAMA. 2002;288(15):1889–97.

132. Graat-Verboom L, Wouters EF, Smeenk FW, van den Borne BE, Lunde R, Spruit MA. Current status of research on osteoporosis in COPD: a systematic review. Eur Respir J. 2009;34(1): 209–18.

133. Biskobing DM. COPD and osteoporosis. Chest. 2002;121(2):609–20.

134. Kanis JA, Johnell O, Oden A, Johansson H, McCloskey E. FRAX and the assessment of fracture probability in men and women from the UK. Osteoporos Int. 2008;19(4):385–97.

135. National Osteoporosis Foundation. Clinician's guide to prevention and treatment of osteoporosis. Washington, DC: National Osteoporosis Foundation; 2010.

136. Yanbaeva DG, Dentener MA, Creutzberg EC, Wesseling G, Wouters EF. Systemic effects of smoking. Chest. 2007;131(5):1557–66.

137. Bauer DC, Browner WS, Cauley JA, Orwoll ES, Scott JC, Black DM, et al. Factors associated with appendicular bone mass in older women. The Study of Osteoporotic Fractures Research Group. Ann Intern Med. 1993;118(9):657–65.

138. Hollenbach KA, Barrett-Connor E, Edelstein SL, Holbrook T. Cigarette smoking and bone mineral density in older men and women. Am J Public Health. 1993;83(9):1265–70.

139. Oncken C, Prestwood K, Kleppinger A, Wang Y, Cooney J, Raisz L. Impact of smoking cessation on bone mineral density in postmenopausal women. J Womens Health (Larchmt). 2006;15(10):1141–50.

140. Cornuz J, Feskanich D, Willett WC, Colditz GA. Smoking, smoking cessation, and risk of hip fracture in women. Am J Med. 1999;106(3):311–4.

141. Ries AL, Bauldoff GS, Carlin BW, Casaburi R, Emery CF, Mahler DA, et al. Pulmonary rehabilitation: joint ACCP/AACVPR evidence-based clinical practice guidelines. Chest. 2007;131(5 Suppl):4S–2.

142. Gillespie LD, Robertson MC, Gillespie WJ, Lamb SE, Gates S, Cumming RG et al. Interventions for preventing falls in older people living in the community. Cochrane Database Syst Rev 2009;(2):CD007146.

143. Feskanich D, Willett W, Colditz G. Walking and leisure-time activity and risk of hip fracture in postmenopausal women. JAMA. 2002;288(18):2300–6.

144. Braith RW, Conner JA, Fulton MN, Lisor CF, Casey DP, Howe KS, et al. Comparison of alendronate vs alendronate plus mechanical loading as prophylaxis for osteoporosis in lung transplant recipients: a pilot study. J Heart Lung Transplant. 2007;26(2):132–7.

145. Mitchell MJ, Baz MA, Fulton MN, Lisor CF, Braith RW. Resistance training prevents vertebral osteoporosis in lung transplant recipients. Transplantation. 2003;76(3):557–62.

146. Wang WQ, Ip MS, Tsang KW, Lam KS. Antiresorptive therapy in asthmatic patients receiving high-dose inhaled steroids: a prospective study for 18 months. J Allergy Clin Immunol. 1998;101(4 Pt 1):445–50.

147. Reid DM, Nicoll JJ, Smith MA, Higgins B, Tothill P, Nuki G. Corticosteroids and bone mass in asthma: comparisons with rheumatoid arthritis and polymyalgia rheumatica. Br Med J (Clin Res Ed). 1986;293(6560):1463–6.

148. Kanis JA, Johansson H, Oden A, Johnell O, de Laet C, Melton III LJ, et al. A meta-analysis of prior corticosteroid use and fracture risk. J Bone Miner Res. 2004;19(6):893–9.

149. Saag KG, Emkey R, Schnitzer TJ, Brown JP, Hawkins F, Goemaere S, et al. Alendronate for the prevention and treatment of glucocorticoid-induced osteoporosis. Glucocorticoid-Induced Osteoporosis Intervention Study Group. N Engl J Med. 1998;339(5):292–9.

150. Shane E, Rivas M, McMahon DJ, Staron RB, Silverberg SJ, Seibel MJ, et al. Bone loss and turnover after cardiac transplantation. J Clin Endocrinol Metab. 1997;82(5):1497–506.

151. Reid IR, Heap SW. Determinants of vertebral mineral density in patients receiving long-term glucocorticoid therapy. Arch Intern Med. 1990;150(12):2545–8.

152. Brown JP, Josse RG. 2002 clinical practice guidelines for the diagnosis and management of osteoporosis in Canada. CMAJ. 2002;167(10 Suppl):S1–34.

153. Recommendations for the prevention and treatment of glucocorticoid-induced osteoporosis: 2001 update. American College of Rheumatology Ad Hoc Committee on Glucocorticoid-Induced Osteoporosis. Arthritis Rheum 2001; 44(7):1496–503.

154. Frediani B, Falsetti P, Bisogno S, Baldi F, Acciai C, Filippou G, et al. Effects of high dose methylprednisolone pulse therapy on bone mass and biochemical markers of bone metabolism in patients with active rheumatoid arthritis: a 12-month randomized prospective controlled study. J Rheumatol. 2004;31(6):1083–7.

155. Van Staa TP, Leufkens HG, Abenhaim L, Zhang B, Cooper C. Use of oral corticosteroids and risk of fractures. J Bone Miner Res. 2000;15(6):993–1000.

156. Hubbard R, Tattersfield A, Smith C, West J, Smeeth L, Fletcher A. Use of inhaled corticosteroids and the risk of fracture. Chest. 2006;130(4):1082–8.

157. Lee TA, Weiss KB. Fracture risk associated with inhaled corticosteroid use in chronic obstructive pulmonary disease. Am J Respir Crit Care Med. 2004;169(7):855–9.

158. Suissa S, Baltzan M, Kremer R, Ernst P. Inhaled and nasal corticosteroid use and the risk of fracture. Am J Respir Crit Care Med. 2004;169(1):83–8.

159. Scanlon PD, Connett JE, Wise RA, Tashkin DP, Madhok T, Skeans M, et al. Loss of bone density with inhaled triamcinolone in Lung Health Study II. Am J Respir Crit Care Med. 2004;170(12):1302–9.

160. Lung Health Study Research Group. Effect of inhaled triamcinolone on the decline in pulmonary function in chronic obstructive pulmonary disease. N Engl J Med. 2000;343(26): 1902–9.

161. Ferguson GT, Calverley PM, Anderson JA, Jenkins CR, Jones PW, Willits LR, et al. Prevalence and progression of osteoporosis in patients with COPD: results from the TOwards a Revolution in COPD Health study. Chest. 2009;136(6):1456–65.

162. de Vries F, Pouwels S, Lammers JW, Leufkens HG, Bracke M, Cooper C, et al. Use of inhaled and oral glucocorticoids, severity of inflammatory disease and risk of hip/femur fracture: a population-based case-control study. J Intern Med. 2007;261(2):170–7.

163. Johannes CB, Schneider GA, Dube TJ, Alfredson TD, Davis KJ, Walker AM. The risk of nonvertebral fracture related to inhaled corticosteroid exposure among adults with chronic respiratory disease. Chest. 2005;127(1):89–97.

164. Pauwels RA, Lofdahl CG, Laitinen LA, Schouten JP, Postma DS, Pride NB, et al. Long-term treatment with inhaled budesonide in persons with mild chronic obstructive pulmonary disease who continue smoking. European Respiratory Society Study on Chronic Obstructive Pulmonary Disease. N Engl J Med. 1999;340(25):1948–53.

165. Heaney RP, Recker RR, Saville PD. Menopausal changes in calcium balance performance. J Lab Clin Med. 1978;92(6):953–63.

166. Ensrud KE, Taylor BC, Paudel ML, Cauley JA, Cawthon PM, Cummings SR, et al. Serum 25-hydroxyvitamin D levels and rate of hip bone loss in older men. J Clin Endocrinol Metab. 2009;94(8):2773–80.
167. Cauley JA, Lacroix AZ, Wu L, Horwitz M, Danielson ME, Bauer DC, et al. Serum 25-hydroxyvitamin D concentrations and risk for hip fractures. Ann Intern Med. 2008;149(4): 242–50.
168. Bischoff-Ferrari HA, Dietrich T, Orav EJ, Dawson-Hughes B. Positive association between 25-hydroxy vitamin D levels and bone mineral density: a population-based study of younger and older adults. Am J Med. 2004;116(9):634–9.
169. Pasco JA, Henry MJ, Kotowicz MA, Sanders KM, Seeman E, Pasco JR, et al. Seasonal periodicity of serum vitamin D and parathyroid hormone, bone resorption, and fractures: the Geelong Osteoporosis Study. J Bone Miner Res. 2004;19(5):752–8.
170. Avenell A, Gillespie WJ, Gillespie LD, O'Connell D. Vitamin D and vitamin D analogues for preventing fractures associated with involutional and post-menopausal osteoporosis. Cochrane Database Syst Rev 2009;(2):CD000227.
171. Buckley LM, Leib ES, Cartularo KS, Vacek PM, Cooper SM. Calcium and vitamin D3 supplementation prevents bone loss in the spine secondary to low-dose corticosteroids in patients with rheumatoid arthritis. A randomized, double-blind, placebo-controlled trial. Ann Intern Med. 1996;125(12):961–8.
172. Sambrook P, Birmingham J, Kelly P, Kempler S, Nguyen T, Pocock N, et al. Prevention of corticosteroid osteoporosis. A comparison of calcium, calcitriol, and calcitonin. N Engl J Med. 1993;328(24):1747–52.
173. Friedman PA. Agents affecting mineral ion homeostasis and bone turnover. In: Brunton LL, Lazo JS, Parker KL, editors. Goodman and Gilman's the pharmacological basis of therapeutics. New York, NY: McGraw-Hill; 2006. p. 1647–78.
174. Black DM, Cummings SR, Karpf DB, Cauley JA, Thompson DE, Nevitt MC, et al. Randomised trial of effect of alendronate on risk of fracture in women with existing vertebral fractures. Fracture Intervention Trial Research Group. Lancet. 1996;348(9041): 1535–41.
175. Harris ST, Watts NB, Genant HK, McKeever CD, Hangartner T, Keller M, et al. Effects of risedronate treatment on vertebral and nonvertebral fractures in women with postmenopausal osteoporosis: a randomized controlled trial. Vertebral Efficacy With Risedronate Therapy (VERT) Study Group. JAMA. 1999;282(14):1344–52.
176. Wells G, Cranney A, Peterson J, Boucher M, Shea B, Robinson V et al. Risedronate for the primary and secondary prevention of osteoporotic fractures in postmenopausal women. Cochrane Database Syst Rev 2008;(1):CD004523.
177. Wells GA, Cranney A, Peterson J, Boucher M, Shea B, Robinson V, et al. Alendronate for the primary and secondary prevention of osteoporotic fractures in postmenopausal women. Cochrane Database Syst Rev 2008;(1):CD001155.
178. Black DM, Schwartz AV, Ensrud KE, Cauley JA, Levis S, Quandt SA, et al. Effects of continuing or stopping alendronate after 5 years of treatment: the Fracture Intervention Trial Long-term Extension (FLEX): a randomized trial. JAMA. 2006;296(24):2927–38.
179. Sawka AM, Papaioannou A, Adachi JD, Gafni A, Hanley DA, Thabane L. Does alendronate reduce the risk of fracture in men? A meta-analysis incorporating prior knowledge of antifracture efficacy in women. BMC Musculoskelet Disord. 2005;6:39.
180. Homik J, Cranney A, Shea B, Tugwell P, Wells G, Adachi R, et al. Bisphosphonates for steroid induced osteoporosis. Cochrane Database Syst Rev 2000;(2):CD001347.
181. Reginster JY, Lecart MP. Efficacy and safety of drugs for Paget's disease of bone. Bone. 1995;17(5 Suppl):485S–8.
182. Cardwell CR, Abnet CC, Cantwell MM, Murray LJ. Exposure to oral bisphosphonates and risk of esophageal cancer. JAMA. 2010;304(6):657–63.
183. Loke YK, Jeevanantham V, Singh S. Bisphosphonates and atrial fibrillation: systematic review and meta-analysis. Drug Saf. 2009;32(3):219–28.

184. Khosla S, Burr D, Cauley J, Dempster DW, Ebeling PR, Felsenberg D, et al. Bisphosphonate-associated osteonecrosis of the jaw: report of a task force of the American Society for Bone and Mineral Research. J Bone Miner Res. 2007;22(10):1479–91.

185. Rossouw JE, Anderson GL, Prentice RL, Lacroix AZ, Kooperberg C, Stefanick ML, et al. Risks and benefits of estrogen plus progestin in healthy postmenopausal women: principal results from the Women's Health Initiative randomized controlled trial. JAMA. 2002;288(3):321–33.

186. Schneider DL, Barrett-Connor EL, Morton DJ. Timing of postmenopausal estrogen for optimal bone mineral density. The Rancho Bernardo Study. JAMA. 1997;277(7):543–7.

187. Greenspan SL, Emkey RD, Bone HG, Weiss SR, Bell NH, Downs RW, et al. Significant differential effects of alendronate, estrogen, or combination therapy on the rate of bone loss after discontinuation of treatment of postmenopausal osteoporosis. A randomized, double-blind, placebo-controlled trial. Ann Intern Med. 2002;137(11):875–83.

188. Lindsay R, Cosman F, Lobo RA, Walsh BW, Harris ST, Reagan JE, et al. Addition of alendronate to ongoing hormone replacement therapy in the treatment of osteoporosis: a randomized, controlled clinical trial. J Clin Endocrinol Metab. 1999;84(9):3076–81.

189. Wimalawansa SJ. A four-year randomized controlled trial of hormone replacement and bisphosphonate, alone or in combination, in women with postmenopausal osteoporosis. Am J Med. 1998;104(3):219–26.

190. Barrett-Connor E, Mosca L, Collins P, Geiger MJ, Grady D, Kornitzer M, et al. Effects of raloxifene on cardiovascular events and breast cancer in postmenopausal women. N Engl J Med. 2006;355(2):125–37.

191. Riggs BL, Hartmann LC. Selective estrogen-receptor modulators – mechanisms of action and application to clinical practice. N Engl J Med. 2003;348(7):618–29.

192. Delmas PD, Bjarnason NH, Mitlak BH, Ravoux AC, Shah AS, Huster WJ, et al. Effects of raloxifene on bone mineral density, serum cholesterol concentrations, and uterine endometrium in postmenopausal women. N Engl J Med. 1997;337(23):1641–7.

193. Luckey M, Kagan R, Greenspan S, Bone H, Kiel RD, Simon J, et al. Once-weekly alendronate 70 mg and raloxifene 60 mg daily in the treatment of postmenopausal osteoporosis. Menopause. 2004;11(4):405–15.

194. Kamischke A, Kemper DE, Castel MA, Luthke M, Rolf C, Behre HM, et al. Testosterone levels in men with chronic obstructive pulmonary disease with or without glucocorticoid therapy. Eur Respir J. 1998;11(1):41–5.

195. Riggs BL, Wahner HW, Seeman E, Offord KP, Dunn WL, Mazess RB, et al. Changes in bone mineral density of the proximal femur and spine with aging. Differences between the postmenopausal and senile osteoporosis syndromes. J Clin Invest. 1982;70(4):716–23.

196. Snyder PJ, Peachey H, Berlin JA, Hannoush P, Haddad G, Dlewati A, et al. Effects of testosterone replacement in hypogonadal men. J Clin Endocrinol Metab. 2000;85(8):2670–7.

197. Amory JK, Watts NB, Easley KA, Sutton PR, Anawalt BD, Matsumoto AM, et al. Exogenous testosterone or testosterone with finasteride increases bone mineral density in older men with low serum testosterone. J Clin Endocrinol Metab. 2004;89(2):503–10.

198. Kenny AM, Prestwood KM, Gruman CA, Marcello KM, Raisz LG. Effects of transdermal testosterone on bone and muscle in older men with low bioavailable testosterone levels. J Gerontol A Biol Sci Med Sci. 2001;56(5):M266–72.

199. Snyder PJ, Peachey H, Hannoush P, Berlin JA, Loh L, Holmes JH, et al. Effect of testosterone treatment on bone mineral density in men over 65 years of age. J Clin Endocrinol Metab. 1999;84(6):1966–72.

200. Snyder PJ. Androgens. In: Brunton LL, Lazo JS, Parker KL, editors. Goodman and Gilman's the pharmacological basis of therapeutics. New York, NY: McGraw-Hill; 2006. p. 1573–86.

201. Bringhurst FR, Demay MB, Kronenberg HM. Hormones and disorders of mineral metabolism. In: Kronenberg HM, Melmed S, Polonsky KS, Larsen PR, editors. Williams textbook of endocrinology. Philadelphia, PA: Saunders Elsevier; 2008. p. 1203–68.

202. Cranney A, Welch V, Adachi JD, Homik J, Shea B, Suarez-Almazor ME, et al. Calcitonin for the treatment and prevention of corticosteroid-induced osteoporosis. Cochrane Database Syst Rev 2000;(2):CD001983.

203. Downs Jr RW, Bell NH, Ettinger MP, Walsh BW, Favus MJ, Mako B, et al. Comparison of alendronate and intranasal calcitonin for treatment of osteoporosis in postmenopausal women. J Clin Endocrinol Metab. 2000;85(5):1783–8.

204. Knopp JA, Diner BM, Blitz M, Lyritis GP, Rowe BH. Calcitonin for treating acute pain of osteoporotic vertebral compression fractures: a systematic review of randomized, controlled trials. Osteoporos Int. 2005;16(10):1281–90.

205. Reginster JY, Franchimont P. Side effects of synthetic salmon calcitonin given by intranasal spray compared with intramuscular injection. Clin Exp Rheumatol. 1985;3(2):155–7.

206. Antonelli Incalzi R, Fuso L, De Rosa M, Forastiere F, Rapiti E, Nardecchia B, et al. Co-morbidity contributes to predict mortality of patients with chronic obstructive pulmonary disease. Eur Respir J. 1997;10(12):2794–800.

207. Crisafulli E, Costi S, Luppi F, Cirelli G, Cilione C, Coletti O, et al. Role of comorbidities in a cohort of patients with COPD undergoing pulmonary rehabilitation. Thorax. 2008;63(6): 487–92.

208. Mannino DM, Thorn D, Swensen A, Holguin F. Prevalence and outcomes of diabetes, hypertension and cardiovascular disease in COPD. Eur Respir J. 2008;32(4):962–9.

209. Gudmundsson G, Gislason T, Lindberg E, Hallin R, Ulrik CS, Brondum E, et al. Mortality in COPD patients discharged from hospital: the role of treatment and co-morbidity. Respir Res. 2006;7:109.

210. Parappil A, Depczynski B, Collett P, Marks GB. Effect of comorbid diabetes on length of stay and risk of death in patients admitted with acute exacerbations of COPD. Respirology. 2010;15(6):918–22.

211. van den Borst B, Gosker HR, Zeegers MP, Schols AM. Pulmonary function in diabetes: a metaanalysis. Chest. 2010;138(2):393–406.

212. Walter RE, Beiser A, Givelber RJ, O'Connor GT, Gottlieb DJ. Association between glycemic state and lung function: the Framingham Heart Study. Am J Respir Crit Care Med. 2003;167(6):911–6.

213. Slatore CG, Bryson CL, Au DH. The association of inhaled corticosteroid use with serum glucose concentration in a large cohort. Am J Med. 2009;122(5):472–8.

214. Faul JL, Wilson SR, Chu JW, Canfield J, Kuschner WG. The effect of an inhaled corticosteroid on glucose control in type 2 diabetes. Clin Med Res. 2009;7(1–2):14–20.

215. Walters JA, Walters EH, Wood-Baker R. Oral corticosteroids for stable chronic obstructive pulmonary disease. Cochrane Database Syst Rev. 2005;20(3):CD005374.

216. Goel A, Suri JC, Aggarwal K. Role of corticosteroids in the management of chronic obstructive lung disease: factors predicting response. Indian J Chest Dis Allied Sci. 1992;34(1): 11–7.

217. Pauwels RA, Buist AS, Calverley PM, Jenkins CR, Hurd SS. Global strategy for the diagnosis, management, and prevention of chronic obstructive pulmonary disease. NHLBI/WHO Global Initiative for Chronic Obstructive Lung Disease(GOLD) Workshop summary. Am J Respir Crit Care Med. 2001;163(5):1256–76.

218. Walters JA, Gibson PG, Wood-Baker R, Hannay M, Walters EH. Systemic corticosteroids for acute exacerbations of chronic obstructive pulmonary disease. Cochrane Database Syst Rev 2009;(1):CD001288.

219. Baker EH, Janaway CH, Philips BJ, Brennan AL, Baines DL, Wood DM, et al. Hyperglycaemia is associated with poor outcomes in patients admitted to hospital with acute exacerbations of chronic obstructive pulmonary disease. Thorax. 2006;61(4):284–9.

220. Chakrabarti B, Angus RM, Agarwal S, Lane S, Calverley PM. Hyperglycaemia as a predictor of outcome during non-invasive ventilation in decompensated COPD. Thorax. 2009;64(10): 857–62.

221. Ceglia L, Lau J, Pittas AG. Meta-analysis: efficacy and safety of inhaled insulin therapy in adults with diabetes mellitus. Ann Intern Med. 2006;145(9):665–75.

222. Petersen AH, Korsatko S, Kohler G, Wutte A, Olschewski H, Sparre T, et al. The effect of terbutaline on the absorption of pulmonary administered insulin in subjects with asthma. Br J Clin Pharmacol. 2010;69(3):271–8.

223. Mudaliar S, Henry RR. Inhaled insulin in patients with asthma and chronic obstructive pulmonary disease. Diabetes Technol Ther. 2007;9 Suppl 1:S83–92.

224. Rosenstock J, Cefalu WT, Hollander PA, Klioze SS, Reis J, Duggan WT. Safety and efficacy of inhaled human insulin (exubera) during discontinuation and readministration of therapy in adults with type 2 diabetes: a 3-year randomized controlled trial. Diabetes Technol Ther. 2009;11(11):697–705.

225. Ang E, Lawrence MK, Heilmann CR, Ferguson JA, Tobian JA, Webb DM, et al. Safety and efficacy of AIR inhaled insulin compared with subcutaneous insulin in patients having diabetes and asthma: a 12-month, randomized, noninferiority trial. Diabetes Technol Ther. 2009;11 Suppl 2:S35–44.

226. Shapiro H, Kagan I, Shalita-Chesner M, Singer J, Singer P. Inhaled aerosolized insulin: a "topical" anti-inflammatory treatment for acute lung injury and respiratory distress syndrome? Inflammation. 2010;33(5):315–29.

227. Berry SJ, Coffey DS, Walsh PC, Ewing LL. The development of human benign prostatic hyperplasia with age. J Urol. 1984;132(3):474–9.

228. Miyazaki H, Suda T, Otsuka A, Nagata M, Ozono S, Hashimoto D, et al. Tiotropium does not affect lower urinary tract functions in COPD patients with benign prostatic hyperplasia. Pulm Pharmacol Ther. 2008;21(6):879–83.

229. Gudmundsson G, Gislason T, Janson C, Lindberg E, Suppli UC, Brondum E, et al. Depression, anxiety and health status after hospitalisation for COPD: a multicentre study in the Nordic countries. Respir Med. 2006;100(1):87–93.

230. Zigmond AS, Snaith RP. The hospital anxiety and depression scale. Acta Psychiatr Scand. 1983;67(6):361–70.

231. Eisner MD, Blanc PD, Yelin EH, Katz PP, Sanchez G, Iribarren C, et al. Influence of anxiety on health outcomes in COPD. Thorax. 2010;65(3):229–34.

232. Lacasse Y, Beaudoin L, Rousseau L, Maltais F. Randomized trial of paroxetine in end-stage COPD. Monaldi Arch Chest Dis. 2004;61(3):140–7.

233. Omachi TA, Katz PP, Yelin EH, Gregorich SE, Iribarren C, Blanc PD, et al. Depression and health-related quality of life in chronic obstructive pulmonary disease. Am J Med. 2009;122(8):778. e9–15.

234. Ng TP, Niti M, Tan WC, Cao Z, Ong KC, Eng P. Depressive symptoms and chronic obstructive pulmonary disease: effect on mortality, hospital readmission, symptom burden, functional status, and quality of life. Arch Intern Med. 2007;167(1):60–7.

235. Argyropoulou P, Patakas D, Koukou A, Vasiliadis P, Georgopoulos D. Buspirone effect on breathlessness and exercise performance in patients with chronic obstructive pulmonary disease. Respiration. 1993;60(4):216–20.

236. Singh NP, Despars JA, Stansbury DW, Avalos K, Light RW. Effects of buspirone on anxiety levels and exercise tolerance in patients with chronic airflow obstruction and mild anxiety. Chest. 1993;103(3):800–4.

237. Silvertooth EJ, Doraiswamy PM, Clary GL, Babyak MA, Wilkerson N, Hellegars C, et al. Citalopram and quality of life in lung transplant recipients. Psychosomatics. 2004;45(3):271–2.

238. Borson S, McDonald GJ, Gayle T, Deffebach M, Lakshminarayan S, VanTuinen C. Improvement in mood, physical symptoms, and function with nortriptyline for depression in patients with chronic obstructive pulmonary disease. Psychosomatics. 1992;33(2):190–201.

239. Gordon GH, Michiels TM, Mahutte CK, Light RW. Effect of desipramine on control of ventilation and depression scores in patients with severe chronic obstructive pulmonary disease. Psychiatry Res. 1985;15(1):25–32.

240. Light RW, Merrill EJ, Despars J, Gordon GH, Mutalipassi LR. Doxepin treatment of depressed patients with chronic obstructive pulmonary disease. Arch Intern Med. 1986;146(7):1377–80.

241. Strom K, Boman G, Pehrsson K, Alton M, Singer J, Rydstrom PO, et al. Effect of protriptyline, 10 mg daily, on chronic hypoxaemia in chronic obstructive pulmonary disease. Eur Respir J. 1995;8(3):425–9.

242. Eisner MD, Trupin L, Katz PP, Yelin EH, Earnest G, Balmes J, et al. Development and validation of a survey-based COPD severity score. Chest. 2005;127(6):1890–7.
243. Smoller JW, Pollack MH, Systrom D, Kradin RL. Sertraline effects on dyspnea in patients with obstructive airways disease. Psychosomatics. 1998;39(1):24–9.
244. Cantor L, Jacobson R. COPD: How to manage comorbid depression and anxiety. J Fam Pract 2003; 2(11). http://www.jfponline.com/Pages.asp?AID=691. Accessed Oct 2011.
245. Brenes GA. Anxiety and chronic obstructive pulmonary disease: prevalence, impact, and treatment. Psychosom Med. 2003;65(6):963–70.
246. Mikkelsen RL, Middelboe T, Pisinger C, Stage KB. Anxiety and depression in patients with chronic obstructive pulmonary disease (COPD). A review. Nord J Psychiatry. 2004;58(1): 65–70.
247. Dunlop BW, Davis PG. Combination treatment with benzodiazepines and SSRIs for comorbid anxiety and depression: a review. Prim Care Companion J Clin Psychiatry. 2008;10(3): 222–8.
248. Lam RW, Kennedy SH, Grigoriadis S, McIntyre RS, Milev R, Ramasubbu R, et al. Canadian Network for Mood and Anxiety Treatments (CANMAT) clinical guidelines for the management of major depressive disorder in adults. III. Pharmacotherapy. J Affect Disord. 2009;117 Suppl 1:S26–43.
249. Goddard AW, Brouette T, Almai A, Jetty P, Woods SW, Charney D. Early coadministration of clonazepam with sertraline for panic disorder. Arch Gen Psychiatry. 2001;58(7):681–6.
250. Yagan MB, White D, Staab J. Sedation of the mechanically ventilated patient. Crit Care Nurs Q. 2000;22(4):90–100.
251. Cox CE, Reed SD, Govert JA, Rodgers JE, Campbell-Bright S, Kress JP, et al. Economic evaluation of propofol and lorazepam for critically ill patients undergoing mechanical ventilation. Crit Care Med. 2008;36(3):706–14.
252. Spiegel DR, Ramdath N. A failed case of weaning from a mechanical ventilator with lorazepam successfully accomplished by ziprasidone. Gen Hosp Psychiatry. 2009;31(5):494–6.
253. Katon WJ. The comorbidity of diabetes mellitus and depression. Am J Med. 2008;121 (11 Suppl 2):S8–15.
254. Ghaeli P, Shahsavand E, Mesbahi M, Kamkar MZ, Sadeghi M, Dashti-Khavidaki S. Comparing the effects of 8-week treatment with fluoxetine and imipramine on fasting blood glucose of patients with major depressive disorder. J Clin Psychopharmacol. 2004;24(4):386–8.
255. Goodnick PJ. Use of antidepressants in treatment of comorbid diabetes mellitus and depression as well as in diabetic neuropathy. Ann Clin Psychiatry. 2001;13(1):31–41.
256. Knol MJ, Derijks HJ, Geerlings MI, Heerdink ER, Souverein PC, Gorter KJ, et al. Influence of antidepressants on glycaemic control in patients with diabetes mellitus. Pharmacoepidemiol Drug Saf. 2008;17(6):577–86.
257. Boyer W. Serotonin uptake inhibitors are superior to imipramine in alleviating panic attacks: a meta-analysis. In: Darcourt G, editor. Current therapeutic approaches to panic and other anxiety disorders. New York, NY: Karger; 1994.
258. Glassman AH, O'Connor CM, Califf RM, Swedberg K, Schwartz P, Bigger Jr JT, et al. Sertraline treatment of major depression in patients with acute MI or unstable angina. JAMA. 2002;288(6):701–9.
259. Alvarez M, Malecot CO, Gannier F, Lignon JM. Antimony-induced cardiomyopathy in guinea-pig and protection by L-carnitine. Br J Pharmacol. 2005;144(1):17–27.
260. Emery CF, Schein RL, Hauck ER, MacIntyre NR. Psychological and cognitive outcomes of a randomized trial of exercise among patients with chronic obstructive pulmonary disease. Health Psychol. 1998;17(3):232–40.
261. de Godoy DV, de Godoy RF. A randomized controlled trial of the effect of psychotherapy on anxiety and depression in chronic obstructive pulmonary disease. Arch Phys Med Rehabil. 2003;84(8):1154–7.
262. Donnelly LE, Tudhope SJ, Fenwick PS, Barnes PJ. Effects of formoterol and salmeterol on cytokine release from monocyte-derived macrophages. Eur Respir J. 2010;36(1):178–86.

263. Remels AH, Gosker HR, van der Velden J, Langen RC, Schols AM. Systemic inflammation and skeletal muscle dysfunction in chronic obstructive pulmonary disease: state of the art and novel insights in regulation of muscle plasticity. Clin Chest Med. 2007;28(3):537–52. vi.

264. Remels AH, Schrauwen P, Broekhuizen R, Willems J, Kersten S, Gosker HR, et al. Peroxisome proliferator-activated receptor expression is reduced in skeletal muscle in COPD. Eur Respir J. 2007;30(2):245–52.

265. Patel HJ, Belvisi MG, Bishop-Bailey D, Yacoub MH, Mitchell JA. Activation of peroxisome proliferator-activated receptors in human airway smooth muscle cells has a superior anti-inflammatory profile to corticosteroids: relevance for chronic obstructive pulmonary disease therapy. J Immunol. 2003;170(5):2663–9.

266. Matera MG, Calzetta L, Cazzola M. TNF-alpha inhibitors in asthma and COPD: we must not throw the baby out with the bath water. Pulm Pharmacol Ther. 2010;23(2):121–8.

267. Rabe KF, Bateman ED, O'Donnell D, Witte S, Bredenbroker D, Bethke TD. Roflumilast – an oral anti-inflammatory treatment for chronic obstructive pulmonary disease: a randomised controlled trial. Lancet. 2005;366(9485):563–71.

268. Calverley PM, Sanchez-Toril F, McIvor A, Teichmann P, Bredenbroeker D, Fabbri LM. Effect of 1-year treatment with roflumilast in severe chronic obstructive pulmonary disease. Am J Respir Crit Care Med. 2007;176(2):154–61.

269. Cazzola M, Picciolo S, Matera MG. Roflumilast in chronic obstructive pulmonary disease: evidence from large trials. Expert Opin Pharmacother. 2010;11(3):441–9.

270. Giamarellos-Bourboulis EJ. Macrolides beyond the conventional antimicrobials: a class of potent immunomodulators. Int J Antimicrob Agents. 2008;31(1):12–20.

271. Seemungal TA, Wilkinson TM, Hurst JR, Perera WR, Sapsford RJ, Wedzicha JA. Long-term erythromycin therapy is associated with decreased chronic obstructive pulmonary disease exacerbations. Am J Respir Crit Care Med. 2008;178(11):1139–47.

272. Cazzola M, Ciaprini C, Page CP, Matera MG. Targeting systemic inflammation: novel therapies for the treatment of chronic obstructive pulmonary disease. Expert Opin Ther Targets. 2007;11(10):1273–86.

273. Barnes PJ. Future treatments for chronic obstructive pulmonary disease and its comorbidities. Proc Am Thorac Soc. 2008;5(8):857–64.

Chapter 14
Pulmonary Rehabilitation: Targeting the Systemic Manifestations of COPD

Linda Nici and Richard ZuWallack

Abstract Optimal clinical management of chronic obstructive pulmonary disease (COPD) requires a comprehensive, integrated approach encompassing both pharmacologic and nonpharmacologic interventions. Pulmonary rehabilitation is an interdisciplinary, patient-centered approach to patient care that complements pharmacological therapy. It has emerged as a standard component of treatment of COPD, and as such, has a prominent place in all its current guidelines.

Keywords Pulmonary rehabilitation • COPD • Systemic manifestations • Pharmacologic intervention • Non-pharmacologic intervention • Pharmacological therapy • Guidelines • Self-management education

Introduction

Optimal clinical management of chronic obstructive pulmonary disease (COPD) requires a comprehensive, integrated approach encompassing both pharmacologic and nonpharmacologic interventions. Pulmonary rehabilitation is an interdisciplinary, patient-centered approach to patient care that complements pharmacological therapy. It has emerged as a standard component of treatment of COPD, and as such, has a prominent place in all its current guidelines [1, 2] (http://www.GOLDCOPD.com).

L. Nici(✉)
The Warren Alpert Medical School of Brown University, Providence, RI, USA

Providence Veterans Affairs Medical Center, Providence, RI, USA
e-mail: linda_nici@brown.edu

R. ZuWallack
University of Connecticut School of Medicine, Hartford, CT, USA

St. Francis Hospital and Medical Center, Hartford, CT, USA
e-mail: rzuwalla@stfranciscare.org

L. Nici and R. ZuWallack (eds.), *Chronic Obstructive Pulmonary Disease: Co-Morbidities and Systemic Consequences*, Respiratory Medicine, DOI 10.1007/978-1-60761-673-3_14, © Springer Science+Business Media, LLC 2012

Definition of Pulmonary Rehabilitation

The 2006 American Thoracic Society and European Respiratory Society Statement on Pulmonary Rehabilitation defines it as, "… an evidence-based, multidisciplinary, and comprehensive intervention for patients with chronic respiratory diseases who are symptomatic and often have decreased daily life activities. Integrated into the individualized treatment of the patient, pulmonary rehabilitation is designed to reduce symptoms, optimize functional status, increase participation, and reduce health care costs through stabilizing or reversing systemic manifestations of the disease" [3]. Pulmonary rehabilitation includes patient assessment, exercise training, self-management education, and psychosocial support. Although these components can (and should) be given as part of standard medical care, an efficient and effective method is bundling these therapies in the form of a comprehensive pulmonary rehabilitation program delivered by an interdisciplinary team in collaboration with the patient and family.

Benefits of Pulmonary Rehabilitation

Of all treatments currently available for COPD, pulmonary rehabilitation provides the greatest benefits in patient-centered outcomes. These include decreased dyspnea and fatigue, increased exercise capacity, improved functional performance, and enhanced health-related quality of life. Pulmonary rehabilitation also reduces healthcare costs in COPD, although the evidence base behind this is not as robust as in patient-centered outcomes. The effect of pulmonary rehabilitation on reducing healthcare utilization associated with the COPD exacerbation should translate into a survival benefit. However, to date, a survival benefit has not been demonstrated, probably because the few studies that evaluated survival in this setting have been underpowered to demonstrate this effect. There are data suggesting that pulmonary rehabilitation beginning at the time of the hospitalization for COPD (when mortality risk is especially high) may increase survival [4]. Table 14.1 lists the benefits from pulmonary rehabilitation and the level of evidence supporting each area.

Rationale Behind the Effectiveness of Pulmonary Rehabilitation

As described above, pulmonary rehabilitation leads to substantial improvements in symptoms, exercise capacity, functional performance, and health-related quality of life. These benefits are realized despite the fact that pulmonary rehabilitation does not improve traditional lung function measurements such as the FEV1. This disconnect is explained by the fact that: (1) COPD has prominent systemic manifestations and frequent comorbid conditions, (2) these contribute substantially to its symptom

Table 14.1 Pulmonary rehabilitation: outcomes in patients with COPD

Outcome	Source	Comments
Cost effectiveness	ACCP/AACVPR	Weak to very weak evidence; weak recommendation
Dyspnea relief	ACCP/AACVPR	Strong evidence, strong recommendation[a]
	ACP	Average effect on dyspnea subscale of the Chronic Respiratory Questionnaire was clinically significant[b]
	Cochrane review	Effect on dyspnea subscale of the Chronic Respiratory Questionnaire was greater than minimum clinically important difference[b], strong support
	Gold	Evidence Grade A[c]
Improved exercise performance	ACCP/AACVPR	Strong evidence, strong recommendation[a]
	ACP	Clinically insignificant difference in six-minute walk distance
	Cochrane review	Clinically insignificant difference in six-minute walk distance
	Gold	Evidence grade A[c]
Improved health-related quality of life	ACCP/AACVPR	Strong evidence, strong recommendation[a]
	ACP	Pooled difference in health status scores on the St. George's Respiratory Questionnaire was less than minimum clinically significant difference[d]
	Cochrane review	Effect on all subscales of the Chronic Respiratory Questionnaire was greater than minimum clinically improved difference, strong support
	Gold	Evidence Grade A[c]
Psychosocial benefits	ACCP/AACVPR	Moderate evidence, weak recommendation
	Gold	Reduced anxiety and depression, evidence Grade A[c]
	Meta-analysis	Small to moderate improvements in anxiety and depression compared to usual care
Reduced health care utilization	ACCP/AACVPR	Moderate evidence, weak recommendation
	ACP	Equivocal for health care utilization outcomes
	Gold	Evidence Grade A[c]
Survival	ACCP/AACVPR	Insufficient evidence; no recommendation provided
	Gold	Evidence Grade B

AACVPR American Association of Cardiovascular and Pulmonary Rehabilitation
ACCP American College of Chest Physicians
ACP American College of Physicians
GOLD Global Initiative for Obstructive Lung Disease
COPD Chronic obstructive pulmonary disease
RCT Randomized controlled trial
[a]Evidence from well-designed RCTs with consistent and directly applicable results; benefits outweigh the risks and burden
[b]The Chronic Respiratory Questionnaire is a health status questionnaire for COPD, with dyspnea, fatigue, emotion, and mastery subscale
[c]Evidence from well-designed RCTs with consistent findings, with a substantial number of studies involving many participants
[d]The St. George's Respiratory Questionnaire is a health status questionnaire for COPD and asthma, with symptom, activity, and impact subscales.
Limited data From Nici et al. [5] Reprinted with permission

burden, morbidity, and mortality, and (3) these are identified, targeted, and treated by pulmonary rehabilitation. Table 14.2 lists some of the frequent systemic manifestations of COPD.

A typical COPD patient referred to pulmonary rehabilitation has airflow limitation, hyperinflation, and gas-exchange abnormalities which cause dyspnea and activity limitation. However, the typical patient also has peripheral muscle dysfunction and muscle wasting resulting from physical inactivity, systemic inflammation, and systemic corticosteroid use. The resulting negative effects on dyspnea and exercise limitation often dwarf those from the respiratory system. The exercise component of pulmonary rehabilitation ameliorates some of the negative effects from peripheral muscle abnormalities. For example, exercise training of the ambulatory muscles leads to less lactate production and a reduction of the ventilatory burden associated with that exercise. A lessened ventilatory burden permits a lower respiratory rate and longer expiratory time, thereby reducing dynamic hyperinflation.

The typical COPD patient is also more likely to have maladaptive behaviors (i.e., smoking), anxiety, depression, poor coping skills, insufficient insight into the disease and its treatment, and poor adherence to therapy. Self-management strategies adopted during pulmonary rehabilitation work in these areas. For example, the implementation of an individualized action plan that addresses the early recognition and treatment of the COPD exacerbation can lessen its effects and potentially reduce hospitalizations and even mortality. Additionally, the psychosocial support provided during pulmonary rehabilitation can lessen the severity and impact of anxiety and depression [20].

The Pulmonary Rehabilitation Team

Pulmonary rehabilitation is delivered by an interdisciplinary team. While the specific makeup of this team varies, depending on the setting and resources of the program, the following are essential members: the medical director and the program coordinator. Most programs also include health care professionals from other disciplines, including nursing, physical therapy, occupational therapy, respiratory therapy, exercise physiology, social work, psychology or psychiatry, and nutrition. The current recommendations for staffing and professional roles and competencies are provided by the American Association of Cardiovascular and Pulmonary Rehabilitation Guidelines for Pulmonary Rehabilitation Programs [21].

Components of Pulmonary Rehabilitation

Pulmonary rehabilitation includes patient assessment, exercise training, self-management education, and psychosocial support [21]. Each of these components is discussed below.

Table 14.2 Systemic manifestations of COPD

Peripheral muscle dysfunction	Respiratory muscle dysfunction	Cardiac abnormalities	Nutritional and body composition abnormalities	Skeletal abnormalities	Psychosocial factors
Atrophy, [6, 7]	Diaphragm mechanical disadvantage from static and dynamic hyperinflation	Cardiovascular deconditioning	Decreased fat-free mass [8, 9]	Decreased bone mineral density in COPD patients [10]	Depression [11, 12]
Decreases in oxidative enzymes [13] and impaired oxidative capacity [6, 13]		Increased right ventricular after-load from hypoxia-mediated pulmonary vasoconstriction			Anxiety
Decreased ratio of type I to type II muscle fibers [6, 14]		Cor pulmonale, reduced stroke volume and increased heart rate [15]			Cognitive defects
Systemic inflammatory process in COPD [16, 17]		Increased right atrial pressure resulting from dynamic hyperinflation			Maladaptive behaviors
Chronic corticosteroid use [18, 19]					Poor coping skills
					Poor adherence to therapy

Patient Assessment

A comprehensive, initial assessment is an essential component of pulmonary rehabilitation. The initial assessment sets the stage for all subsequent treatment and serves several purposes, including determining the appropriateness of the referral; assessing physiologic and functional impairments; identifying relevant comorbid conditions; identifying exercise, educational, nutritional, and psychosocial needs; recognizing safety issues; creating an initial exercise prescription; setting realistic and achievable goals; and establishing lines of communication among the patient, family, and professional staff. The assessment includes a history and physical and any testing necessary to define physiologic and functional impairments. The patient assessment may also include a maximal cardiopulmonary exercise test, which can assess the safety of exercise and the factors contributing to exercise limitation [22]. The exercise test can also aid in developing the exercise prescription.

Referral to pulmonary rehabilitation is indicated for patients with dyspnea, fatigue, and/or functional limitations despite otherwise standard medical therapy. Contraindications to pulmonary rehabilitation include any condition that would place the patient at increased risk during rehabilitation or any condition that would interfere with the rehabilitative process. This decision is made by the pulmonary rehabilitation medical director in collaboration with the patient's primary health care providers.

Pulmonary rehabilitation guidelines state that specific thresholds of pulmonary function, such as the FEV1, are not of paramount importance in determining the need for pulmonary rehabilitation. This is due to the fact that the overall morbidity of COPD is influenced by considerably more than airflow limitation alone [23]. However, symptoms and functional status limitation are typically seen in patients with disease severity of moderate to severe, and current Medicare policy reflects this.

Exercise Training

Exercise training, including upper and lower extremity endurance training and strength training, is a necessary and highly effective component of pulmonary rehabilitation [24]. Its effectiveness reflects the importance of peripheral muscle dysfunction in COPD [25–28]. Exercise training adheres to the general principles of *intensity*: higher levels produce greater results; *specificity*: only those muscles trained show an effect; and *reversibility*: its effects lessen with cessation [29]. Patients with COPD are capable of exercising for prolonged periods of time at levels close to their peak exercise capacity [30]. Higher levels of exercise are associated with increased physiologic training effects [31, 32], however, patients who cannot tolerate high levels of exercise training also benefit [33]. Strength training yields additive benefits [34].

The type, intensity, and duration of training are based on the patient's limitations to exercise, which may include, in addition to skeletal muscle dysfunction, ventilatory limitations, gas-exchange abnormalities, dynamic hyperinflation, and respiratory muscle dysfunction. Exercise training leads to decreased breathlessness [35]. It may also have additional beneficial effects, including increased motivation for exercise, reduced mood disturbance [36, 37], and improved cardiovascular function.

The optimal frequency and duration of exercise training are not known, and, indeed, probably depend on the individual patient's unique needs. In general, longer programs yield better results [38–40]. Patients should perform exercise at least three times per week under direct supervision [41, 42]. However, if program constraints exist, twice-weekly supervised exercise training plus one or more unsupervised sessions at home is an acceptable alternative. Maximizing bronchodilation, interval training (alternating high and low intensities), and oxygen supplementation may allow for higher exercise training intensity in some COPD patients [43–48].

Self-management Education

Education is also an integral component of all comprehensive pulmonary rehabilitation programs [3]. Rather than simply providing didactic education, education in pulmonary rehabilitation must promote self-efficacy, the belief that one's action will influence outcome. This is generally achieved through teaching self-management skills [49–51] and fostering collaborative self-care [52, 53]. A typical self-management education program emphasizes practice and problem solving. An important focus of self-management education is the development and implementation of an action plan for early recognition and treatment of exacerbations. This has proven to be highly effective in improving health status and reducing health care costs [54]. Advance directives should also be addressed [55, 56].

Psychosocial Support

Anxiety, depression, cognitive defects, inadequate coping mechanisms, and poor self-management skills all contribute to the burden of COPD [57–60]. Indeed, gains made from participation in a pulmonary rehabilitation program may be limited if existing significant psychosocial issues are not addressed. These are addressed by the psychosocial component of pulmonary rehabilitation. This should include psychological screening and educational sessions and support groups to assist patients in developing coping strategies, and relaxation and stress-management techniques. Progressive muscle relaxation, identification of stressors, and panic control may reduce not only anxiety but dyspnea as well. Participation by family members and friends in pulmonary rehabilitation support groups is encouraged and may provide additional emotional support to patients and their families. Individuals with substantial psychiatric illness are referred for appropriate professional care outside of the pulmonary rehabilitation program.

Exercise training itself is one of the best interventions for the symptoms of anxiety and depression, and stress relief. Even a short course of pulmonary rehabilitation may result in improvements in psychological outcomes [61]. However, it appears that exercise training has little effect on cognitive dysfunction in hypoxic COPD [26].

Other Aspects of Pulmonary Rehabilitation

Nutritional Intervention

Abnormalities in body composition, especially decreases in body weight and muscle mass, are prevalent in COPD [62–65]. Reductions in muscle mass are often present even in normal weight patients. Reductions in body mass index (BMI, the weight in kg divided by the height in meters squared) or recent weight loss (>10% in the past 6 months or >5% in the past month) are important predictors of morbidity and mortality. Decreased fat-free or lean body mass also factor in exercise limitation, reduced health status, increased health care utilization, and reduced survival [66–69].

Since body weight and body composition abnormalities are common and are associated with poor outcomes, it is reasonable to include their treatment in a comprehensive pulmonary rehabilitation program. Interventions that may potentially improve body weight and composition abnormalities include calorie replacement, [70, 71] strength training, [72, 73] and anabolic hormonal therapy [74, 75]. Whether these interventions will translate into functional benefits and/or increased survival remains to be determined.

Supplemental Oxygen

While long-term oxygen therapy prolongs survival in COPD patients with severe hypoxemia [76, 77], supplemental oxygen therapy can also be used as an adjunct to exercise training in pulmonary rehabilitation. Oxygen therapy allows for greater intensity of exercise training in symptom-limited COPD patients [78]. The mechanisms behind this exercise-enhancing effect are not completely clear, but probably include the reduction in stimulation of peripheral chemoreceptors; resultant decreased respiratory rate, more time for exhalation, and less dynamic hyperinflation. These effects are present even in exercising nonhypoxemic COPD patients [79, 80].

Pulmonary Rehabilitation and the Acute Exacerbation

The COPD exacerbation is associated with prolonged deteriorations of functional status and health-related quality of life, increased health care costs, and a higher mortality risk [81]. Additionally, frequent exacerbators have an accelerated decline in lung function.

Pulmonary rehabilitation in stable COPD patients may directly or indirectly reduce the frequency and/or severity of subsequent exacerbations through several mechanisms. Most importantly, the development and implementation of the individualized, collaborative action plan leads to the early recognition and treatment of the exacerbation, thereby lessening its impact. Inhaled corticosteroids and long-acting bronchodilators are associated with fewer COPD exacerbations [82, 83]. Pulmonary rehabilitation promotes adherence to this pharmacologic therapy, and thereby should indirectly reduce exacerbation rates. Additionally, higher levels of physical activity resulting from pulmonary rehabilitation may result in fewer hospitalizations [84].

During hospitalization for an exacerbation, exercise training can lessen the deleterious effects of inactivity and systemic inflammation on muscle function. In addition, the hospitalization may represent a teachable moment (and a captive audience) for self-management education.

In the immediate posthospitalization period, symptoms remain increased, physical activity is dramatically limited, health care needs are substantial, and patients are at considerable risk for rehospitalization. Pulmonary rehabilitation can facilitate the transition to the home setting through developing an individualized plan of care, and providing the framework (i.e., the pulmonary rehabilitation program) for sharing this plan with the patient, family, and all health care providers [85]. This is integrated care, and it has been demonstrated to have substantial positive effects [86].

Sustaining the Benefits from Pulmonary Rehabilitation

As stated earlier, pulmonary rehabilitation improves dyspnea, increases exercise capacity, improves functional status, and enhances health-related quality of life. These benefits may gradually decrease over time [87]. While this gradual decrease in benefit probably has multiple causes, the failure to adhere to the healthy behavior change promoted in pulmonary rehabilitation is considered most important. Thus, some patients decrease their physical activity and exercise levels over time. This is most acute in the period following the exacerbation, when patients are highly symptomatic and prone to revert to a more sedentary lifestyle [88]. Longer duration formal pulmonary rehabilitation [89], readily available and inexpensive maintenance programs, repeated courses (booster shots), and regular reinforcement by health care professionals may help maintain benefits. Efforts at promoting and optimizing patient self-efficacy will probably ultimately have the greatest success in this important area.

Summary

Pulmonary rehabilitation has ascended to the status of a standard of care for patients with COPD. It has proven benefits across multiple areas, including dyspnea, exercise tolerance, functional performance, health-related quality of life, and health care utilization. Furthermore, its utilization following a hospitalization for an exacerbation may reduce morbidity and mortality. The rationale behind these impressive benefits rests on the fact that systemic effects of COPD are common, play a major role in the morbidity of the disease, are targeted by this intervention, and often respond to treatment.

Pulmonary rehabilitation is an important component of the integrated care of the COPD patient, and should be considered for those who remain symptomatic or have decreased functional status despite otherwise optimal medical management. Components of comprehensive pulmonary rehabilitation include assessment, exercise training, self-management education, and psychosocial support. Sustaining the long-term benefits of pulmonary rehabilitation is an ongoing area of investigation, but in all likelihood this will depend in large part on the ability to foster self-efficacy in patients with this complex, chronic disease.

References

1. American Thoracic Society and European Respiratory Society. Standards for the diagnosis and management of patients with COPD 2004; http://www.thoracic.org.
2. Ries AL, Bauldoff GS, Carlin BW, Casaburi R, Emery CF, Mahler DA, et al. Pulmonary rehabilitation. Joint ACCP/AACVPR evidence-based clinical practice guidelines. Chest. 2007;131: 4S–42S.
3. Nici L, Donner C, ZuWallack R, Wouters E, et al. The ATS/ERS statement on pulmonary rehabilitation. Am J Respir Crit Care Med. 2006;173:1390–414.
4. Puhan MA, Scharplatz M, Troosters T, Steurer J. Respiratory rehabilitation after acute exacerbation of COPD may reduce risk for readmission and mortality – a systematic review. Respir Res. 2005;6:54.
5. Nici L, Lareau S, ZuWallack R. Pulmonary Rehabilitation in the treatment of COPD. Am Fam Phys. 2010;82(6):655–60.
6. Mador MJ, Bozkanat E. Skeletal muscle dysfunction in chronic obstructive pulmonary disease. Respir Res. 2001;2(4):216–24.
7. Bernard S et al. Peripheral muscle weakness in patients with chronic obstructive pulmonary disease. Am J Respir Crit Care Med. 1998;158(2):629–34.
8. Vermeeren MA et al. Prevalence of nutritional depletion in a large out-patient population of patients with COPD. Respir Med. 2006;100(8):1349–55.
9. Schols A. Nutritional modulation as part of the integrated management of chronic obstructive pulmonary disease. Proc Nutr Soc. 2003;62(4):783–91.
10. Jorgensen NR et al. The prevalence of osteoporosis in patients with chronic obstructive pulmonary disease-A cross sectional study. Respir Med. 2007;101(1):177–85.
11. Guell R et al. Impact of pulmonary rehabilitation on psychosocial morbidity in patients with severe COPD. Chest. 2006;129(4):899–904.
12. Light RW et al. Prevalence of depression and anxiety in patients with COPD. Relationship to functional capacity. Chest. 1985;87(1):35–8.
13. Maltais F et al. Oxidative enzyme activities of the vastus lateralis muscle and the functional status in patients with COPD. Thorax. 2000;55(10):848–53.
14. Maltais F et al. Altered expression of myosin heavy chain in the vastus lateralis muscle in patients with COPD. Eur Respir J. 1999;13(4):850–4.
15. Berger HJ et al. Memorial Award Paper. Comparison of exercise right ventricular performance in chronic obstructive pulmonary disease and coronary artery disease: noninvasive assessment by quantitative radionuclide angiocardiography. Invest Radiol. 1979;14(5):342–53.

16. Schols AM et al. Evidence for a relation between metabolic derangements and increased levels of inflammatory mediators in a subgroup of patients with chronic obstructive pulmonary disease. Thorax. 1996;51(8):819–24.

17. Spruit MA et al. Muscle force during an acute exacerbation in hospitalised patients with COPD and its relationship with CXCL8 and IGF-I. Thorax. 2003;58(9):752–6.

18. Decramer M et al. Corticosteroids contribute to muscle weakness in chronic airflow obstruction. Am J Respir Crit Care Med. 1994;150(1):11–6.

19. Rahman I, Skwarska E, MacNee W. Attenuation of oxidant/antioxidant imbalance during treatment of exacerbations of chronic obstructive pulmonary disease. Thorax. 1997;52(6): 565–8.

20. Kayahan B et al. Psychological outcomes of an outpatient pulmonary rehabilitation program in patients with chronic obstructive pulmonary disease. Respir Med. 2006;100(6):1050–7.

21. American Association of Cardiovascular & Pulmonary Rehabilitation. Guidelines for pulmonary rehabilitation programs. 3rd ed. Chicago, IL: American Association of Cardiovascular & Pulmonary Rehabilitation; 2004.

22. Human Kinetics, American Thoracic Society/American College of Chest Physicians. ATS/ACCP statement on cardiopulmonary exercise testing. Am J Respir Crit Care Med. 2003;167:211–77.

23. Celli BR, Cote CG, Marin JM, Casanova C, Montes de Oca M, Mendez RA, et al. The body mass index, airflow obstruction, dyspnea and exercise capacity index in chronic obstructive pulmonary disease. N Engl J Med. 2004;350:1005–12.

24. American Thoracic Society, European Respiratory Society. ATS/ERS statement on skeletal muscle dysfunction in chronic obstructive pulmonary disease. Am J Respir Crit Care Med. 1999;159:S1–S40.

25. Bernard S, Leblanc P, Whittom F, et al. Peripheral muscle weakness in patients with chronic obstructive pulmonary disease. Am J Respir Crit Care Med. 1998;158(2):629–34.

26. Engelen MP, Schols AM, Does JD, et al. Skeletal muscle weakness is associated with wasting of extremity fat-free mass but not with airflow obstruction in patients with chronic obstructive pulmonary disease. Am J Clin Nutr. 2000;71(3):733–8.

27. Gosselink R, Troosters T, Decramer M. Peripheral muscle weakness contributes to exercise limitation in COPD. Am J Respir Crit Care Med. 1996;153:976–80.

28. Sala E, Roca J, Marrades RM, Alonso J, Gonzalez de Suso JM, Moreno A, et al. Effects of endurance training on skeletal muscle bioenergetics in chronic obstructive pulmonary disease. Am J Respir Crit Care Med. 1999;159:1726–34.

29. American college of sports medicine. Position stand. The recommended quantity and quality of exercise for developing and maintaining cardiorespiratory and muscular fitness in healthy adults. Med Sci Sports Exerc. 1990;22:265–74.

30. Maltais F, LeBlanc P, Jobin J, et al. Intensity of training and physiologic adaptation in patient with chronic obstructive pulmonary disease. Am J Respir Crit Care Med. 1997;155:555–61.

31. Casaburi R, Patessio A, Ioli F, Zanaboni S, Donner CF, Wasserman K. Reductions in exercise lactic acidosis and ventilation as a result of exercise training in patients with obstructive lung disease. Am Rev Respir Dis. 1991;143:9–18.

32. Normandin EA, McCusker C, Connors ML, Vale F, Gerardi D, ZuWallack RL. An evaluation of two approaches to exercise conditioning in pulmonary rehabilitation. Chest. 2002;121: 1085–91.

33. Puente-Maestu L, Sanz ML, Sanz P, de Ona JM Ruiz, Rodriguez-Hermosa JL, Whipp BJ. Effects of two types of training on pulmonary and cardiac responses to moderate exercise in patients with COPD. Eur Respir J. 2000;15:1026–32.

34. Bernard S, Whittom F, LeBlanc P, Jobin J, Belleau R, Berube C, et al. Aerobic and strength training in patients with chronic obstructive pulmonary disease. Am J Respir Crit Care Med. 1999;159:896–901.

35. O'Donnell DE, McGuire M, Samis L, Webb KA. The impact of exercise reconditioning on breathlessness in severe chronic airflow limitation. Am J Respir Crit Care Med. 1995;152: 2005–13.

36. Emery CF, Leatherman NE, Burker EJ, MacIntyre NR. Psychological outcomes of a pulmonary rehabilitation program. Chest. 1991;100:613–7.
37. Emery CF, Schein RL, Hauck ER, MacIntyre NR. Psychological and cognitive outcomes of a randomized trial of exercise among patients with chronic obstructive pulmonary disease. Health Psychol. 1998;17:232–40.
38. Green RH, Singh SJ, Williams J, Morgan MD. A randomised controlled trial of four weeks versus seven weeks of pulmonary rehabilitation in chronic obstructive pulmonary disease. Thorax. 2001;56:143–5.
39. Rossi G, Florini F, Romagnoli M, Bellatone T, Lucic S, Lugli D, et al. Length and clinical effectiveness of pulmonary rehabilitation in outpatients with chronic airway obstruction. Chest. 2005;127:105–9.
40. Lacasse Y, Brosseau L, Milne S, Martin S, Wong E, Guyatt GH, et al. Pulmonary rehabilitation for chronic obstructive pulmonary disease. Cochrane Database Syst Rev. 2002;3:CD003793.
41. Ringbaek TJ, Broendum E, Hemmingsen L, Lybeck K, Nielsen D, Andersen C, et al. Rehabilitation of patients with chronic obstructive pulmonary disease. Exercise twice a week is not sufficient! Respir Med. 2000;94:150–4.
42. Puente-Maestu L, Sanz ML, Sanz P, Cubillo JM, Mayol J, Casaburi R. Comparison of effects of supervised versus self-monitored training programs in patients with chronic obstructive pulmonary disease. Eur Respir J. 2000;15:517–25.
43. Casaburi R, Kukafka D, Cooper CB, Witek TJ, Kesten S. Improvement in exercise tolerance with the combination of tiotropium and pulmonary rehabilitation in patients with COPD. Chest. 2005;127:809–17.
44. Vogiatzis I, Nanas S, Roussos C. Interval training as an alternative modality to continuous exercise in patients with COPD. Eur Respir J. 2002;20:12–9.
45. O'Donnell DE, D'Arisigny C, Webb KA. Effects of hperoxia on ventilatory limitation during exercise in advanced chronic obstructive pulmonary disease. Am J Respir Crit Care Med. 2001;163:892–8.
46. Coppoolse R, Schols AMWJ, Baarends EM, et al. Interval versus continuous training in patients with severe COPD: a randomized clinical trial. Eur Respir J. 1999;14:258–63.
47. Somfay A, Porszasz J, Lee SM, et al. Dose-response effect of oxygen on hyperinflation and exercise endurance in nonhypoxaemic COPD patients. Eur Respir J. 2001;18:77–84.
48. Emtner M, Porszasz J, Burns M, et al. Benefits of supplemental oxygen in exercise training in nonhypoxemic chronic obstructive pulmonary disease patients. Am J Respir Crit Care Med. 2003;168:1034–42.
49. Ries AL, Moser KM, Bullock PJ, Limber TM, Myers R, Sassi-Dambron DE, et al., editors. Shortness of breath: a guide to better living and breathing. St. Louis, MO: Mosby; 1996.
50. Ries AL. Pulmonary rehabilitation. In: Tierney DF, editor. Current pulmonology. St. Louis, MO: Mosby; 1994. p. 441–67.
51. Von Korff M, Gruman J, Schaefer J, Curry SJ, Wagner EH. Collaborative management of chronic illness. Ann Intern Med. 1997;127:1097–102.
52. Gilmartin ME. Patient and family education. Clin Chest Med. 1986;7:619–27.
53. Neish CM, Hopp JW. The role of education in pulmonary rehabilitation. J Cardiopulm Rehabil. 1988;11:439–41.
54. Bourbeau J, Julien M, Maltais F, et al. Reduction of hospital utilization in patients with chronic obstructive pulmonary disease: a disease-specific self-management intervention. Arch Intern Med. 2003;163(5):585–91.
55. Heffner JE, Fahy B, Barbieri C. Advance directive education during pulmonary rehabilitation. Chest. 1996;109(2):373–9.
56. Heffner JE, Fahy B, Hilling L, Barbieri C. Outcomes of advance directive education of pulmonary rehabilitation patients. Am J Resp Crit Care Med. 1997;155(3):1055–9.
57. Agle DP, Baum GL. Psychosocial aspects of chronic obstructive pulmonary disease. Med Clin North Am. 1977;61:749–58.
58. McSweeny AJ, Grant I, Heaton RK, Adams KM, Timms RM. Life quality of patients with chronic obstructive pulmonary disease. Arch Intern Med. 1982;142:473–8.

59. Kaplan RM, Ries AL, Prewitt LM, Eakin E. Self-efficacy expectations predict survival for patients with chronic obstructive pulmonary disease. Health Psychol. 1994;13:366–8.
60. Mauer J et al. Anxiety and depression in COPD: current understanding, unanswered questions, and research needs. Chest. 2008;134:43S–56S.
61. Kozora E, Tran ZV, Make B. Neurobehavioral improvement after brief rehabilitation in patients with chronic obstructive pulmonary disease. J Cardiopulm rehabil. 2002;22:426–30.
62. Engelen MPKJ, Schols AMWJ, Baken WC, Wesseling GJ, Wouters EF. Nutritional depletion in relation to respiratory and peripheral skeletal muscle function in outpatients with COPD. Eur Respir J. 1994;7:1793–7.
63. Schols AMWJ, Soeters PB, Dingemans AMC, Mostert R, Frantzen PJ, Wouters EF. Prevalence and characteristics of nutritional depletion in patients with stable COPD eligible for pulmonary rehabilitation. Am Rev Respir Dis. 1993;147:1151–6.
64. Schols AMWJ, Fredrix EW, Soeters PB, Westerterp KR, Wouters EFM. Resting energy expenditure in patients with chronic obstructive pulmonary disease. Am J Clin Nutr. 1991;5:983–7.
65. Engelen MPKJ, Schols AMWJ, Heidendal GAK, Wouters EFM. Dual-energy X-ray absorptiometry in the clinical evaluation of body composition and bone mineral density in patients with chronic obstructive pulmonary disease. Am J Clin Nutr. 1998;68:1298–303.
66. Mostert R, Goris A, Weling-Scheepers C, Wouters EF, Schols AM. Tissue depletion and health related quality of life in patients with chronic obstructive pulmonary disease. Respir Med. 2000;94(9):859–67.
67. Schols AM, Slangen J, Volovics L, Wouters EF. Weight loss is a reversible factor in the prognosis of chronic obstructive pulmonary disease. Am J Respir Crit Care Med. 1998;157(6 Pt 1): 1791–7.
68. Wilson DO, Rogers RM, Wright EC, Anthonisen NR. Body weight in chronic obstructive pulmonary disease. The National Institutes of Health Intermittent Positive-Pressure Breathing Trial. Am Rev Respir Dis. 1989;139(6):1435–8.
69. Landbo C, Prescott E, Lange P, Vestbo J, Almdal TP. Prognostic value of nutritional status in chronic obstructive pulmonary disease. Am J Respir Crit Care Med. 1999;160(6):1856–61.
70. Steiner MC, Barton RL, Singh SJ, Morgan MD. Nutritional enhancement of exercise performance in chronic obstructive pulmonary disease: a randomised controlled trial. Thorax. 2003;58(9):745–51.
71. Efthimiou J, Fleming J, Gomes C, Spiro SG. The effect of supplementary oral nutrition in poorly nourished patients with chronic obstructive pulmonary disease. Am Rev Respir Dis. 1988;137(5):1075–82.
72. Franssen FM, Broekhuizen R, Janssen PP, Wouters EF, Schols AM. Effects of whole-body exercise training on body composition and functional capacity in normal-weight patients with COPD. Chest. 2004;125(6):2021–8.
73. Bernard S, Whittom F, Leblanc P, Jobin J, Belleau R, Berube C, et al. Aerobic and strength training in patients with chronic obstructive pulmonary disease. Am J Respir Crit Care Med. 1999;159(3):896–901.
74. Schols AM, Soeters PB, Mostert R, Pluymers RJ, Wouters EF. Physiologic effects of nutritional support and anabolic steroids in patients with chronic obstructive pulmonary disease. A placebo-controlled randomized trial. Am J Respir Crit Care Med. 1995;152:1268–74.
75. Casaburi R, Bhasin S, Cosentino L, Porszasz J, Somfay A, Lewis MI, et al. Effects of testosterone and resistance training in men with chronic obstructive pulmonary disease. Am J Respir Crit Care Med. 2004;170(8):870–8.
76. The Nocturnal Oxygen Therapy Group. Continuous or nocturnal oxygen therapy in hypoxemic chronic obstructive lung disease. Ann Intern Med. 1980;93:391–8.
77. Medical Research Council Working Party. Long term domiciliary oxygen therapy in chronic hypoxic cor pulmonale complicating chronic bronchitis and emphysema. Lancet. 1981;8222: 681–6.
78. O'Donnell DE, D'Arisigny C, Webb KA. Effects of hyperoxia on ventilatory limitation during exercise in advanced chronic obstructive pulmonary disease. Am J Respir Crit Care Med. 2001;163:892–89.

79. Somfay A, Porszasz J, Lee SM, Casaburi R. Dose-response effect of oxygen on hyperinflation and exercise endurance in nonhypoxemic COPD patients. Eur Respir J. 2001;18:77–84.
80. Emtner M, Porszasz J, Burns M, Somfay A, Casaburi R. Benefits of supplemental oxygen in exercise training in nonhypoxemic chronic obstructive pulmonary disease patients. Am J Respir Crit Care Med. 2003;168:1034–42.
81. Celli BR, Barnes PJ. Exacerbations of chronic obstructive pulmonary disease. Eur Respir J. 2007;29:1224–38.
82. Burge PS, Calverley PM, Jones PW, Spencer S, Anderson JA, Maslen TK. Randomised, double-blind, placebo-controlled study of fluticasone propionate in patients with moderate to severe chronic obstructive pulmonary disease: the ISOLDE trial. BMJ. 2000;320:1297–303.
83. Tashkin DP, Celli B, Senn S, Burkhart D, Kesten S, Menjoge S, et al. UPLIFT Study Investigators. A 4-year trial of tiotropium in chronic obstructive pulmonary disease. N Engl J Med. 2008;359:1543–54.
84. Garcia-Aymerich J, Hernandez C, Alonso A, Casas A, Rodriguez-Roisin R, Anto JM, et al. Effects of an integrated care intervention on risk factors of COPD readmission. Respir Med. 2007;101(7):1462–9.
85. Casas A, Troosters T, Garcia-Aymerich J, Roca J, Hernandez C, Alonso A, et al. Integrated care prevents hospitalisations for exacerbations in COPD patients. Eur Respir J. 2006;28:123–30.
86. Puhan M, Scharplatz M, Troosters T, Walters EH, Steurer J. Pulmonary rehabilitation following exacerbations of chronic obstructive pulmonary disease. Cochrane Database Syst Rev. 2009;1:005305.
87. Ries AL, Kaplan RM, Limberg TM, Prewitt LM. Effects of pulmonary rehabilitation on physiologic and psychosocial outcomes in patients with chronic obstructive pulmonary disease. Ann Intern Med. 1995;122:823–32.
88. Brooks D, Krip B, Mangovski-Alzamora S, Goldstein RS. The effect of postrehabilitation programmes among individuals with chronic obstructive pulmonary disease. Eur Respir J. 2002;20:20–9.
89. Troosters T, Gosselink R, Decramer M. Short- and long-term effects of outpatient rehabilitation in patients with chronic obstructive pulmonary disease: a randomized trial. Am J Med. 2000;109(3):207–12.

Chapter 15
Disease Management and Integrated Care

Emiel F.M. Wouters and Ingrid M.L. Augustin

Abstract One of the greatest challenges that will face health systems globally in the twenty-first century will be the increasing burden of chronic diseases. Greater longevity, increasing exposure to many chronic disease risk factors such as tobacco consumption, and the growing ability to intervene with new treatments to keep alive those who previously would have died, have changed the burden of diseases. Chronic conditions are defined by the World Health Organization as requiring ongoing management over a period of years or decades. These conditions require a complex response over an extended period of time that involves coordinated input from a wide range of health professionals and access to essential medicine and monitoring systems. The goals of chronic care are not to cure but rather to enhance functional status, minimize distressing symptoms, prolong life, and to enhance quality of life. It is clear that these goals are difficult to achieve by means of the traditional approach to health care that focuses on individual organ-directed diseases and that is built around an acute, episodic model of care and a relationship between the individual patients and the doctor.

Keywords COPD • Disease management • Integrated care • Chronic disease • Definitions • Disease-management programs • Patient-related intervention • Professional-directed intervention • Organizational intervention

E.F.M. Wouters (✉)
Department of Respiratory Medicine, Maastricht University Medical Center, Maastricht,
The Netherlands
e-mail: e.wouters@mumc.nl

I.M.L. Augustin
CIRO, Center of Expertise for Chronic Organ Failure, Horn, The Netherlands
e-mail: ingridaugustin@ciro-horn.nl

L. Nici and R. ZuWallack (eds.), *Chronic Obstructive Pulmonary Disease: Co-Morbidities and Systemic Consequences*, Respiratory Medicine, DOI 10.1007/978-1-60761-673-3_15, © Springer Science+Business Media, LLC 2012

Introduction

One of the greatest challenges that will face health systems globally in the twenty-first century will be the increasing burden of chronic diseases. Greater longevity, increasing exposure to many chronic disease risk factors such as tobacco consumption, and the growing ability to intervene with new treatments to keep alive those who previously would have died, have changed the burden of diseases. Chronic conditions are defined by the World Health Organization (WHO) as requiring ongoing management over a period of years or decades. These conditions require a complex response over an extended period of time that involves coordinated inputs from a wide range of health professionals and access to essential medicines and monitoring systems. The goals of chronic care are not to cure but to enhance functional status, minimize distressing symptoms, prolong life, and to enhance quality of life [1]. It is clear that these goals are difficult to achieve by means of the traditional approach to health care that focuses on individual organ-directed diseases and that is built around an acute, episodic model of care and a relationship between the individual patients and the doctor.

Many chronic conditions require significant participation by informed patients. Chronic illness confronts patients with a spectrum of needs that requires them to alter their behavior and engage in activities that promote physical and psychological well-being, to interact with healthcare providers and adhere to treatment regimens, to monitor their health status and make associated decisions, and to manage the impact of the illness on physical, psychological, and social functioning [2]. This requires healthcare providers to inform and enable patients to self-manage their illness and necessitates an ongoing collaborative process between patients and professionals. This patient-centered approach requires a model of care taking into account, a partnership with the patient and other health care personnel. Furthermore, patients vary in their preferences for care and the importance they place on health outcomes. The ability of the empowered patient to develop individualized treatment plans will be very important for effective care over a prolonged period of time.

Effective management of chronic diseases cannot be achieved by trying harder within the current care systems but demands the creation of new complex systems that bridge the different disciplinary perspectives and empower the patient to achieve individualized management goals. This increasing organizational complexity is paralleled with an increasing scientific and problem complexity of patients with chronic conditions.

Disease Management and Integrated Care

Chronic illness requires complex models of care, involving collaboration among professionals and institutions that have traditionally been separate. Instead of stimulating competition on value between providers and institutions in the acute care model, there is pressing need to bridge the boundaries between professions, providers, and institutions through the development of more integrated and coordinated approaches to care delivery [3]. Alongside the relative paucity of empirical evidence on the consequences of different forms of integration, coordination and care models, there is a plethora of terminologies and an academic quagmire of definitions and concept analyses surrounding the notion of integration [4]. This lack in specificity and clarity has significantly hampered the systematic understanding of integrated care and related notions [5].

Disease Management: Definitions

Originally, disease management is focused on targeted persons with a single disease or condition. Historically, disease-management programs provided narrowly tailored medical solutions focused on one dominant health problem [6]. Disease management was initially used mainly by pharmaceutical companies to promote medication adherence and behavior change among patients with chronic conditions [7]. More recently, second-generation disease-management programs provide a more integrated approach to care by addressing the multiple needs of patients with comorbidities and multiple conditions [6]. Disease management was put forward as an approach to patient care that coordinates medical resources for patients across the entire delivery system [8].

The Disease Management Association of America (DMMA) defined disease management as a system of coordinated health care interventions and communications for populations with conditions in which patient self-care efforts are significant [9]. These disease-management programs support the use of multiple interventions, defined as combinations of at least two of three types of intervention: patient-related, professional-directed, and organizational interventions [10]. Although the boundaries between disease management and integrated care have become increasingly blurred, disease-management programs are normally limited to linkages within the health care sector.

The Effectiveness of Disease Management Interventions in COPD

Disease management, which combines different approaches and targets different barriers to improvement, has been introduced as the answer to handle the needs of patients with COPD. Lemmens et al. recently reported a systematic review of integrated use of disease-management interventions in asthma and COPD. They identified 36 studies fulfilling the criteria of multiple interventions: 17 studies used both patient-related and organizational interventions and another 19 studies used triple interventions (patient related, professional-directed, and organizational). Twenty-two of these studies included COPD patients. Meta-analyses demonstrated statistically significant improvements in health status in cases of multiple interventions as well as significant reductions in the number of patients with one or more hospital admissions within triple interventions. No effects were found in emergency department visits per person. The authors report little evidence to support nurse-led management of COPD patients in the community [11]. The authors concluded that estimates of the effectiveness of multifaceted interventions are limited by the wide range of outcomes measured, the diverging combinations of interventions, the different study designs, and the many different settings in which care was delivered [11].

Recently, a randomized, blinded, controlled one-year trial reported the effects of a simplified disease-management program in severe COPD patients. The intervention consists of a single 1–1.5 h educational session, an action plan for self-management of exacerbations, and monthly follow-up calls from a case manager. After one year, the mean cumulative frequency of COPD-related hospitalizations and emergency department visits was significantly reduced in the intervention group as well as hospitalizations for cardiac or pulmonary conditions other than COPD. Interestingly, this study was restricted to relatively high-risk COPD patients [12].

Integrated Care: Taxonomies

The term integration was initially used in economics to describe a way of thinking about a range of approaches to increase coordination, cooperation, continuity, collaboration, and networking across different components of a certain system: integration aims to make a whole out of different parts. In health care, many providers are involved: hospitals, clinics, physician groups, and individual physicians are all central actors in the current health care system. They all operate in very complex health care structures and the health care delivered is highly fragmented [13]. Different frameworks and delivery models are described in chronic care in order to achieve this integration of health care. In order to understand and interpret integrative health care systems, it will be very important to distinguish the different dimensions of integration: the type, the breath, the degree, and the process. The literature differentiates different types of integration: functional, organizational, professional, and clinical integration [14, 15]. The breadth of integration could be horizontal or vertical: horizontal integration takes place between organizations or organizational units at the same level of delivery while vertical integration refers to integrative activities between organizations at different levels. The degree of integration can vary from collaboration to full integration. The process of integration distinguishes structural integration, cultural integration, and social integration [16]. Therefore, integration may occur in different and complex structural configurations [17].

Integrated Care: Delivery Models in Chronic Care

Integrated Framework

The integration framework, proposed by Leutz in 1999, describes three levels of integration which are set against the dimensions of service users' need and operational domains of systems in order to enable a comprehensive approach responding to the needs of persons with chronic conditions [18]. Dimensions of need were defined in terms of stability and severity of the patient's conditions, duration of illness, urgency of the intervention, scope of the services required, and the user's capacity for self-direction.

Service users were divided into three categories: those with mild-to-moderate but stable conditions, those with moderate levels of need, and the third group with long-term, severe, unstable conditions, who frequently require urgent intervention from various sectors and who have a limited capacity for self-direction. Leutz argued that the first group would be likely served sufficiently by relative simple structures of existing health and social services systems while the last subgroup was likely to benefit most from a high level of integration of the different service domains [18]. Bodenheimer et al. describes a population management care model that divides the population with chronic conditions into three district groups based on their degree of need [19]. Patients at the lowest level had a relatively low level of need for healthcare: the chronic condition is reasonably under control, with support of self-management provided by the primary care setting. This population is assumed to constitute the majority of the population with chronic conditions. The next level is patients at increased risk because their condition is unstable or because they could deteriorate unless they have structured support through specialist disease management. Finally, the third group includes those persons with highly complex needs and/or a high intensity of unplanned secondary care: these patients require active management through case managers.

Chronic Care Model

Recognizing the failures of health systems that remain largely built on an acute, episodic model of care with little emphasis on patient self-management, Wagner and colleagues developed the chronic care model (CCM) aimed to provide a comprehensive framework for the organization of health care to improve outcomes for people with chronic conditions [20]. This concept is based on the premise that high-quality chronic care is characterized by productive interactions between the practice team and patients, involving assessment, self-management support, optimization of therapy, and follow-up. The CCM compromises four interacting system components that are considered key to providing good chronic care: self-management support, delivery system design, decision support, and clinical information systems (Fig. 15.1).

What is the evidence of CCM in COPD? Adams et al. published a systematic review of the CCM in COPD prevention and management: they included 20 randomly controlled trials, five controlled clinical trials, and seven before/after studies [21]. They reported that symptoms, quality of life, lung function, and functional status were not significantly different between the intervention and control groups. Their review suggested that an effective preventative strategy to reduce health care costs (unscheduled/emergency center visits, number of hospitalizations, and hospital length of stay) for patients with COPD requires implementation of 2 or more

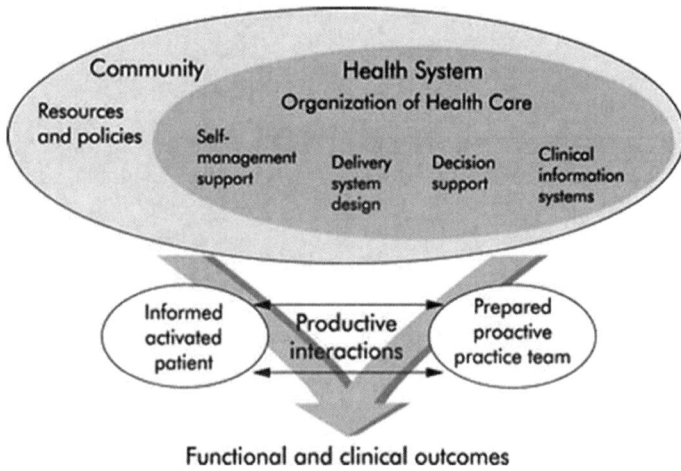

Fig. 15.1 The Chronic Care Model (CCM) compromises four interacting system components that are considered key to providing good chronic care: self-management support, delivery system design, decision support, and clinical information systems

CCM components. Trials resulting in reduced health care use provided the implementation of an extensive self-management program with an individualized action plan, advanced access to care which consisted of a knowledgeable health care provider, guideline-based therapy, and a clinical registry system. As judged by the published literature, the evidence remains inconclusive on the impact of applying CCM in COPD management. Furthermore, as in other chronic conditions, most studies have not focused on individuals with coexisting conditions or multiple health problems and research has concentrated on relatively short-term outcomes.

Integrated Practice Units and Care Delivery Value Chain

In their book *Redefining Health Care: Creating Value based Competition on Results*, Porter and Teisberg advocate that moving to value-based competition presents a formidable agenda for health care [22]. They put forward that value-based competition requires a profound transformation of health care delivery. Care needs to become organized around medical conditions, and medically integrated across specialties, treatments, and services, and over time. Dedicated teams need to utilize facilities designed for maximum value in care delivery for the medical condition being addressed. Care over the full care cycle is tightly coordinated, and patient information is extensively and seamlessly shared. Results need to be measured, analyzed, and reported. Porter and Teisberg put forward the value chain as the framework to implement this new model of care delivery: the value chain is based on the observation that delivering any product or service consists of performing numerous discrete activities [22]. The choices made about how these activities are configured and integrated drive

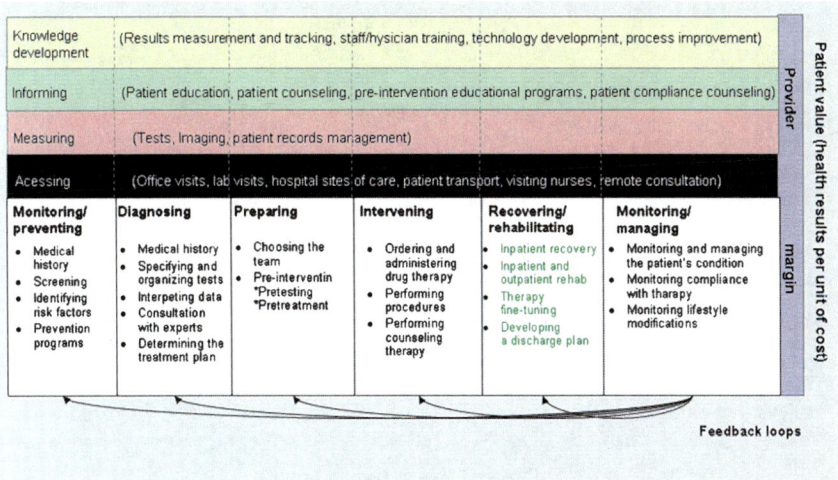

Knowledge development	(Results measurement and tracking, staff/hysician training, technology development, process improvement)
Informing	(Patient education, patient counseling, pre-intervention educational programs, patient compliance counseling)
Measuring	(Tests, Imaging, patient records management)
Acessing	(Office visits, lab visits, hospital sites of care, patient transport, visiting nurses, remote consultation)

Monitoring/ preventing	Diagnosing	Preparing	Intervening	Recovering/ rehabilitating	Monitoring/ managing
• Medical history • Screening • Identifying risk factors • Prevention programs	• Medical history • Specifying and organizing tests • Interpeting data • Consultation with experts • Determining the treatment plan	• Choosing the team • Pre-interventin *Pretesting *Pretreatment	• Ordering and administering drug therapy • Performing procedures • Performing counseling therapy	• Inpatient recovery • Inpatient and outpatient rehab • Therapy fine-tuning • Developing a discharge plan	• Monitoring and managing the patient's condition with tharapy • Monitoring compliance • Monitoring lifestyle modifications

Feedback loops

Patient value (health results per unit of cost)

Provider margin

Fig. 15.2 The care delivery value chain (CDVC) depicts the types of activities involved in caring for patients with a particular medical condition over the entire cycle of care

value, and should guide the organizational structure. The care delivery value chain (CDVC) depicts the types of activities involved in caring for patients with a particular medical condition over the entire cycle of care (Fig. 15.2).

Every care delivery chain begins with monitoring and prevention. The CDVC progresses through diagnosing, preparing, intervening, and rehabilitating, and ends with monitoring and managing. Three additional cross-cutting activities complete the CDVC: accessing, measuring, and informing. Accessing refers to the steps involved in gaining access to the patient, and other means of access such as remote monitoring and internet consultations. Measuring refers to the measurement of the patient's medical circumstances and informing encompasses the activities involved in notifying, educating, and coaching the patient. These activities are considered as the glue that binds the care cycle together and are considered very important to patient value and to prevention and management. Finally, knowledge development is a crucial enabler of value-based competition: the set of activities involved in learning how to improve care processes and outcomes. The authors put forward that the CDVC is an important tool to minimize iteration in health care delivery as much of today's iteration is caused by mistakes, poor processes, and inattention to the full care cycle.

The CDVC is considered the premier tool for designing integrated practice units (IPU) in the health care reform put forward by Porter and Teisberg [22]. They argue that the typical organizational structure of health care providers is a functional, supply driven structure organized around types of skills and facilities. Like other domains of organizations, these functional structures need to be replaced by business unit structures, organized around products or service lines. An IPU includes the full range of medical expertise, technical skills, and specialized facilities needed to

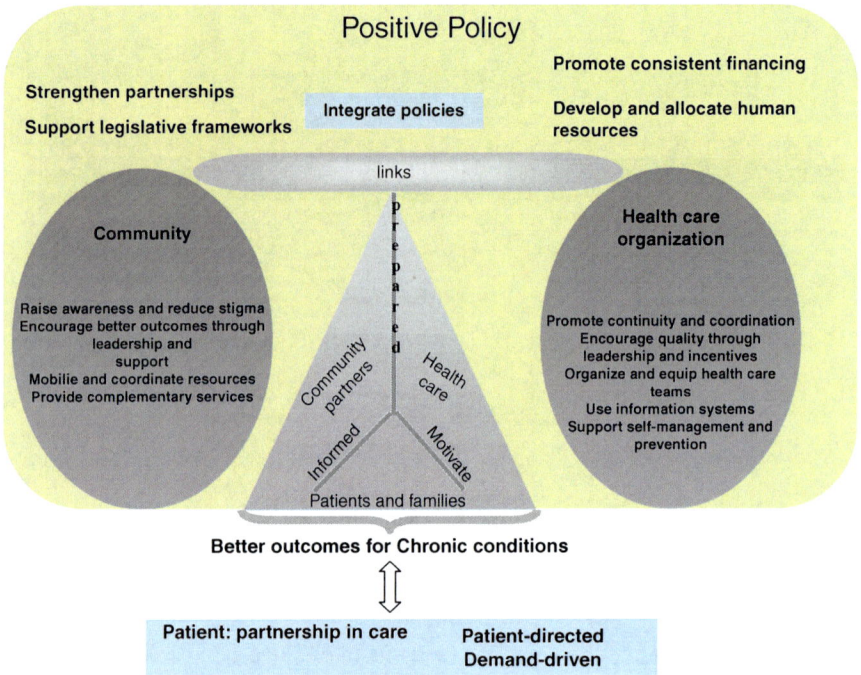

Fig. 15.3 In order to create a well functioning health care system to improve care for patients with chronic conditions, the World Health Organization (WHO) has provided a conceptual framework to address the pressing need of improving care for chronic conditions, the Innovative Care for Chronic Conditions (ICCC) Framework, an expanded, internationalized adaptation of the earlier Chronic Care Model (CCM) [23]

address a medical condition or set of related medical conditions over the cycle of care. The IPU is patient-centric and results-driven and embodies the growing recognition of the importance of multidisciplinary approaches to diagnosis, treatment, and disease management. In the IPU model, care is provided by a team and individuals and facilities are dedicated. Porter and Teisberg put forward that within the IPU structure, significant benefits can be achieved from organizing diagnosis as a distinct function, rather than co-mingled with treatment [22].

World Health Organization (WHO) Model of Integrated Care

In order to create a well-functioning health care system to improve care for patients with chronic conditions, the WHO has provided a conceptual framework to address the pressing need of improving care for chronic conditions, the Innovative Care for Chronic Conditions (ICCC) Framework [23]. This ICCC framework is an expanded, internationalized adaptation of the earlier CCM (Fig. 15.3).

The framework outlines the components necessary to improve care for patients across multiple levels of the health care system: the general policy environment, the health-care organization and community, and the patient-care level. The micro level or the patient-care level emphasizes the partnership between patients and families, the healthcare teams, and the community partners. The meso level refers to the health care organization and community: the health care organization needs to promote continuity and coordination, to encourage quality of care, to organize and equip health care teams, to support self-management and prevention, and to apply information systems. At the community level, the WHO framework stresses the importance to raise the awareness and reduce the stigmatization of patients with chronic conditions, to mobilize and coordinate resources, and to mobilize complementary services in order to achieve better outcomes. The macro level of the ICCC framework emphasizes the need to create a positive policy environment by the promotion of consistent financing, by support of legislative frameworks, and by development and allocation of human resources.

Coordination in Care Delivery

All the structured care models identify that the lack of coordination is one of the major obstacles to better care for patients with chronic conditions. The observational study "Tackling chronic disease in Europe," published by the European Observatory on health systems and policies, identifies five important dimensions of coordination in chronic care; [24]

- *Getting in*: getting access to appropriate care
- *Fitting in*: adapting the care to the requirements
- *Knowing what is going on*: receiving information
- *Continuity:* of staff and coordination and communication among professionals
- *Difficulties in making progress through the system*

The same document refers to the framework of Boon and colleagues identifying seven types of provision with varying degrees of coordination: at the one end of the spectrum is the strict solo provision, at the other end the full integration of disciplines for curative, rehabilitative, and preventive services (Fig. 15.4) [25].

In parallel, practice practitioners work independently while in consultative practice information on patients is shared informally, case by case. In coordinated practice, the exchange of data on patients is related to particular diseases and therapies are administered though a formal structure. An advanced model of coordinated practice is the multidisciplinary team, which is composed of more team members while in the interdisciplinary team group, decisions will be made, shared policies will be developed, and regular face-to-face meetings will be organized. Multidisciplinarity can be defined as a non-integrative mixture of disciplines in that each discipline retains its methodologies and assumptions without change or development from

Types of care provision with varying degrees of coordination

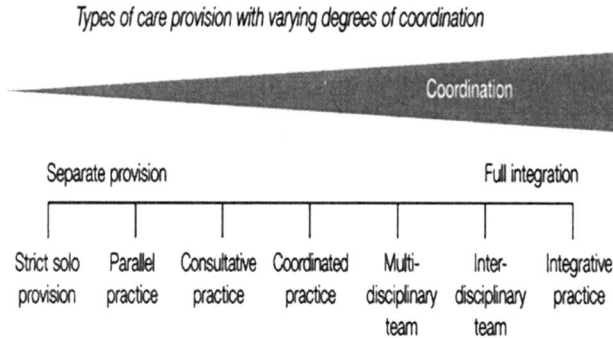

Fig. 15.4 Seven types of provision with varying degrees of coordination: at the one end of the spectrum is the strict solo provision, at the other end the full integration of disciplines for curative, rehabilitative, and preventive services [25]

other disciplines within the multidisciplinary relationship. Multidisciplinarity in the context of health care means that health care providers from different disciplines work together to collaboratively provide diagnoses, assessments, and treatment within their scope of practice and areas of competence. Interdisciplinarity involves approaching a subject from various angles and methods, eventually cutting across disciplines and forming a new method of understanding the subject. The integrative practice is based on a shared vision and provides a seamless continuum of decision making and patient-centered care and support. Nolte and McKee [17] identified many structural barriers in the current health care system:

(a) Competing operating cultures and management approaches in different sectors
(b) Different ownership structures
(c) Separate and competing providers with no incentives to cooperate
(d) Rivalries between professional groups
(e) Lack of clarity about competencies and accountability
(f) Integrated care for patient: partnership in care

Integrated Care for the Patient: Partnership in Care

Health care for patients with chronic conditions is a complex interaction of health care providers and other factors around the patient. Individualization is considered a key factor in the management of chronic conditions as COPD. Individualization requires that the workforce is organized to offer health care around the patient: the workforce needs to adopt a patient-centered approach. Individualization of the program in a patient-centered approach needs to consider the patient as a partner in the program: information about treatment, goals, and outcomes is shared with patients to prepare them to take greater responsibility in health care decision making.

A patient-centered integrated care approach needs to consider core competencies applying to all members of the workforce caring for these patients. Competencies are the skills, abilities, knowledge, behaviors, and attitudes that are instrumental in the delivery of desired results, and, consequently of job performance [26]. Competencies add further definition to any job by their focus on how work is done and what work is done. Core competencies in the management of chronic conditions are part of the WHO report "Preparing a health care workforce for the 21st century" [26]. Five core competencies are formulated to complement existing ones for caring patients with chronic conditions. First, the workforce needs to organize care around the patient. Second, providers need communication skills that enable them to collaborate with others. Third, the workforce needs skills to ensure that the safety and quality of patient care are continuously improved. Fourth, the workforce needs skills that assist them in monitoring patients across time. Finally, the workforce needs to consider patient care and the provider's role in that care from the broadest perspective, multiple levels of the health care system, and the care continuum [26].

Partnering skills is considered as a core competency to enhance care coordination and health outcomes. Health care providers need to develop skills to set-up partnerships with the patient and with other providers. Providers need communication skills that allow them to share power and involve patients in all aspects of health care decision making. Partnering requires that health care providers transform their core business in terms of relationships, behavior, processes, communication, and leadership. Partnering takes a collaborative approach to achieve shared objectives. The shared objective health care providers involved in the management of COPD patients is to return the patient to the highest possible capacity and to contribute to achieve the individual's maximum level of independence and functioning in the community. Communication is considered as the essential element in successful partnership. Communication skills include the ability to negotiate, share decisions, solve problems collectively and establish goals, implement action, identify strengths and weaknesses, clarify roles and responsibilities, and evaluate progress [26].

Summary

It is widely accepted that the traditional acute episodic model of care is ill-equipped to meet the long-term needs of patients with chronic illness and that an effective response will only be possible in a health system that facilitates the development and implementation of structured approaches of these conditions. Collaboration and cooperation among professions and institutions that have traditionally worked separately are characteristics of these new service delivery models in order to really realize coordination of care [17]. In response to the experienced growing needs in chronic care, a myriad of concepts have been developed, contributing to further fragmentation and blurring in this field.

Initiatives for integration and coordination of care need to analyze and identify the major barriers of integration. Barriers in setting up integrated health care may be structural, procedural, financial, professional, or status and legitimacy related [27]. Overcoming these challenges will result in a unique structural organization reflecting the diverse environments and historical paths taken by health systems. Generic models can offer guidance in the realization of this unique structure. In the transition from the traditional model of care to a more integrated care structure, Nolte and McKee identified four crucial conditions to become successful: the provision of adequate finances, the creation of an appropriately trained and motivated workforce, information technology to support the new approaches to care, and systems that enable effective self-management of patients [17]. The increasing organizational complexity of chronic care needs to be integrated with the increasing scientific complexity of the chronic conditions themselves. Making integrated care happen poses the greatest challenge of the health care system in this century! Success is possible but requires an overall vision and commitment of health policy makers.

References

1. Grumbach K. Chronic illness, comorbidities, and the need for medical generalism. Ann Fam Med. 2003;1(1):4–7.
2. Clark NM. Management of chronic disease by patients. Annu Rev Public Health. 2003;24:289–313.
3. Plochg T, Klazinga NS. Community-based integrated care: myth or must? Int J Qual Health Care. 2002;14(2):91–101.
4. Howarth M, Haigh C. The myth of patient centrality in integrated care: the case of back pain. Int J Integr Care. 2007;7:e27.
5. Kodner D, Spreeuwenberg C. Integrated care: meaning, logic, applications, and implications: a discussion paper. Int J Integr Care. 2002;2:e12.
6. Krumholz HM, Currie PM, Riegel B, et al. A taxonomy for disease management: a scientific statement from the American Heart Association Disease Management Taxonomy Writing Group. Circulation. 2006;114(13):1432–45.
7. Bodenheimer T. Disease management–promises and pitfalls. N Engl J Med. 1999;340(15): 1202–5.
8. Ellrodt G, Cook DJ, Lee J, Cho M, Hunt D, Weingarten S. Evidence-based disease management. JAMA. 1997;278(20):1687–92.
9. DMAA. Disease Management Program Evaluation Guide Online.
10. EPOC. http://www.epoc.cochrane.org. Accessed 16 July 2008.
11. Lemmens KM, Nieboer AP, Huijsman R. A systematic review of integrated use of disease-management interventions in asthma and COPD. Respir Med. 2009;103(5):670–91.
12. Rice KL, Dewan N, Bloomfield HE, et al. Disease management program for chronic obstructive pulmonary disease: a randomized controlled trial. Am J Respir Crit Care Med. 2010; 182(7):890–6.
13. IOM. Institute of Medicine. Crossing the quality chasm: a new health system for the 21st century. Committee on the quality of health care. 2000;Executive summary:1–22.
14. Delnoij D, Klazinga N, Glasgow IK. Integrated care in an international perspective. Int J Integr Care. 2002;2:e04.
15. Simoens S, Scott A. Towards a definition and taxonomy of integration in primary care. Aberdeen: University of Aderdeen; 1999.
16. Fabbricotti I. Taking care of integrated care: integration and fragmentation in the development of integrated care arrangements. Rotterdam: Erasmus University; 2007.

17. Nolte E, McKee M, eds. Caring for people with chronic conditions. A health system perspective. Berkshire: Open University Press; 2008. Figueras J, McKee M, Mossialos E, Saltman R, eds. European observatory on health systems and policies series.
18. Leutz WN. Five laws for integrating medical and social services: lessons from the United States and the United Kingdom. Milbank Q. 1999;77(1):77–110. iv-v.
19. Bodenheimer T, Wagner EH, Grumbach K. Improving primary care for patients with chronic illness: the chronic care model, Part 2. JAMA. 2002;288(15):1909–14.
20. Wagner EH, Davis C, Schaefer J, Von Korff M, Austin B. A survey of leading chronic disease management programs: are they consistent with the literature? Manag Care Q. 1999;7(3): 56–66.
21. Adams SG, Smith PK, Allan PF, Anzueto A, Pugh JA, Cornell JE. Systematic review of the chronic care model in chronic obstructive pulmonary disease prevention and management. Arch Intern Med. 2007;167(6):551–61.
22. Porter M, Teisberg E. Redefining health care. Creating value-based competition on results. Boston, MA: Harvard Business School Press; 2006.
23. WHO. Innovative care for chronic conditions: building blocks for action. Geneva: World Health Organization; 2002.
24. Busse R, Blümel M, Scheller-Kreinsen D, Zentner A. Tackling chronic disease in Europe. http://www.euro.who.int/__data/assets/pdf_file/0008/96632/E93736.pdf. Copenhagen: WHO; 2010.
25. Boon H, Verhoef M, O'Hara D, Findlay B. From parallel practice to integrative health care: a conceptual framework. BMC Health Serv Res. 2004;4(1):15.
26. WHO. Preparing a health care workforce for the 21st century. The challenge of chronic conditions. http://www.who.int/chp/knowledge/publications/workforce_report/en/: World Health Organization; 2005.
27. Hardy B, Mur-Veemanu I, Steenbergen M, Wistow G. Inter-agency services in England and The Netherlands. A comparative study of integrated care development and delivery. Health Policy. 1999;48(2):87–105.

.

Index

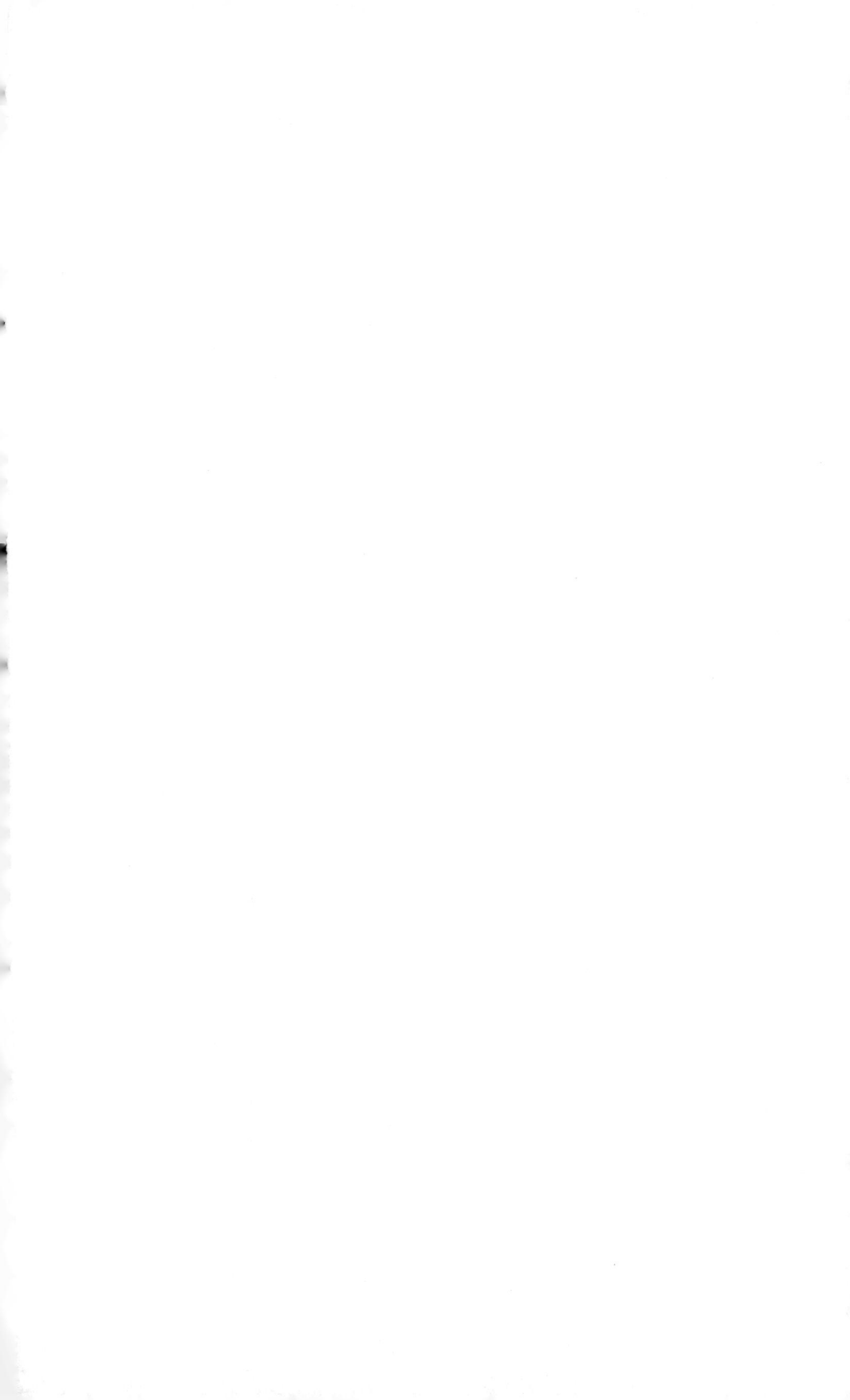